Sociocultural Psychology of the Lifecourse

Series Editor
Tania Zittoun
Institute of Psychology and Education
University of Neuchâtel
Neuchâtel, Switzerland

The Sociocultural Psychology of the Lifecourse book series seeks to further our knowledge of the development of people in their complex sociocultural worlds, both empirically and theoretically. Its sociocultural psychological perspective proposes to account for the development of people as unique persons, with their perspective and subjectivity, within the social and cultural environments that guide them and yet which they can themselves transform. The book series showcases works that provide a complex understanding of development in the lifecourse, contribute to the theorization of the lifecourse and present original data – based on case studies, segments of lives, or trajectories of living. It will also include books which present synthetic theoretical, epistemological or methodological contributions. By documenting the richness of lives and developing the relevant theoretical tools, books in this series will make a unique contribution to sociocultural, developmental psychology, and to the study of the courses of lives.

Biljana Stanković

Giving Birth To A Subject

Transition To Motherhood As An Embodied & Technologically Mediated Experience

palgrave
macmillan

Biljana Stanković
Faculty of Philosophy
University of Belgrade
Belgrade, Serbia

ISSN 2946-4617 ISSN 2946-4625 (electronic)
Sociocultural Psychology of the Lifecourse
ISBN 978-3-031-77235-1 ISBN 978-3-031-77236-8 (eBook)
https://doi.org/10.1007/978-3-031-77236-8

This Palgrave Macmillan imprint is published by the registered company Springer Nature Switzerland AG.
The registered company address is: Gewerbestrasse 11, 6330 Cham, Switzerland

To Iskra

Foreword of the Series' Editor

Giving Birth to a Subject: Bringing the Body Back to Theory

Sociocultural psychology of the lifecourse examines the social and cultural embeddedness of the trajectories of living of unique persons (de Saint-Laurent, 2020; Rosa & Valsiner, 2018). Together with lifecourse studies, it acknowledges the importance of understanding courses of life in their cultural and historical environments, and the role of transitions within (Levy et al., 2005). Its specificities are in emphasising people's unique experiences of living, and the sense they confer to it (Valsiner et al., 2016; Zavershneva & Van der Veer, 2018).

Studies in sociocultural psychology of the lifecourse mostly chose between studying the course of one or many courses of life over a longer period of time, either reconstructively (Mayer et al., 2021) or longitudinally (Wagoner et al., 2015; Zittoun et al., 2023), or alternatively, focusing on one specific transition in the life of people (Adams & Fleer, 2017; Märtsin, 2019). The study of transitions is important to apprehend dynamics of the lifecourse both because these may dramatically reorient the course of a life (Crafter et al., 2019; Sato, 2017) and because they constitute naturally occurring laboratories to study human development (Zittoun, 2009). Indeed, they can be seen as catalysed occasions for change and development (Cabell & Valsiner, 2014), and when thoroughly analysed, they give a unique entry in the complex processes by which the sociocultural environment guides people's becoming, and by which people may object, resist or recreate their living conditions (Chaudhary et al., 2017; Lawrence et al., 1992).

This book collection offers authors the space to examine one specific aspect of human development from a sociocultural perspective, and working through case studies, put to the fore some of the intricacies of the processes at stake. In the last two volumes, identity dynamics have been examined from a semiotic perspective in young people's international transitions (Märtsin, 2019), and through biographical analysis from a more longitudinal approach to the life of people (Mayer et al., 2021). In this third volume, we come back to the study of a specific transition, yet from a new theoretical perspective.

In "Giving birth to a subject. Transition to motherhood as an embodied and technologically mediated experience", Biljana Stanković takes very seriously the sociocultural call to examine the social and historical situation of people's life, as well as the necessity to preserve the person's unique experience. The transition to parenthood is probably one of the most significant lifecourse transitions, both culturally and personally (Crosnoe & Elder, 2002, 2004; Lévi-Strauss, 1981), and, together with adolescence, one of the most documented in psychology (Cabell et al., 2015; LaRossa & LaRossa, 1981; Michaels & Goldberg, 1988; Stern et al., 1998). However, authors interested in going beyond the medical dimension of this transition to apprehend its experiential aspects, usually focus on verbal, narrative material, that is, on declarative knowledge (Bastos, 2016; Pontecorvo et al., 2001; Zittoun, 2004, 2011). Of course, a focus on the symbolic aspects of becoming a father or a mother makes sense: sociocultural psychology has always been close to the social sciences, and especially anthropology (Boesch, 1991; Cole, 1996; Obeyesekere, 1990; Stenner, 2017; Valsiner, 2000), domains interested in the cultural birth of the child and the parent, complementing the biological birth. In effect, birth rituals, naming, baptism, circumcision are some of the many cultural rituals by which a newly living organism is accepted in a community of humans and turned into one of its members, and by which (young) adults are turned into parents—a liminal experience, and a turning point in the order of generations and cultural (re)production (Edwards et al., 2006; Moro, 2001; Nathan, 1993; Stenner, 2017; Van Gennep, 1909). But what about the actual process and experience of birth-giving? Can it be understood fully from a sociocultural psychological perspective, without reducing it to its symbolic or biological aspects?

This is the small revolution that Biljana Stanković proposes in this book. In effect, she starts with the assumption that in order to analyse the sociocultural becoming of a mother, one needs to account for the materiality of both the environment in which the transition takes place and the embodied nature of the absolute specific experience of giving birth. Yet materiality and embodiment were, one must admit with the author, traditionally the blind spots of psychology, and are still, the poor parents even of sociocultural psychology. Biljana Stanković thus expands the theoretical scope of her enquiry; she explores the material turn in the social sciences, and especially actor-network theory (whose blind spot is the absence of the subject), which she complements with phenomenology. Her theoretical synthesis brings her to "approach the early transition to motherhood—during the period of pregnancy and childbirth—as a technologically mediated, embodied experience embedded in a specific cultural-historical, discursive and material context" (Stanković, 2024, p. 31). More specifically, she proposes a double approach: from the outside, or from a third-person perspectives, she accounts for the national (Serbia), legal, social, institutional, architectural, material, power-laden, environment of the transition to motherhood—including routine echography made by doctors whose eyes never cross these of the pregnant woman, or maternity wards where women giving birth are kept alone, in lines of glass boxes, bodies exposed to the gaze of doctors. This is completed by a first-person perspective, where it is women's very specific embodied experience that is captured, and for which Biljana Stanković became sensitive not only to what is said, but to body movements and positions, cries and emotional outbursts, as she writes:

> I have tried to be very sensitive to pre-reflective layers of experience that exist prior and (at least partly) independent of our narrative understanding and meaning construction and are not easily shareable with others. Thus,

> my analysis generally focuses on the embodied self—understood as an embodied and singular first-person perspective—rather than the narrative autobiographical self, which implies a reflective and storied accumulated articulation of oneself as a particular kind of person (Stanković, 2024, p. 31).

The book itself is based on an in-depth longitudinal ethnographic study in Serbia, during which Biljana Stanković followed women before, during and after birth, observing them, interviewing them and interviewing doctors and professionals around women, their pregnancy, and the process of childbirth. Her original analysis is both phenomenological and critical-discursive. The book is articulated in three main chronological movements, also combining in different manners her first- and third-person perspectives. First, it presents the cultural-historical context of the transition into motherhood, and the two main social representations—or cultural narratives translated into material arrangements and practices (Marková, 2023; Moscovici, 2008)—to which women will be exposed. On the one side, women are conceived of, and treated as, bodies that need to be monitored and controlled by the mainly men-led medical institution, to the risk of denying any legitimacy to their subjective experience; on the other, women are exposed to the normative ideal of a "natural" pregnancy and birth. Biljana Stanković notes that both are equally misleading, as no human pregnancy or birth can ever occur without being already culturally mediated and shaped—in social, symbolic and material terms. The second movement of the analysis mainly focuses on the phenomenological experiences of women, and especially, their "interoception"—the perception of movements occurring inside their body. It follows the chronology of the transition to parenthood from the discovery of the pregnancy to the identification of another being inside of oneself, and to the transformation of one's body. Here too, it reveals the important mediating role of the medical personnel and technologies for these processes. The third movement now fully combines these two perspectives—considering both the socio-materiality of the situation and the subjective, embodied experience—to examine the process of childbirth. It demonstrates how much it is necessarily mediated by strong technical, social and symbolic constraints, which may result in a person's alienation, but which equally can enable women to recover a sense of creative agency.

With this very sketchy summary, I wish to highlight two of the main contributions of the volume. First, Biljana Stanković present us with a unique, in-depth case study of the transition to motherhood in contemporary Serbia. The contribution of this case study goes far beyond the Serbian case. Indeed, it demonstrates how much a contemporary society, at least as much as a supposedly traditional one, set the norms, values and discourses framing its own reproduction. The volume demonstrates, with explicit references to both Foucault and Latour, that producing babies is a heavily regulated process, constrained and guided by a distributed institution. It could be said that this institution is of a transformative type (Scott, 2011)—it transforms free, independent, educated women, into parturient bodies, now completed by a new being. As did Goffman's (1961) *Asylum* study, such an analysis is likely to inspire many other studies not only of the transition to motherhood, but probably, on other lifecourse transitions (e.g., the entry into school, the military, or the transition to retirement homes, etc.). More generally, case-studies are ground for theoretical generalisation (Cornish, 2020; Demuth, 2018; Salvatore & Valsiner, 2010).

Hence, the second great contribution of the volume to sociocultural psychology of the lifecourse is theoretical. Biljana Stanković offers us a long-awaited, groundbreaking theoretical proposition to address people's subjective, embodied experience. Of course, embodiment has been searched for repeatedly in various orientations of social and/or cultural psychology (Brown et al., 2011; Fonagy, 2007; Gfeller, 2017), and is debated in various interdisciplinary domains of enquiry relevant to psychology, such as science learning (de Saint-Georges, 2014; Shvarts & Abrahamson, 2023), or critical ageing studies (Gilleard & Higgs, 2015). Yet the risk is always to focus on the bodily experience and to forget its social embeddedness, and the fact that it is never cultural-free. It needed the strength of Biljana Stanković's theoretical construct, and the subtlety of her analysis, to bring to the fore this paradoxical evidence: even the most basic embodied experience, felt below symbolisation, is already highly culturally guided. Her coup de force is to show that human development happens also and foremost as an embodied experience, and this embodied experience is paradoxically both hyper culturally—socially, symbolically, technically—mediated, AND that still it can be experienced in a pre-semiotic manner. Here, as in many other developmental routes (Zavershneva & Van der Veer, 2018), human development and creativity entail re-creating for oneself what has been socio-culturally guided, and that this re-creation is both the condition of one's emancipation—inner freedom, social independence—and possibly, of social change.

Altogether, thus, this third volume of the series *Sociocultural psychology of the lifecourse* brings us one step ahead in the understanding of the dynamics of human development: after identity and meaning-making, we can now embrace both the socio-material environment, and the embodied nature of people's unique lived experiences. Understanding human lifecourse in changing societies requires complex thinking, and Biljana Stanković elegantly and vividly invites us to move forward in that direction.

Champp-du-Moulin, Switzerland Tania Zittoun
August 2024

References

Adams, M., & Fleer, M. (2017). International transitions: Generating subjective sense and subjective configuration in relation to the development of identity. *Mind, Culture, and Activity*, *0*(0), 1–15. https://doi.org/10.1080/10749039.2017.1346686

Bastos, A. C. de S. (2016). Shadow trajectories: The poetic motion of motherhood meanings through the lens of lived temporality. *Culture & Psychology*, 1354067X16655458. https://doi.org/10.1177/1354067X16655458

Boesch, E. E. (1991). *Symbolic action theory and cultural psychology* (Vol. ix). Springer-Verlag Publishing.

Brown, S. D., Cromby, J., Harper, D. J., Johnson, K., & Reavey, P. (2011). Researching "experience": Embodiment, methodology, process. *Theory & Psychology*, *21*(4), 493–515. https://doi.org/10.1177/0959354310377543

Cabell, K. R., Marsico, G., Cornejo, C., & Valsiner, J. (Eds.). (2015). *Making meaning, making motherhood*. Information Age Publishing.

Cabell, K. R., & Valsiner, J. (Eds.). (2014). *The catalyzing mind—Beyond models of causality*. Springer.

Chaudhary, N., Hviid, P., Marsico, G., & Villadsen, J. (Eds.). (2017). *Resistance in everyday life: Constructing cultural experiences*. Springer Singapore. Retrieved from https://www.springer.com/in/book/9789811035807

Cole, M. (1996). *Cultural psychology. A once and future discipline*. The Belknap Press of Harvard University Press.
Cornish, F. (2020). Communicative generalisation: Dialogical means of advancing knowledge through a case study of an 'unprecedented' disaster. *Culture & Psychology, 26*(1), 78–95. https://doi.org/10.1177/1354067X19894930
Crafter, S., Maunder, R., & Soulsby, L. (2019). *Developmental transitions: Exploring stability and change through the lifespan*. Routledge. https://doi.org/10.4324/9781315625263
Crosnoe, R., & Elder, G. H. (2002). Life course transitions, the generational stake, and grandparent-grandchild relationships. *Journal of Marriage and Family, 64*(4), 1089–1096.
Crosnoe, R., & Elder, G. H. (2004). From childhood to the later years: Pathways of human development. *Research on Aging, 26*(6), 623–654. https://doi.org/10.1177/0164027504268491
de Saint-Georges, I. (2014). Mediated Discourse Analysis, 'embodied learning' and emerging social and professional identities. In S. Norris & C. D. Maier (Eds.), *Interactions, images and texts. A reader in multimodality* (pp. 349–356). Walter de Gruyter. Retrieved from http://orbilu.uni.lu/handle/10993/17506
de Saint-Laurent, C. (2020). Sociocultural psychology. In *Social thinking and history: A sociocultural psychological perspective on representations of the past* (1st ed., pp. 6–26). Routledge. https://doi.org/10.4324/9780429465116
Demuth, C. (2018). Generalization from single cases and the concept of double dialogicality. *Integrative Psychological and Behavioral Science, 52*(1), 77–93. https://doi.org/10.1007/s12124-017-9399-1
Edwards, C. P., Knoche, L., Aukrust, V., Kumru, A., & Kim, M. (2006). Parental ethnotheories od child development. Looking beyond independence and individualism in American belief systems. In M. Kim, K.-S. Yang, & K. Hwang (Eds.), *Indigenous and cultural psychology. Understanding people in context* (pp. 141–162). Springer.
Fonagy, P. (2007). Embodied cognition? Commentary. In L. Mayes, P. Fonagy, & M. Target (Eds.), *Developmental science and psychoanalysis. Integration and innovation* (pp. 39–43). Karnac.
Gfeller, F. (2017). Imagination as embodied activity? Combining Zittoun's 'Imaginary loop model' with Schuetz' 'provinces of meaning'. In G. Sullivan, J. Cresswell, B. D. Ellis, M. Morgan, & E. Schraube (Eds.), *Resistance and renewal in theoretical psychology* (pp. 136–144). Captus University Publications.

Gilleard, C., & Higgs, P. (2015). Aging, embodiment, and the somatic turn. *Age, Culture, Humanities: An Interdisciplinary Journal, 2*, 17–33. https://doi.org/10.7146/ageculturehumanities.v2i.130485

Goffman, E. (1961). *Asylums: Essays on the social situation of mental patients and other inmates*. Anchor books.

LaRossa, R., & LaRossa, M. M. (1981). *Transition to parenthood.* Sage Publications.

Lawrence, J. A., Benedikt, R., & Valsiner, J. (1992). Homeless in the mind: A case-history of personal life in and out of a close orthodox community. *Journal of Social Distress and the Homeless, 1*(2), 157–176.

Lévi-Strauss, C. (1981). *Les structures élémentaires de la parenté* (Original 1949). Mouton.

Levy, R., Ghisletta, P., Le Goff, J.-M., Spini, D., & Widmer, E. (Eds.). (2005). *Towards an interdisciplinary perspective on the life course*. Elsevier.

Marková, I. (2023). *The making of a dialogical theory: Social representations and communication.* Cambridge University Press. https://doi.org/10.1017/9781009295000

Märtsin, M. (2019). *Identity development in the lifecourse: A semiotic cultural approach to transitions in early adulthood.* Palgrave Macmillan. https://doi.org/10.1007/978-3-030-27753-6

Mayer, C.-H., Fouché, P., J. P., & Van Niekerk, R. (Eds.). (2021). *Psychobiographical illustrations on meaning and identity in sociocultural contexts.* Springer International Publishing. https://doi.org/10.1007/978-3-030-81238-6

Michaels, G. Y., & Goldberg, W. A. (Eds.). (1988). *The transition to parenthood. Current theory and research*. Cambridge University Press.

Moro, M.-R. (2001). *Parents en exil: Psychopathologie et migrations* (2e éd.). Presses Universitaires de France.

Moscovici, S. (2008). *Psychoanalysis. Its image and its public* (G. Duveen, Ed.; D. Macey, Trans.). Polity Press.

Nathan, T. (1993). *Le sperme du diable: Éléments d'ethnopsychothérapie*. Presses Universitaires de France—PUF.

Obeyesekere, G. (1990). *The work of culture: Symbolic transformation in psychoanalysis and anthropology.* University of Chicago Press.

Pontecorvo, C., Fasulo, A., & Sterponi, L. (2001). Mutual apprentices: The making of parenthood and childhood in family dinner conversations. *Human Development, 44*(6), 340–361.

Rosa, A., & Valsiner, J. (Eds.). (2018). *The Cambridge handbook of sociocultural psychology* (2nd ed.). Cambridge University Press. https://doi.org/10.1017/9781316662229

Salvatore, S., & Valsiner, J. (2010). Between the general and the unique: Overcoming the nomothetic versus idiographic opposition. *Theory & Psychology, 20*(6), 817–833. https://doi.org/10.1177/0959354310381156

Sato, T. (2017). *Collected papers on trajectory equifinalty approach*. Chitose Press.

Scott, S. (2011). *Total institutions and reinvented identities* (2011 ed.). Palgrave Macmillan.

Shvarts, A., & Abrahamson, D. (2023). *Coordination dynamics of semiotic mediation: A functional dynamic systems perspective on mathematics teaching/learning*. Retrieved from https://www.semanticscholar.org/paper/Coordination-Dynamics-of-Semiotic-mediation%3A-A-on-Abrahamson-Shvarts/ccc133b93eb568aee290655b16b794056e541ae9

Stanković, B. (2024). *Giving birth to a subject. Transition to motherhood as an embodied and technologically mediated experience*. Palgrave.

Stenner, P. (2017). *Liminality and experience. A transdisciplinary approach to the psychosocial*. Palgrave Macmillan.

Stern, D. N., Bruschweiler-Stern, N., & Freeland, A. (1998). *The birth of a mother. How the experience of motherhood changes you forever*. Basic Bks.

Valsiner, J. (2000). *Culture and human development*. Sage.

Valsiner, J., Marsico, G., Chaudhary, N., Sato, T., & Dazzani, V. (Eds.). (2016). *Psychology as the science of human being: The Yokohama Manifesto*. Springer International Publishing. Retrieved from http://link.springer.com/10.1007/978-3-319-21094-0

Van Gennep, A. (1909). *Les rites de passage. Etude systématique des rites de la porte et du seuil, de l'hospitalité; de l'adoption, de la grossesse et de l'accouchement; de la naissance, de l'enfance, de la puberté; de l'initiation, de l'ordination, du couronnement; des fiancailles et du marriage; des funérailles, des saisons, etc.* Editions A. & J. Picard.

Wagoner, B., Chaudhary, N., & Hviid, P. (Eds.). (2015). *Integrating experiences: Body and mind moving between contexts*. Information Age Publishing.

Zavershneva, E., & Van der Veer, R. (2018). *Vygotsky's notebooks. A selection*. Springer.

Zittoun, T. (2004). Symbolic competencies for developmental transitions: The case of the choice of first names. *Culture & Psychology, 10*(2), 131–161. https://doi.org/10.1177/1354067X04040926

Zittoun, T. (2009). Dynamics of life-course transitions—A methodological reflection. In J. Valsiner, P. C. M. Molenaar, M. C. D. P. Lyra, & N. Chaudhary (Eds.), *Dynamic process methodology in the social and developmental sciences* (pp. 405–430). Springer.

Zittoun, T. (2011). A girl like a will-o'-the wisp. Listening to reports of cultural experiences as methodological mean to access to preconscious dynamics of sense making. In S. Salvatore & T. Zittoun (Eds.), *Cultural psychology and psychoanalysis in dialogue. Issues for constructive theoretical and methodological Synergies.*

Zittoun, T., Gillespie, A., & Bernal Marcos, M. J. (2023). Development and vulnerability across the lifecourse. Culture & Psychology, 1354067X231201384. https://doi.org/10.1177/1354067X231201384

Acknowledgements

This book would not have been possible without the generosity and commitment of the women who shared their stories, experiences, feelings and time with me. Many of them opened their homes and spent hours talking to me, even in the midst of pressing personal challenges. Their honesty, humour and resilience have deeply enriched this work. I am also profoundly grateful to the women who spoke to me in maternity hospitals, sometimes in very delicate states. Even though their voices may not be that explicitly present in this book, their experiences helped me immensely to piece together a complex picture of how giving birth and becoming a mother feels like within the local medical and institutional context. I extend my sincere thanks to the few medical practitioners who, despite their busy schedules, showed good will and found time to talk to me and allow me to observe their activities. Even if our views did not often align, their insights were invaluable in providing a well-rounded perspective on the topic.

Although the idea for this book was conceived years ago, it would likely not have come to fruition without the support of the series editor, Tania Zittoun. She recognised the potential of my study and believed that, despite its somewhat unorthodox approach, it could be a meaningful addition to a sociocultural book series. I am immensely grateful to her for her encouragement and unwavering support throughout this process and for her kind offer to write the foreword to this book.

I would also like to thank the production team at Palgrave Macmillan and Springer for their understanding, enormous patience and efficiency in guiding this book through the publication process.

Above all, I owe my deepest gratitude to my partner Rade for his insightful reading and invaluable feedback on the manuscript, for his endless and loving support over the years, and for taking on a disproportionate share of everyday parenting tasks while I was finishing the book. Finally, a heartfelt thank you to our daughter Iskra for her patience, which has been as great as can be expected from a preschooler, and with a big apology for missing some of our time together over the final months of writing. She has been both my everyday inspiration and my favourite distraction.

Certain parts of the analysis in this book, based on my PhD thesis, draw on work previously published in both English (Stankovic, 2017a, 2017b) and Serbian (Stanković, 2014, 2016; Stanković et al., 2017). I would like to thank Springer Nature for granting me permission to reproduce parts of my article: Stankovic, B. (2017a). Women's experiences of childbirth in Serbian public healthcare institutions: A qualitative study. *International Journal of Behavioral Medicine, 24*(6), 803–814. All previous articles dealt exclusively with the intricacies of the childbirth experience and medical care, unlike the broader exploration of pregnancy and the transition to motherhood presented in this book.

References

Stanković, B. (2014). Woman as a subject of childbirth: Physical, technological and institutional aspects. *Sociologija, 56*(4), 524–544. https://doi.org/10.2298/SOC1404524S

Stanković, B. (2016). Kritički prikaz istorije medikalizacije i maskulinizacije staranja o ženskom reproduktivnom telu. In N. Sekulić & M. Radoman (Eds.), *Izabrani radovi iz studija roda* (pp. 82–109). Institut za sociološka istraživanja Filozofskog fakulteta u Beogradu.

Stankovic, B. (2017a). Women's experiences of childbirth in Serbian public healthcare institutions: A qualitative study. *International Journal of Behavioral Medicine, 24*(6), 803–814. https://doi.org/10.1007/s12529-017-9672-1

Stankovic, B. (2017b). Situated technology in reproductive health care: Do we need a new theory of the subject to promote person-centred care? *Nursing Philosophy, 18*(1), e12159. https://doi.org/10.1111/nup.12159

Stanković, B., Skočajić, M., & Đorđević, A. (2017). Upravljanje porođajem u Srbiji: Medicinske intervencije i porođajna iskustva. *Limes Plus: Journal of Social Science and Humanities, 14*(2), 197–225.

Contents

1 **Introduction** 1
- 1.1 Early Transition to Motherhood as a Hybrid Process 3
- 1.2 Navigating the Theoretical Landscape 12
- 1.3 Introducing the Project 33
- References 52

2 **Situated Subjects: Cultural-Historical Contextualisation of Transition into Motherhood** 67
- 2.1 Medicalisation of the Transition into Motherhood 69
- 2.2 Alternative Discourses and Practices: The Naturalness Ideal 99
- 2.3 Medical & Natural Models: Mutually Exclusive or Complementary? 117
- References 125

3 **Embodied Subjects: Phenomenological Reconstruction of the Process of Becoming a Mother** 133
- 3.1 Phenomenology of the Reproductive Body: Hermeneutic and Practical Challenges 134
- 3.2 Uncertain Beginnings 141

3.3 Identification with Pregnancy and Individuation of the Baby: Pregnant Embodiment and the Role of Medical Knowledge/Technology 155
3.4 Ambivalent Role of Medical Technology in the Embodied Experience of Pregnancy 193
References 216

4 Distributed Subjects: Losing and Reclaiming Maternal Agency Under the Alienating Conditions of Local Institutional Practice 221
4.1 The Emergence of the Body-in-Labour: Institutional Resolution of Embodied Uncertainty 222
4.2 Transforming Embodied Subjects into Objects of Care 228
4.3 Broken Connections 236
4.4 Alienated Birth: Disrupted Embodied Subjectivity as a Consequence of Medical Interventions 250
4.5 Women as Embodied Agents Across Socio-material Networks 278
References 296

5 Conclusion 301
5.1 Maternal Embodiment 303
5.2 Technological Mediatedness 311
5.3 Socio-material Embeddedness 327
5.4 A Revised Theory of Subjectivity and Ethical-Political Consequences 333
References 344

References 349

Index 375

1
Introduction

As a pioneering author on motherhood, Ann Oakley, rightly suggests—"the choice of research topic amongst social scientists reflects a mixture of the personal and the professional" (Edmonds & Warburton, 2013), and I am no exception. Growing up in a post-socialist country in the Balkans that in the 1990s upheld the traditionalist and patriarchal aspects of its pre-Yugoslavian past (Blagojević, 1997; Vujadinović & Stanimirović, 2017), I was more than ambivalent when it came to the expected roles and responsibilities of women—motherhood being one of the most prominent. Entering academia and embracing the feminist ideals only fortified this resistance. But subscribing to various forms of discursive and constructivist thinking just left me perplexed when faced with my own experience—the fascination with the generative capacities of the female body and the (ambivalent) desire to bear a child, as well as the constant reminders of my own female/reproductive corporeality long before I had a child of my own.[1] I struggled to approach the subject in such a way as to avoid simplification and to engage also with the aspects

[1] As Jane Ussher states in the Preface to her book "Managing the monstrous feminine" (2006): "the relationship between the construction and materiality of the reproductive body and my own subjectivity is a relationship I cannot ignore".

B. Stanković, *Giving Birth To A Subject*, Sociocultural Psychology of the Lifecourse,
https://doi.org/10.1007/978-3-031-77236-8_1

that seemed the most elusive and challenging. I wanted to explore the early stages of the transition to motherhood—namely pregnancy and childbirth—as embodied experiences that are fundamentally shaped by the constructions, representations, practices, technologies and institutional and material conditions governing contemporary femininity and motherhood in the local context.

This book analyses how women, during a life stage of intense changes and ruptures, navigate their personal worlds that are embedded in a complex and rapidly changing sociocultural context of a post-socialist society. Transition into first-time motherhood is recognised as a unique non-pathological phase in adult development that brings about an abundance of profound psychosocial and bodily changes for a person. The aim was to study those changes from a first-person perspective and with a particular attention to those dimensions of personal experience and functioning that are usually neglected in psychological (even sociocultural) scholarship—their embodiment and techno-material mediatedness. The experiences of pregnancy, childbirth and the immediate postpartum, as crucial early stages of the transition into motherhood, are treated as paradigmatic showcases for these neglected aspects. While some parts of this book may seem strangely detached from the usual considerations of maternal identity and transition to motherhood (e.g. Laney et al., 2015; Smith, 1999), I want to suggest that some crucial aspects of this peculiar, complex and ambivalent experience emerge in the early stages of adjustment to living with and caring for another being recognised as one's own. Furthermore, I firmly believe that a study of the lived experience of motherhood cannot be separated from the study of female reproduction and gendered embodiment, so I will draw on authors and traditions that are not common in psychological studies of developmental processes or social identities. Therefore, I will be primarily committed to the topic I am engaging with and not to disciplinary boundaries or the usual genres in the field.

The aim of exploring the processes of technologically mediated embodied subjectivity embedded in the vicissitudes of the local institutional and social environment calls for a range of theoretical and methodological resources. To account for this multi-layered, complex and contextualised phenomenon, I outline a theoretical framework that connects sociocultural psychology with phenomenology and science and technology studies, and I approach the topic empirically through both a phenomenological and a critical-discursive methodological lens. Hopefully, this pluralistic and interdisciplinary approach will help me move forward the way we think not only about women's experiences, pregnant and birthing bodies and medical practices, but also the way we think about subjects, their embodied conditions of existence and their entanglements with socio-material aspects of culture.

The focus on experiential female subjectivity is not accidental—it is grounded in both my theoretical/political commitments and my own lived experience. And it is further encouraged by the subtle, yet persistent dominance of the male norm in both psychology and the common imagination when thinking about subjects. This norm, both productive and oppressive, firmly rooted in the gender and sexual difference (re)produced by patriarchal society, shapes female bodies and minds, their conduct and relationships. It also becomes especially visible and damaging when it comes to the issue of reproduction. This is why the choice of topic was not solely grounded in my lived experience as a woman of reproductive age. I recognised it as particularly suitable for exploring different issues that lie at the convergence of various contemporary theoretical and political interests and fascinations.

This introductory chapter has three aims: to outline the complex and dynamic nature of the topic that I will try to elaborate in the remainder of the book, to position it in the conversation with different theoretical traditions and to provide an insight into the aspects of its empirical investigation.

1.1 Early Transition to Motherhood as a Hybrid Process

In Serbia, where the study that forms the empirical basis of this book takes place, it is customary to refer to pregnancy as "*drugo stanje*"—"the other state" or "the other condition". There is no English equivalent for this idiom and yet it adequately describes the peculiarity of the process a woman undergoes in the early stages of the transition to motherhood.

In a short period of just nine months, enormous changes occur in the psychophysical functioning of a woman's body. Extensive physiological, metabolic, anatomical and biochemical changes are part of the process of adapting a woman's body to a new state. Many of them begin immediately after conception and continue throughout pregnancy, and the body only returns to its previous state after childbirth or even after cessation of breastfeeding. As a result of these changes, all organ systems function at an increased level: the total amount of blood raises, so the heart works faster and the pressure in the blood vessels increases; the need for oxygen increases, so breathing accelerates and deepens; the total amount of fluid in the body increases, so the excretory system works under a greater load; the functioning of the glands with internal secretion changes, so the levels of certain hormones increase up to several tens of thousands of times, while others are almost completely absent (Cunningham et al., 2010, p. 107–131). This description exemplifies a scientific and at the same time quite common way of depicting pregnancy and birth. They are represented as spontaneous and objectively determined processes in which a woman's subjectivity has no role at all. Based on such a representation of pregnancy and childbirth, which has acquired not only a dominant but also an indisputable status in modern age, it seems as if the pregnant body is the sole bearer of these processes—like a hidden *laboratory* or *factory* in which the process of natural reproduction takes place. But this peculiar representation is historically relatively recent, and both metaphors in the previous sentence were deliberately chosen to reflect the kind of transformation—*scientific* and *technological*—that pregnancy and childbirth have undergone and which have enabled their identification with the biological process of foetal development. This transformation had a profound impact on female experiential subjectivity and shaped a historically specific process of transition into motherhood.

At the same time, from a psychosocial perspective, pregnancy represents a significant and complex transitional phase in which a woman's experience of herself and others, her interactions, functioning, imagining of the future change, sometimes in a radical manner (Cabell et al., 2015; Darvill et al., 2010; Gross & Pattison, 2007; Smith, 1999; Stern et al., 1998). The above medical description is therefore limited, as it considers the location and cause of the changes to be exclusively internal—in the spontaneity and inevitability of the bodily changes and the accompanying psychological transformations. However, once a woman becomes pregnant, a whole set of social expectations and rules apply to her, under the influence of which she reshapes her daily life in various ways—her eating habits and medication intake, sleeping patterns, daily activities, exercising and so on. This is a consequence of the fact that pregnancy and childbirth are not only private events, developmental stages important for an individual subject, nor are they only physiological processes that can be objectively observed and regulated. They have also been the subject of various sociocultural representations, practices, norms and taboos throughout history (Duby & Perrot, 1992; Martin, 1992; McGrath, 2002; Rich, 1986b; Riggs & Bartholomaeus, 2023, etc.).

For centuries, all around the world, certain cultural attitudes and practices have surrounded pregnancy and childbirth. "Nowhere is the pregnant woman taken for granted", and the associations and regulative practices directed at her "culminate in the birth itself" (Rich, 1986b, p. 162). The cultural regulation of female reproduction, particularly childbirth, is of particular importance because of the social function of initiating "the new social members that will ensure the future of the society into which they are born" (Davis-Floyd, 1994, p. 1125). Pregnancy and childbirth are associated with crucial transitional phases—with entry into life, but also with death, which in the past was a frequent outcome of these events, which were therefore subject to the strictest taboos (de Beauvoir, 2011). The way in which women are treated at this stage of their lives has depended crucially on historically specific representations of their reproductive bodies.[2]

[2] This book deals with a phenomenon that is culturally and historically constituted, and I believe that it cannot be adequately understood without at least a partial reconstruction of its sociogenesis and historical roots. The interpretation of history has implications for how we understand the present situation and how we ask and answer ethical and political questions, hence "we need a historical awareness of our current circumstances" (Foucault, 1982, p. 778). On the one hand, it is unproblematic and self-evident to claim that the forms of representation and treatment of (female reproductive) bodies have changed throughout history. On the other hand, it is less self-evident to claim that this also applies to our intimate experience of our own corporeality (Duden, 1991; Kukla, 2005; Kuriyama, 1999; Porter, 2003). Without at least a cursory insight into their historical genesis, it would be difficult to distance ourselves from contemporary hegemonic representations of the body or to adequately understand all the meanings associated with these representations with-

Reproductive processes and women as subjects/objects of these processes figure in various ways in numerous discourses—medical, neoliberal, feminist, religious, psychological, etc. This creates a situation of occasionally incommensurable constructions that coexist in a dynamic space of contemporary culture, while their voices, more or less loud and articulated, shape everyday practice, behaviour and relationships. The concrete female experience is thus constituted by a whole system of cultural beliefs and practices related to the notion of a woman, a pregnant woman, a mother, originating in a variety of social institutions at a given historical moment. As Adrienne Rich argues: "As soon as a woman knows that a child is growing in her body, she falls under the power of theories, ideals, archetypes, descriptions of her new existence, almost none of which have come from other women (though other women may transmit them) and all of which have floated invisibly about her since she first perceived herself to be female, and therefore potentially a mother" (1986b, p. 61–62). A woman's experience is simultaneously enabled and constrained by certain representations of pregnancy and childbirth that she encounters "in the booklet in her obstetrician's waiting room, the novels she had read, her mother-in-law's approval, her memories of her own mother, the Sistine Madonna or Michelangelo's Pietà (...)" (Rich, 1986b, p. 39). Most of the time, however, these "archetypal mothers, Italian Madonnas" that capture our imagination stand in stark contrast to our own experience, which remains "blind and dumb, unspoken" (Griffin, 2001, p. 35).

Moreover, no other period in a woman's development is as rich in cultural stereotypes as pregnancy, and these stereotypes have often been a major source of discrimination against women (DiQuinzio, 1999; Leifer, 1980). The existence of contraception and the legalisation of abortion put pregnancy (and motherhood) in a unique position compared to all other (biologically conditioned) developmental states—they become a matter of choice and are determined by numerous sociocultural and situational circumstances, thus also acquiring a great political potential (Philipp & Carr, 2001). Therefore, reproductive issues have been and

---

out knowledge of their aetiology. It would be even more difficult to distance ourselves from our immediate embodied experience, which serves us as an inevitable normative ideal.

continue to be the target of political regulation and state intervention in various historical circumstances (Duby & Perrot, 1992; McLaren, 1999). The public interest in the seemingly private matter of becoming a mother is realised not only through cultural representations and normative expectations, but also through numerous practices of surveillance and regulation involving various actors, a range of technologies and the material aspects of the (mostly institutional) environment.

This complex landscape that regulates and shapes the process of becoming a mother for contemporary women reveals the hybrid nature of the phenomenon itself (Latour, 1993)—it is physiological, embodied, deeply emotional and personal yet distinctively public, constituted and reproduced through a number of discursive-material practices. Pregnancy thus entails an array of ambivalences for a woman. It is a process that takes place both inside and outside—as an internal process mediated and regulated by external means. A woman is confronted with a twofold set of changes—those that happen to her body (both in its depths and on the surface) and those that take place in her environment as a result of her changed status. These changes profoundly shape her experience, her relationship to herself and her own body, as well as her everyday practices and functioning. While a woman certainly undergoes a series of *spontaneous* transformations, she is also the one who monitors and takes care of her pregnancy while relying on the prevailing social norms and the culturally available resources. The ambivalent situation in which a woman finds herself implies a complex dynamic of passivity and agency, spontaneity and effort. Partly in continuation with *ambiguous transcendence* that was already a dominant modality of her female embodied existence (Young, 2005a),[3] some new challenges emerge during this phase of her life. While I will explore this dynamic later through discussion of the concrete empirical material, in the next section I will provide a brief

[3] In her seminal essay on feminine body comportment and motility, Iris Marion Young (2005a) proposes ambiguous transcendence as one of the modalities of feminine embodiment. Instead of being primarily open and oriented towards the world and acting in it, women are simultaneously oriented towards their bodies as objects in that world: "Rather than simply beginning in immanence, feminine bodily existence remains in immanence or, better, is overlaid with immanence, even as it moves out toward the world" (Young, 2005a, p. 36). Women are thus never merely lived bodies or embodied subjects, but objectify aspects of their own embodied existence (often by focusing on its aesthetic and erotic qualities).

overview of the central tension that I believe lies at the heart of these ambivalences—the fact that women have historically been both subjects and objects of pregnancy, childbirth and motherhood.

1.1.1 Complementary Processes of the Objectification of the Reproductive Body and the Privatisation of the Female Experience

For more than two thousand years, the female body was constantly portrayed as changeable and unpredictable. Its reproductive capacity was associated with special powers, but also with the risk that these powers could be disrupted and perverted, which is why women's bodies must be subjected to surveillance and control (Kukla, 2005).[4] Until the seventeenth century, the womb was represented as a mysterious, irrational force that was unpredictable and dangerous.[5] It was imagined as a fascinating organ, capable of creating life and sustaining it, but, due to its unpredictability and permeable and changeable nature, also of deforming and endangering the life within.[6] For this reason, across history and cultures, the uterus, and with it the (pregnant) woman, was seen as something to be monitored and protected from harmful influences. Anything could pose a potential danger to the foetus—what a pregnant woman eats, drinks, breathes in, what she thinks or dreams about, what she craves (Kukla, 2005). Outside of the Western tradition, it was also believed that a woman was particularly vulnerable and susceptible to negative influences and occult forces during pregnancy and childbirth, so the practices of isolating women and purification rituals were common in many cultures around the world (Rich, 1986b, p. 163). While the distrust of

[4] Hippocrates believed that women's skin is spongy and permeable, which is why they are much more susceptible to all external influences (King, 1998).

[5] Hippocrates and Plato began a very long tradition of understanding the uterus as an autonomous organ with its own passions and aspirations. Not only was it capable of expanding and contracting, but it also had the ability to wander around the body and cause various diseases and disorders (Platon, 1995, p. 164–165).

[6] This type of representation extended to more than just the uterus—the entire interior of the female body was seen as a fluid space in which the organs moved and in which bodily fluids (milk, blood, pus) could transform into one another and emerge from any opening on the body (Duden, 1991).

the female reproductive body and the accompanying need to monitor and regulate it show a remarkable historical continuity, there has also been an important break with the way this body has been represented and treated.

For centuries, the pregnant body was understood as "a tree that bears fruit", and it was not until the second half of the eighteenth century that it began to be interpreted as "a machine that reproduces the species" (Shaw, 2012, p. 110). It is usually assumed that during this period there was a fundamental shift in the way women were represented and treated in relation to their reproductive states, particularly pregnancy and childbirth (Kukla, 2005; Moscucci, 1990). This transformation is regularly associated, on the one hand, with advances in science, especially medicine, and on the other with changes in the political and social sphere. As Barbara Duden (1993, p. 95) puts it: "Science discovers and professionals control and mediate her womb as a public space. Her flesh becomes the forum whose proceedings are of immediate interest to the state and society". The woman's body thus becomes public, both as an object of observation and medical intervention and as an object of social and institutional management.

The emergence of the hegemonic scientific model, on the one hand, led to a fundamental change at the level of language and the verbal representation of the body—an abundance of local labels for body parts and body processes disappeared and were replaced by medical terminology (Duden, 1991). On the other hand, research by historians of medicine shows that until the end of the seventeenth century, various types of healers operated on a fairly equal footing. Trained physicians (*medici*) offered their services in addition to barbers, midwives, chiropractors, herbalists, sorcerers, etc. (Pelling & Webster, 1979). Apparently all of them took care of the same object—the patient's body—but since this object was not yet defined in a monopolistic way by one discipline, different professions were needed for its care: "The real and symbolic multiformity of the body had its counterpart in the multiformity of the social body of the healers" (Duden, 1991, p. 26). Only the emergence of a new representation of the physical body given by modern science has enabled medicine to have a monopoly on everything that concerns the body.

Today, when we refer to a (reproductive) body, we imply a material object that has a certain shape, occupies a certain space and whose interior is filled with organs that function according to natural laws. The process of "discovering" or constituting this body has been carried out since the eighteenth century by biology and made possible by the epistemological shift in medicine (Foucault, 2003). Knowledge of the illness based on patients' reports has been replaced by the analysis of tissues and organs, and in particular by post-mortem analysis, which entails the most radical absence of the patient's subjectivity: "The power of the anatomical-pathological model, as it emerged from Paris hospitals in the late eighteenth century, lays in its capacity to strip away individual differences, affective and material, so as to perceive the essence of health or disease in organ tissues. The autopsy, not the interview, was the moment of truth" (Laqueur, 1990, p. 188). The emergence of the hospital, with its objective practices and examination techniques—that enabled the naturalisation of the human body—also transformed the patient's experience into a private affair (Mol & Law, 2004). This complementary process of naturalisation of the body and privatisation of experience seems to be an essential characteristic of the specifically modern transformation of human existence, which has also heavily influenced the situation in the field of female reproduction. Namely, since the beginning of the modern era, pregnancy and birth have been constituted as purely physical and therefore natural processes that could not only be objectively described by the apparatus of the natural sciences, but also *technologically* regulated. As a consequence, the subjective, experiential aspect of these processes and the psychosocial transformation that women go through are relocated and transferred to the private sphere.[7]

---

[7] Numerous studies point to this split and duality, although they are often not recognised as a specific consequence of modern transformation, nor is their complementarity reflected upon. Authors who have analysed discourses on pregnancy and childbirth have identified a tension between two models of these processes in Western societies. On the one hand, their biological nature and the need for medical monitoring and regulation are emphasised, and on the other, their psychological significance for women, their identity and their relationships with others (Woollett & Marshall, 1997). Both models are reflected in women's experiences. Women often rely on medical concepts of risk and safety to justify the decision to use technology to monitor pregnancy and childbirth, but they also want to experience their pregnancy and childbirth as natural and emotionally fulfilling (Martin, 1992).

This process of privatisation and psychologisation is of course not limited to the realm of reproductive experience, but is also evident in many other areas of life and plays a decisive role in the genesis of the modern subject, who has become the exclusive bearer of its own activities and states.[8] I am inclined to see the emergence and proliferation of discourses on personal experiences of pregnancy and childbirth as one of the consequences of this specific modern form of sociocultural regulation, which removes pregnancy and childbirth from the public sphere and transforms them into private and psychic experiences. This is particularly true of the contemporary era and the rise of numerous websites, forums and blogs where thousands of anonymous women narrate their pregnancy and birth experiences and share them with others.[9] This has created a complementary sphere to the exclusively physical and medically regulated one.

It seems, however, that an insurmountable gap remains between them, as each sphere is associated with a corresponding public space as well as with different norms, discourses, practices and actors. This divide, as we will see in detail, is reflected both in the literature, which operates within clear disciplinary boundaries, and in practice, particularly in the institutional conditions of maternity hospitals, where doctors are exclusively responsible for reproductive bodies, but not for the subjects who inhibit those bodies. I will discuss this point in detail later in the book, but here is a brief illustration: the typical response of doctors to my question about whether administering hormones during labour increases pain is that it accelerates and intensifies uterine contractions and that pain is a "subjective category". They clearly draw a demarcation line between the objective and the subjective, positioning themselves as responsible only for the former. Relying on experience is seen as inappropriate and as having no place in the evaluation of medical practices and techniques that deal

[8] For example, the practice of suppressing the public expression of pain and the obligation to mourn the deceased in solitude has led to a privatisation of the feelings caused by loss. In this way, mourning after the death of loved ones has been transformed from a public to an intimate family act (Arijes, 1989).

[9] Foucault (1988) emphasised the verbalisation of one's own inner states as one of the most significant technologies of the self, which enables a person to become their own hermeneut (Foucault, 1988). The hermeneutics of the self, an interpretative analysis of oneself by the individual (for oneself and for others), begins with the transformation of the ancient imperative *know thyself* into the Christian imperative *confess thy thoughts*. Foucault considers this transformation to be essential for the development of modern subjectivity.

exclusively with the objective (i.e. objectified) bodies of women. This divide also becomes apparent to a woman herself whenever the objective representation or treatment of her body and the way she experiences it differ significantly. As we will see in the course of the analysis, it can prove particularly difficult to negotiate and bring these two aspects together.

The aim so far has been to introduce various aspects that jointly shape the transitory paths and experiences of mothers-to-be and which I will elaborate in detail in the following chapters. Now I will critically examine how these topics are usually addressed in different areas of psychology, where their hybrid character is regularly neglected with some aspects missing completely, especially those related to women's embodied subjectivity. I will then present my research project, which aims to redress this theoretical and empirical myopia in psychology. Finally, I will provide an overview of the remainder of the book.

1.2 Navigating the Theoretical Landscape

For the positioning of this study, it is relevant to note that although the discourse of personal experience is very present in the public sphere, it cannot be said that this tendency is sufficiently reflected in academic research, especially not in psychology, where one might expect it first. Nearly forty years ago, Iris Marion Young (2005b) concluded that for most disciplines and experts dealing with pregnancy, it is a state during which the foetus develops, an objective process accessible to scientific observation. Treated in this way, "pregnancy does not belong to the woman herself" (Young, 2005b, p. 46), as it is reduced to the natural environment in which prenatal development takes place. Since "discourse on pregnancy omits subjectivity, for the specific experience of women has been absent from most of our culture's discourse about human experience and history", Young (2005b, p. 46) sets as her goal to "let women speak in their own voices". Analysis of the literature available at the time showed that pregnancy almost never appears as a process "concerned with the subject, the mother as the site of her proceedings" (Kristeva, 1990, p. 441). It is precisely this critical project of second-wave feminist authors that has been instrumental in changing the situation considerably, and for this reason we will begin this theoretical positioning with it.

1.2.1 Feminist Appropriation of Female Reproduction and Motherhood

At the beginning of the second wave of feminism, in which issues of women's reproductive rights and birth control occupy a significant place, feminists regarded pregnancy and motherhood as primary factors in the oppression of women and as an important field of political struggle. Simone de Beauvoir (2011) attempts to denaturalise pregnancy and motherhood and to distance women from their reproductive role in order to create space for the conceptualisation of female subjectivity outside of patriarchal discourse. She explicitly understands reproduction as a biological process, a matter of the species, but her theoretical approach and discursive strategies show how it is possible to conceptualise nature not only as normal or productive, but also as invasive, entrapping and castrating (Zerilli, 1992).

Pregnancy is described as a process that inevitably leads to alienation: "inhabited by another who is nourished by her substance, the female is both herself and other than herself during the whole gestation period" (de Beauvoir, 2011, p. 63). However, the alienating and oppressive outcome is not only associated with pregnancy, but also with other reproductive processes: "Childbirth itself is painful; it is dangerous. This crisis shows clearly that the body does not always meet the needs of both the species and the individual (...) Breastfeeding is also an exhausting servitude"; as a consequence "from puberty to menopause she is the principal site of a story that takes place in her and does not concern her personally" (de Beauvoir, 2011, p. 68). Nevertheless, it is important to point out that de Beauvoir introduces a crucial distinction when it comes to recognising the source of women's oppression. Although the woman is "the prey of the species", the extent of this subjugation is not conditioned by biology, but by the social norms, practices and institutions that regulate female reproduction: "It is not possible to measure in the abstract the burden of the generative function for woman (...) it is undefined for woman; only society can decide" (de Beauvoir, 2011, p. 76).

Simone de Beauvoir's critical move opened up a space for the conceptualisation of female subjectivity independently of the patriarchal discourse of *natural* motherhood, and this space could be occupied by different (even completely opposing) theoretical and political strategies.

One current of feminist authors pursued the path of further distancing women from their reproductive capacities and conceptualising their nature as non-specific, i.e. no different from that of men, and based the project of political equality between women and men on this non-difference. They believed that "women are silenced most effectively by their association with maternity" (Walker, 1998, p. 1), because "women's inequality and oppression are related to the social assignment of mothering to women" (DiQuinzio, 1999, p. 13). In contrast, another current saw in de Beauvoir's denaturalisation and distancing an opportunity to affirm women's reproductive powers and motherhood as personal and political capacities on which feminist theory and activism could be based (Rich, 1986b; Young, 2005b; Zerilli, 1992). This affirmation would be impossible within a theoretical and political space where the patriarchal discourse of natural motherhood holds hegemony, as such an affirmation would merely reproduce this discourse. Thus, following a wave of unproblematic and unequivocally critical understandings of reproductive states such as pregnancy and childbirth, voices emerged that attempted to acknowledge these states through a predominantly phenomenological lens in an affirmative tone. The re-affirmation of pregnancy and motherhood becomes one of the goals of feminist theory, repositioning women as subjects of their own reproductive and mothering experiences (O'Reilly, 2004; Rich, 1986b; Young, 2005b). The aim is to transform a patriarchal institution into a rewarding and empowering experience for women. The authors of this current see motherhood as an opportunity for each woman's individualisation and creativity, something that not only distinguishes women from men, but also puts them in a privileged position.[10]

As a consequence of feminist considerations of this topic, recent decades have seen an increasing number of academic references dealing

[10] The description of the specificity of female psychosexuality by Julia Kristeva (2009) is illustrative of this stance: "Far from being as narcissistic as people say and, on the whole, less narcissistic than men, women are straightaway involved in relationships with others: to live means to live for the other, including, and above all, when this is impossible and traumatizing. Far from locking themselves into the obsessional palace of pure thought, thinking, for women, cannot be shut off from carnal sensoriality: the metaphysical body/soul dichotomy is, in these women, unbearable; they describe thought as physical happiness, eros for them is not dissociable from agape and vice versa. Their time is necessarily punctuated by a concern for finitude, but without being haunted by the race to death, and it is calmed by the miracle of birth, a kind of opening out".

with pregnancy, childbirth and motherhood in various fields of the social sciences and humanities—most notably in gender studies, but also in anthropology, sociology, science and technology studies, history and cultural studies. While contemporary critical approaches still follow the crucial distinction between the institution of motherhood and the experience/practice of mothering (Rich, 1986b), they do so in theoretically and politically diverse ways and often through the lenses of intersectionality (Baraitser, 2009; Buchanan, 2013; DiQuinzio, 1999; Hays, 1998; Mack, 2018; O'Reilly, 2004). These issues are approached as complex, situated and highly ambivalent, since motherhood is often seen as both a potential resource of empowerment and a source of gender oppression.

As we shall see, psychology turned to these topics neither early nor readily. Despite the increasing presence of the discourse on pregnancy and childbirth in academia, some aspects remain systematically excluded, at least in psychology. An overview of the literature shows that few studies focus on the subjectivity of women (Chadwick, 2009). Reproductive processes and motherhood are rarely considered from the *embodied* and *first-person* perspectives of pregnant or birthing women. It is characteristic of psychology to ignore and omit concrete subjective experiences (Nicolson, 2010), particularly those concerning bodily states, and addressing women's experiences has historically had an additionally marginalised and contested status.

1.2.2 Psychology on Women, Reproduction and Motherhood

Research into specifically female developmental phases, processes and experiences such as pregnancy, birth, motherhood, menstruation and menopause, which are related to the reproductive potential of women, has only emerged in psychology in recent decades. This is not surprising given the historical androcentrism of psychology, which for a long time was reflected in the fact that women were generally not included in psychological research in any way (Unger, 2001).[11] Furthermore, the

[11] Murray and Allport, for example, based their psychological theories of personality on studies that included only men in the sample (Marecek et al., 2003, p. 252).

theories were formulated under the influence of patriarchal prejudices—the normative model of female functioning was defined from the perspective of a middle-class white male. Any deviation from this model observed in women's behaviour was attributed to biological rather than social factors (Weisstein, 1968). The primary goal of the *psychology of women* program, which emerged under the influence of second-wave feminism (Denmark et al., 2008), was therefore to show that there is no substantial asymmetry in cognitive abilities, emotions, personality traits, values and inclinations between men and women, and that the differences that sometimes manifest are the result of social pressures on women's behaviour—in a discriminatory environment of a patriarchal society, they are a normal adaptive function. It was not until the 1980s that the focus of research shifted from comparing men and women to highlighting the particularity of feminine psychological qualities—specifically female emotions, identities and needs (Marecek et al., 2003). The aim was to revalue and affirm those characteristics of women that had been neglected, rejected or considered signs of weakness and lesser value. This shift allowed women's experiences related to their reproductive capacities to become a topic of study.

The oppression of women has historically and cross-culturally been associated with the reproductive functions of the female body. Until the end of the nineteenth century, it was believed that a change in women's role in society—which would imply better education, greater economic independence, a wider range of professional and personal choices and more political power—would threaten what essentially defines a woman, namely her reproductive potential.[12] Not only would they endanger themselves as individuals—because after compromising their primary function, they would have difficulty finding their identity and maintaining their mental health and well-being—but the survival of society would also be at risk. This belief has long been reproduced by male psychologists, especially within clinical psychology (Weisstein, 1968). Therefore,

[12] In the nineteenth century, doctors still claimed that the uterus competed with the brain for a sufficient blood supply, so that any effort a woman made in terms of education or career was seen as something that would be at the expense of her fertility and primary reproductive role (Endžier, 2010, p. 104). Psychologists also based their recommendations regarding the education of girls on such ideas (Hall, 1904, Chapter XVII).

the preoccupation with the women's reproductive function was both theoretically and politically relevant for feminist projects aimed at the emancipation of women. According to some contemporary feminists (members of the so-called third wave), the preoccupation with reproductive capacities can be seen as problematic because it confirms claims about the difference between women and men and even implies that these differences are biological in nature (Wilson, 1998). However, the fact is that psychology has long ignored and devalued the specific experiences of women, and if this were to continue within the psychology of women, it would only confirm that they are less relevant and suitable for serious research because, among other things, the findings cannot be generalised to men (Ussher, 1990). The importance of addressing these issues is also evident from the fact that in many areas of psychology that have included them in their agenda, research tends to take place within a framework that reproduces the traditional pattern and still leads to pathologisation of women's reproductive capacities.

Thus, within *developmental psychology*, under the influence of psychoanalysis, pregnancy and transition to motherhood are traditionally seen as a period of *crisis* during which a woman faces a series of developmental tasks. She is depicted primarily as a future mother who is in the process of adapting to a new role (Gloger-Tippelt, 1983; Leifer, 1977; Smith, 1999; Valentine, 1982). Research maps the development of women's feelings during pregnancy—their emotional stability, the extent of their anxiety and the transformation of relationships with close persons—partner, mother, etc. (Gerson et al., 1984). Developmental outcomes are assessed by measuring maternal attitudes and competencies, coping mechanisms, attachment patterns, etc. (Alhusen, 2008; Camberis et al., 2014; Cannella, 2005; DiPietro, 2010). The psychoanalytic legacy in this area can also be found in the individualisation of responsibility (and blame)[13] for potential failure in this process of adaptation—it is seen as the result of the woman's inability to resolve her intrapsychic conflicts (Leifer, 1980), and in the fact that the optimal psychological outcome of pregnancy is typically seen as an adjustment to the traditionally defined role of the mother.

[13] It should be noted that the tendency towards individualisation is a much broader trend that has followed mainstream psychology throughout its entire history (Hider, 1978).

Within clinical psychology, in line with the psychopathological heritage, female reproductive processes are only treated to the extent that they appear as potential causes of psychological disturbances. Research therefore focuses on phenomena such as premenstrual syndrome (PMS), menopause, etc. (Chadwick, 2006; Nicolson, 1998; Ussher, 2006). Moreover, there is a particular interest in women whose transition to motherhood is perceived as problematic or dysfunctional. Thus, postpartum depression has been a very common subject of numerous studies and therapeutic treatments (Stanton et al., 2002). As might be expected, clinical psychology shares with developmental psychology the approach that implies the individualisation of pathology, so that the psychological difficulties of postpartum women are not related to the social context in which a woman becomes a mother. Authors such as Paula Nicolson (1998), who come from a critical and feminist-oriented psychology of women, offer an alternative perspective that does not pathologise or individualise phenomena related to motherhood and reproductive processes. Thus, postpartum depression is not recognised as a pathological phenomenon, but as a normal psychological reaction to the realisation that real motherhood differs from the patriarchal myth of natural, instinctive, fulfilling motherhood. This author also notes that women are not allowed to have a "normal" feeling of grief over numerous losses and deficiencies compared to the life they had before having a child—the lack of independence, time, control over their lives, sexuality, etc.—and they are expected to always be content and fulfilled.

Within clinical psychology, psychological studies on *childbirth* can also be found. Until recently, research into birth experiences was a real rarity in psychology. Given the presumed strictly biological nature of this process, the psychology of childbirth would almost represent an inherent contradiction (Chadwick, 2006; Stanton et al., 2002). As might be expected, existing research on childbirth focuses on this process as a possible cause of psychological disorders and pathological conditions. There are a considerable number of recent studies on post-traumatic stress disorder and postnatal depression that develop after childbirth (Bailham & Joseph, 2003; Creedy et al., 2000; Czarnocka & Slade, 2000; Lyons, 1998; Olde et al., 2005; Soet et al., 2003). These studies focus primarily on identifying *individual* risk factors that could explain why some women react so negatively to childbirth, while the potentially distressing or oppressive aspects of medical treatment and the institutional environment are rarely considered empirically.

However, since a number of studies indicate that psychological aspects of childbirth and the quality of childbirth experience are relevant for postpartum outcomes (Bielinski-Blattmann et al., 2016; Creedy et al., 2000; Elmir et al., 2010; Olde et al., 2005; Soet et al., 2003; Thomson & Downe, 2008), this has led to women's perspectives and personal needs being recognised as important in the evaluation and improvement of medical practice in diverse institutional contexts (Chadwick et al., 2014; Hodnett, 2002; Larkin et al., 2012; Pittrof et al., 2002; WHO, 2018). This is a promising change, as traditionally childbirth has been judged primarily by its end result—in terms of mortality rates or physical indicators of maternal and infant health, while the subjective aspect of the process has been largely omitted or deemed irrelevant (Baker et al., 2005). However, attempts to grasp the perspective of women giving birth are often done by assessing simple and superficial aspects—such as measures of satisfaction with the birth experience or the maternal services provided. Some authors report that quantitative measures of birth satisfaction can be biased and skewed towards positive evaluations, so they can differ considerably from the findings of qualitative research (Chadwick et al., 2014).[14] Since the birth experience, as we will see, is very complex and ambiguous, a qualitative analysis that starts from the women's perspective and explores personal meanings, embodied experiences, as well as concrete institutional contexts, is expected to offer more accurate and relevant insights.

Research on reproductive experiences in Serbia was practically non-existent until recently.[15] However, while the process and experience of pregnancy is still conspicuously neglected, during the last decade there emerged a number of studies focusing on the quality of and access to

[14] There is evidence indicating that measures of patient satisfaction provide only a limited and possibly overly optimistic picture of their experience of care (Jenkinson et al., 2002). It is therefore suggested that a more nuanced and detailed exploration of service users' birth experiences would likely provide a more appropriate picture.

[15] There have been previous studies dealing with reproductive rights and population policies in Serbia (e.g. Bracewell, 1996; Djoric & Gavrilovic, 2006; Shiffman et al., 2002).

maternity care and women's birth experiences, but mostly from a sociological and anthropological perspective (Arsenijevic et al., 2014; Matejić et al., 2014; Pantović, 2021, 2022; Sekulić, 2016; Stanković, 2014; 2017; Stanković et al., 2017).

In sum, despite advances in the field and greater inclusion of topics related to women's reproductive experiences and processes, mainstream psychology can be criticised for systematically individualising blame for their "dysfunctional" outcomes. Furthermore, despite the increase in qualitative research, the vast majority of *psychological* studies still do not sufficiently include the perspectives of women themselves and their interpretation of pregnancy or motherhood, with all the potentially contradictory and ambivalent aspects of these processes. Most striking is the lack of inclusion of material and embodied aspects that are central to the topic of female reproduction and the early transition to motherhood.

1.2.3 Towards a Paradigm Shift: The Emergence of Material-Discursive Approaches

As mentioned above, the theme of a specifically female transition and the gendered aspects of experiences, representations and practices position this study within the psychology of women field. However, due to my particular interest in embodied aspects of pregnancy and birth, as well as the role of medical institutions and technologies, another relevant reference point for me is critical health psychology. And it is precisely in this area that we often find a different approach to the study of women's reproductive processes, starting from feminist and some other critical perspectives.[16]

In health psychology, the critical approach was initially directed towards questioning Engel's biopsychosocial model, which took into account not only biological, but also psychological and sociological

[16] Considering that one of the primary goals of the psychology of women has been to integrate women and gender aspects into research belonging to the mainstream areas of psychology—such as general, developmental, social, clinical and health psychology—it is viewed more as a research programme rather than a distinct discipline (Denmark et al., 2008). The field of critical health psychology is exemplary of this (see e.g. Riley et al., 2019; Ussher, 2006).

factors (Engel, 1977). This model itself represented a revision and critique of the reductionist biomedical model that had prevailed until then, which viewed states of illness and health as purely objective phenomena that could be fully explained by biological facts. The biomedical model is particularly relevant to my study because, as will be discussed in the following chapters, it still underpins prevailing discourses and practices related to pregnancy and childbirth today: they are treated as purely biological events centred on the development and delivery of the foetus. Under the influence of this model, research on pregnancy has focused primarily on the hormonal changes in the woman's body during the nine months and research on childbirth on the physiological factors that determine the birth outcomes.

While the biopsychosocial model offered a more comprehensive picture than the biomedical model (although some authors point to its underdevelopment and lack of theoretical grounding, Stam, 2000), critiques based on the constructivist and discursive turn in psychology emerged in the late 1980s and early 1990s. According to these critiques, Engel merely introduced a new set of "objective" variables that reified psychosocial phenomena, and empirical research merely correlated quantitative scores on scales of behaviour, beliefs, values or personality traits with indicators of the presence or intensity of symptoms (Yardley, 1997). This did not challenge the firm boundary of medicine as a science, which was established against all other (non-medical and non-scientific) knowledge and practices, as it in no way problematised the nature of medical knowledge, privileged precisely on the false assumption that it is essentially different (Berg & Mol, 1998). Most research in mainstream health psychology still operates within this framework (Stam, 2000), while critiques have been directed at the positivist nature of this model, pointing to sociocultural and discursive aspects as constitutive of bodily states.

In the first half of the 1990s, however, new critiques emerged that are particularly relevant to the position of this study (Yardley, 1996, 1997; Sims-Schouten et al., 2007; Ussher, 2008). It has been argued that constructivist reform actually led to a new form of reductionism in the approach to health and illness. *Materialistic* reductionism was now replaced by *idealistic* reductionism, in which "the physical dimension of health and illness seems strangely absent from many discursive explorations of the personal and social meaning of symptoms" (Yardley, 1997, p. 9). She notes that this exclusion of the body from analysis paradoxically enabled the reproduction of the dualism that underpinned the pre-critical, biomedical model of health and illness. However, "if social scientists concern themselves solely with the personal, social and linguistic context and meaning of health-related issues" (Yardley, 1997, p. 10), the body as a whole is left to the natural scientists. The criticism was accompanied by the emergence of the so-called material-discursive approach in research, whose main task is to correct precisely this shortcoming of the purely discursive approaches. The innovation of the new approach is not in returning to pre-critical materialism, but in acknowledging the materiality of the body while conceptualising this materiality as always mediated by culture, language and politics (Ussher, 2008, p. 1782). For example, although pain is a bodily sensation, it is not semantically neutral, but its meaning does not depend on our conscious reflection either. It represents a pre-reflective reaction whose meaning is protest and rejection (Yardley, 1997, p. 11). I will return to this point when analysing the empirical material later.

The main difference between the material-discursive and the discursive approach lies in the emphasis on the inseparable intertwining of physical and social aspects of human experience: "Because we are intrinsically social and embodied beings, the material dimension of human lives is always socialised—mediated by language and consciousness and modified by social activity—while the discursive dimension is inevitably physically manifested, in our speech and behaviour, institutions and technology" (Yardley, 1997, p. 15). This further implies that discourse does not operate in a vacuum, which does not only mean that creating a new discourse is not sufficient for creating a new experience, but also that the material aspects of experience have a certain autonomy from discourse.

I believe that by following the material-discursive approach I would be able to compensate for both the theoretical and the political deficiency. Theoretical—because the sole focus on language and constructions cannot account for embodied experience and activity, which is crucial when addressing reproductive phenomena. Political—because when we "blame" constructions and representations, we imply that they are changeable at the level of language or even cognition, which is an idealistic (and unrealistic) assumption that leaves many individuals responsible for their own well-being.[17] When we try to encompass the material nature of our bodies and our surroundings, we recognise the common, historically solidified and hardly changeable (albeit still changeable) determinants of our experience and action, which has a political potential for imagining strategies of resistance. In the next section I will attempt to illuminate how, i.e. relying on what theoretical resources, I have tried to pursue this material-discursive direction.

1.2.4 Positioning This Study and Defining the Subject: A Take on Theoretical Synthesis

The brief overview of the literature suggests that the topic of transition into motherhood, and especially experiences during pregnancy, childbirth and the immediate postpartum, are relatively often explored in recent scholarship and from many angles. However, as we have seen, psychology retains many of its traditional blind spots. While reproductive experiences are shared by most women of reproductive age worldwide, I have been intrigued by the contrast between the apparent ordinariness and the factual extraordinariness of the phenomenon, the seeming polyphony of its representations and the frequent lack of an integrative account. I will try to reconstruct a complex process that led me to attempt a theoretical synthesis when approaching this topic.

Even a superficial acquaintance with the situation in which contemporary women undergo pregnancy and childbirth as early stages of the transition to motherhood foregrounds the mediation of these processes by numerous representations and techniques available both within and outside the institutional framework that has become the "natural" environment in which female reproduction takes place. Perhaps this focus would

[17] I completely agree here with Jane Ussher (2006, p. Preface) who writes that she is "being troubled by theories which deny the materiality of the body, which leave my own experiences of embodied change unexplained; as well as discomfort with the wholesale rejection of professional intervention implicit in many feminist and post-modern critiques (Fee, 2000; Rose, 1996). Where does this leave a woman who experiences distress, which she locates in the fecund body, and who comes forward for professional help? Offering only a theoretical deconstruction of her problem, as I once thought we could (Ussher, 1989), is nothing short of insulting".

not be so obvious if I had not been already interested in the role of tools—symbolic means and material artefacts—in human functioning. Or, in more general terms, interested in the relationship between subjectivity and technology. This general theoretical and research interest was informed by the cultural-historical tradition which for me was (and still is) the only theoretical framework in psychology that can account for the complexity and dynamics of people's lives in the equally complex cultural contexts. My background was in one of the dominant contemporary approaches known as cultural psychology (Cole, 1996; Valsiner, 2004, 2007), which focuses on humans as meaning-making beings, social and cultural factors as constitutive of subjectivity and the mediatedness of all our processes and actions. Culture is recognised as a mediator, which, in the process of constituting individual experience and personal history, offers symbolic means that both support and constrain this process, with particular emphasis on the active role of the individual as a central agent (Boesch, 2001; Lawrence & Valsiner, 2003; Markus & Hamedani, 2007; Shweder et al., 2006; Valsiner, 1997). Although restricting (and enabling) aspects of context are always recognised in theory or declaratively, they are rarely explored in detail empirically. What I found to be a limitation of this approach was that the emphasis was almost exclusively on the symbolic aspect of culture or cultural resources/tools—primarily defined in terms of shared meanings, symbols, concepts, narratives, values and representations that are socially constructed[18]—leading to a lack of recognition of the (limiting) impact of material aspects of the environment, tools and institutional conditions, as well as an often unequal distribution of power and privilege (Ratner, 1999). These aspects are sometimes acknowledged in principle, but rarely analysed in detail, resulting in neglecting materiality of the environment, but also the materiality of our tools (especially relevant for tools in the narrower sense, such as medical technology). And, I would add also the materiality of subjects, i.e. human beings—who are corporeal and more than just discursively mediated.

[18] The social environment is seen as a "toolbox" that provides the individual with means for personal constructions, and cultural psychology research attempts to elaborate in detail the functions that these cultural resources fulfil in the personal biographical constellations of individuals (Valsiner, 2012; Zittoun, 2006).

Authors from the sociocultural field recognise the relevance, even the fundamentality of the topic of motherhood,[19] and they tend to approach it in a processual manner, as a question of transition and becoming. However, as already claimed, they seem to share a blind spot with many other areas of psychology—in not analysing this process of transition as *embodied*[20] and *materially embedded*. The embodied aspects of the experience of becoming a mother—particularly the embodied aspects of pregnancy and childbirth—are largely absent from the analysis of cultural representations, dominant discourses and psychological aspects of reproductive phenomena. But this also applies to many other topics and phenomena, since the dominant traditions within sociocultural psychology "almost entirely fail to address our embodied and pre-reflective experiences. The preverbal, pre-reflective embodied landscape of experience is a blind spot in the sociocultural tradition, from its founding to the present day" (Køster & Winther-Lindqvist, 2018, p. 539). And this neglected aspect does not fall outside the disciplinary boundaries of sociocultural tradition, for our embodied experiences and practices are shaped not only by symbolic messages and cultural representations, but also by the practical ways in which we are handled, beginning in our infancy—the way we are cuddled, dressed, played with, fed and so on. Through childhood and growing up we take part in a multitude of culturally structured activities through which social norms and messages, many of them *gendered*, get bodily incorporated (Butler, 2004; Wehrle, 2017; Young, 2005a). We also *incorporate tools* that are culturally shaped thus extending the limits of our body and our sensorimotor repertoire (Leder, 1990; Merleau-Ponty, 2005).[21] The body, in this sense, is not "static"—it is not "made up

[19] In explaining why the topic of motherhood was chosen for the "firstborn" in the Annals of Cultural Psychology book series, editors point out that: "The topic chosen for the first volume is perhaps the most fundamental of all—motherhood. (…) We the editors feel it is the topic that links our existence with one of the universals of human survival as a species" (Cabell et al., 2015).

[20] However, there are some exceptions to this conclusion, such as the study by Reis and Santos (2015) and the analysis by Frazier et al. (2015, p. 146), who even advocate "foregrounding the body as a unit of analysis".

[21] Phenomenologically speaking, there is no fundamental difference between the part of the body we use and the tools we use. Mastering a part of the body is no less demanding than mastering a tool. Moreover, when we have already mastered the use of a tool, it "falls into oblivion" no less than the parts of the body we use, and only becomes an explicit issue for us when it is broken. As long as it works properly, we focus on what we are doing and not on what we are doing it with. However,

of a fixed mass of organs and abilities" (Leder, 1990, p. 30). All this shapes our pre-reflective experience and reaction to the world making embodiment "inherently sociocultural" (Køster & Winther-Lindqvist, 2018, p. 541).

Thus, the sociocultural approach partly shares with mainstream psychology some of the traditional myopias—the material situatedness of both our self and our environment is rarely theorised or empirically grasped. This has led me to explore additional theoretical resources that might complement this tradition and that seem indispensable if we are to consider the early stages of the transition to motherhood as a processual, (technologically) mediated and embodied phenomenon.

Relatively recent *material* turn[22] in the social sciences and humanities (Barad, 2003, 2007; Coole & Frost, 2010; Haraway, 1991b), which emerged in response to the privileging of the symbolic, discursive aspect of culture over the previous decades, has proved to be a fruitful resource for an empirical approach within psychology that pays attention to the material aspects of the social environment, the bodily situatedness of subjects and the institutional-technological practices through which they are constituted.[23] For instance, actor-network theory (ANT) developed within science and technology studies as an expression of this broader tendency adopts a processual and relational standpoint in which each phenomenon (social formation, technological object or psychological subject) is heterogeneously constructed and only ever locally and temporarily constituted (Latour, 1999, 2005; Law, 1992, 1999).[24] According to this stance, there are nothing but multiple distributions of subjects and multiple distributions of objects, and these distributions are co-constitutive (Law, 2002, p. 65). Hence, both objects and subjects

this analogy between a body and a tool does not imply an instrumental relationship towards our body, but rather that a tool, through its use, becomes like "a second sort of body, incorporated into and extending our corporal powers" (Leder, 1990, p. 179).

[22] This shift in approach to phenomena is sometimes referred to as material-semiotic, posthumanist, relational-materialist or simply new materialism (Kontopodis, 2012).

[23] It is still recognised that institutional-technological practice is a social practice, but it is assumed that it cannot be reduced to social interactions and representations (Berg & Akrich, 2004).

[24] It seemed to me that ANT was particularly suitable as a framework because of its explicitly empirical orientation, in contrast to the primarily theoretical preoccupations in some other parts of this community.

represent unstable categories through space and time—they are constantly re-established as a result of a continuous process of relating to various human and non-human actors. They are in fact effects generated through heterogeneous networks and have no inherent properties, so they acquire their attributes and form as a result of their inter-relations. Therefore, since their nature is never predetermined it can only be established empirically, and only under certain circumstances they are subject to and undergo relativisations.[25] This perspective therefore advocates relational and contextual explanations not only of objects in the environment, but also subjects. It assumes that abilities and competencies are not located within individuals but are distributed in an environment shaped and equipped with techniques that support and enable them, but also limit them. The setting, i.e. the specific constellation of conditions, the arrangement of objects, the availability or absence of certain resources, determines the possible ways of reacting and experiencing.

The understanding of the subject as multiple, potentially incoherent, processual (unfolding over time and through various practices) and as a product of relationships is known and accepted by some authors in psychology close to the sociocultural paradigm (e.g., Benson, 2001; Gergen, 2009; Harré, 2001; van Langenhove & Harré, 1999). The main difference lies in the fact that, according to these positions, subjectivity is exclusively or at least predominantly *discursively* produced in relation to *others* in the social environment. Following Foucault's understanding of the subject and the materially oriented approaches that I recognise as successors to this tradition, I have started from the assumption that subjects are not only positioned in a discourse, but in a reality that is both discursive and material. They are positioned in relation to objects, not only to real or imaginary others, i.e. subjects. This standpoint is in line with another cultural-historical tradition in psychology—activity theory (Engeström, 1987; Kaptelinin & Nardi, 2006; Leontyev, 1978), which promotes the notion of a human subject that is not complete and delimited by its bodily boundaries, but is distributed and mediated to a

[25] This is an important addition, because socio-technological networks (such as the network of hospital birth) are often very resistant and rigid, and it takes a lot to challenge and relativise them (see Halfon, 2010), as the analysis in the following chapters will show.

considerable extent by technological means (for a detailed comparison see Miettinen, 1999; Spinuzzi, 2008). The concept of activity also involves double mediation—"as a process mediated by tools (in the broad sense) and at the same time mediated socially" (Leont'ev, 1981, p. 208), which is particularly relevant for the analysis of female subjectivity in (potentially) collaborative situations such as institutionalised childbirth. However, the focus on the activity system is not compatible with the situation of pregnancy, especially when observing the woman during everyday life outside the medical institution. Moreover, for the activity theory authors relevant objects are primarily *tools*, which excludes all other material aspects of the environment that are not part of the means to achieve ends, whereas it seemed to me necessary to adopt a broader understanding of mediators and material factors.

However, the aforementioned advantages of the actor-network approach come at a certain price. The recourse to an explicitly non-psychological theoretical framework brought numerous difficulties that I managed to overcome, after much wandering, only by departing considerably from this framework itself, or perhaps better said, by flexibly appropriating some of its aspects.[26] The main problem lays in the fact that ANT committed me to a third-person perspective. In studies based

[26] Although ANT will not represent the primary conceptual framework for analysis in this book, I believe it has significantly shaped my approach, as it has continued to function in some sense as a general methodological framework. Inspired by it, I have tried to recognise how experience is constituted through the interaction of various elements present in the local situation, and I have become sensitive to the role of the material environment and objects within it. In addition, the insights from ANT, especially regarding the complex and situated nature of technology, have been a significant resource. Therefore, even though this framework is not as explicitly present as I had initially envisioned, I believe it is implicitly present to a significant extent and has opened up a perspective that I did not have before.

It was probably wrong to initially consider ANT as a theoretical framework that would provide me with conceptual resources for approaching and analysing the phenomenon. Latour emphasises that ANT is not simply a theoretical framework into which we can fit our facts and relationships (Latour, 1999). Rather, it is a method, a way of tracing the production of facts, or perhaps just a set of attitudes that we take for granted when researching. Even the idiosyncratic terms Latour introduces (actor, translation, network) do not denote what they refer to, i.e. the nature of the phenomenon, but the way in which it is possible to map this phenomenon, i.e. how we should approach it (Latour, 2005, p. 174), which also points to the methodological nature of this standpoint. ANT concepts are first and foremost a way of approaching the material, rather than a ready-made interpretative scheme into which concrete empirical material can be fitted. Therefore, many empirical studies from this tradition are not immediately recognisable because they do not rely on a common set of concepts.

on this theory, the interactions and co-productions of subjects and objects in a given context are typically examined from an external, objectivist perspective. Given that I based my research on the subjective, i.e. first-person experiences of women, when analysing the empirical material it often felt as if I was committing hermeneutical injustice (Fricker, 2007) by looking at their experiences through the ANT lens. Due to this fixation on the third-person perspective, I was also inclined to reify subjectivity, to imagine it as an object among other objects and to question its characteristics. In fact, subjectivity is not a thing in the world, but the way all other things appear. Understood from the first-person perspective, subjectivity is inevitably experiential and has a reflexive structure. I am primarily interested in how something appears *to a woman*, so I endeavour to reconstruct the early transition to motherhood, i.e. the situation of pregnancy and birth from her first-person perspective. To understand this, I am certainly also concerned with how the woman and her body are treated, positioned and represented, because these aspects of *objective* treatment are constitutive of her *subjective* experience. Therefore, I follow the Foucauldian tradition, i.e. the critical-discursive approach to analysis, but I still consider the reconstruction and understanding of the first-person perspective to be central.

In his book *We Have Never Been Modern*, Latour (1993) emphasises that actor-network researchers are not concerned with technological or scientific objects per se, but with how these objects are involved in communities and human subjects. Also, they are not concerned with subjects, social context, power and political interests as such, but with how these are involved in the world of objects. In reality, however, researchers from this tradition were almost exclusively concerned with the latter aspect. Most of the studies came from the socio-anthropological tradition of science and technology studies (STS), so the research phenomena concerned mainly technological and scientific objects and not persons, i.e. subjects. As a result, much less attention has been given to the reliance of subjectivity on technology than to the reliance of science and technology on social, individual and political factors. Consequently, unlike "unblackboxing"[27] of technology, this approach, despite all its potential, lacks adequate conceptual resources for "unblackboxing" of subjectivity.

In an attempt to compensate for this deficiency and to address subjectivity (and not only technology) in a situated manner, I have introduced an additional *phenomenological* theoretical framework that allows for a differentiated conceptual reconstruction of the embodied experience of the subject (Leder, 1990; Merleau-Ponty, 2005; Sartre, 2003; Young, 2005a).[28] In view of the specific topic I am dealing with, there is another reason for this choice of theory. Unlike many other types of technology, *medical* technology mediates not only the relationship between the subject and the world, but also between the subject and her own body, as a very specific part of that world. I believe that focusing on embodied experience and drawing on phenomenology as a resource can enable us as sociocultural psychologists to understand why we choose certain tools as mediators, what role they play and what meaning they have, especially in a specific situation where the mediated relationship is one between our (embodied) self and our body.[29]

The phenomenological framework also helped me to conceptualise the subject as embodied, rather than considering the body as an independent actor in the situation, which would only reproduce the Cartesian

[27] When something is considered as a "black box", it is only seen with regard to its inputs and outputs—its inner workings, its connections with other subjects/objects and its embeddedness in a socio-political context are ignored. In the case of health technology, for example, opening this black box or "unblackboxing" process entails understanding how the technology works and examining how its power lies in its connection with different individuals and groups both inside and outside medical institutions (Lehoux, 2006, p. 51).

[28] An indicator that ANT is not sufficiently equipped to deal with subjects and their experiences is the fact that authors working within this framework also tend to rely on phenomenological resources in research focused on subjectivity (see Akrich & Pasveer, 2004; Mol & Law, 2004).

[29] Authors belonging to the sociocultural tradition elaborate in detail hierarchically arranged processes of symbolic mediation that both enable the attribution of meaning to immediate experience and constrain the construction of that meaning by higher-level symbolic constructs (Valsiner, 2002). It is assumed that semiotic mediation takes place on hierarchically different levels of generalisation and that this determines the role and influence of the symbolic resource. It is thus possible to distinguish between mediation at the level of immediate perception and unelaborated feelings and mediation by more stable symbolic categories that emerge over longer periods of time as regulators of behaviour, as well as the establishment of an abstract, generalised symbolic complex (such as worldviews or core beliefs) that governs lower-level functioning and behaviour (Zittoun, 2006, p. 41). I would argue that mediation is also determined from below, i.e. from the pre-reflective level of our embodied experience (see also Køster, 2017).

dichotomy. In contemporary literature that draws on the materialist tradition, particularly literature dealing with health and reproductive issues, it has actually become quite common to write about bodies rather than subjects (e.g. Chadwick, 2018; Kukla, 2005). Although I draw on some of the insights and a shift in emphasis that materialist approaches bring, since I start from the embodied female perspective, I have avoided talking about bodies, as this choice of terminology has led me to a third-person perspective. Women are indeed bodies, but *lived bodies* (Young, 2005a), and this distinction is crucial to my analysis. I believe that the decision to write about "embodied subjects" rather than "bodies" is consistent with Adrienne Rich's invitation to put "a moratorium on saying 'the body'", because talking about bodies invites abstractions. She suggests that to "write 'my body' plunges me into lived experience, particularity" (Rich, 1986a), and it is precisely the particularity of lived experience that I am after.

To summarise, I have tried to approach the early transition to motherhood—during the period of pregnancy and childbirth—as a technologically mediated, embodied experience embedded in a specific cultural-historical, discursive and material context. This articulation of the phenomenon emphasises the dramatic bodily changes that bring embodied women's subjectivity to the fore. At other stages of life and under different circumstances, this embodied aspect can remain implicit and it usually is so, as explained in the phenomenological literature (Leder, 1990; Merleau-Ponty, 2005). To account for it, I have tried to be very sensitive to pre-reflective layers of experience that exist prior to and (at least partly) independent of our narrative understanding and meaning construction and are not easily shareable with others. Thus, my analysis generally focuses on the embodied self—understood as an embodied and singular first-person perspective—rather than the narrative autobiographical self, which implies a reflective and storied accumulated articulation of oneself as a particular kind of person.[30] For this reason, the analysis may seem oddly displaced from the usual accounts of lifecourse

[30] A similar distinction is made by Køster and Winther-Lindqvist (2018, p. 539) when differentiating between the "Self" and the "Person": "Whereas the self designates the pre-reflective, embodied, and personal being-in-the-world, the person refers to the autobiographical actualization of the self".

transitions, as it will be directed at temporally limited and often liminal phases of subjective experience in specific life circumstances.

By now, it became clear that my attention would be focused on both the experience of pregnancy and the experience of childbirth. The reason lies in my inclination to see childbirth, despite all its specificities, as the final stage of a long process of transformations during pregnancy. Although it is in many ways a unique event, the experience of childbirth is determined by various occurrences that a woman has lived through during pregnancy—especially the experiences she has had in medical institutions, the knowledge and skills she has acquired over the preceding period and the relationship with her own body that she has developed over the nine months (and all the previous years of her life), which enables only certain positionings and defines her needs and preferences during childbirth. The actual outcomes, however, will largely depend on the material and symbolic characteristics of the institutional environment in which childbirth takes place. Thus, while the experience of pregnancy is oriented towards childbirth and involves various preparations for that event, the experience of childbirth is shaped by, among other things, the embodied and mediated experiences during pregnancy. In this sense, I am inclined to recognise a continuity between pregnancy and birth. Not all authors dealing with the reproductive processes of women agree with this position. Some consider childbirth to be a temporally limited event and argue that it is more relevant to focus on long-term experiences, such as pregnancy and motherhood (Mullin, 2005), because childbirth is "almost surreally severed from the narrative of the rest of life both before and after" (Kukla, 2005, p. 25). Based on my research, it seems to me that such a stance does not correspond to the actual experience of women, in whose narratives childbirth appears as a highly significant event that is interpreted in accordance with previous life experiences and provides a framework for making sense of future experiences (e.g. considering having another child). Although there are many studies on both pregnancy and childbirth, it is interesting to note that those dealing with both experiences are extremely rare. It seems that this has contributed to an unwarranted separation of these phenomena and a missed opportunity to recognise them as phases in a single life flow and as important interconnected aspects of becoming a mother. At the same time, although I have chosen to focus on pregnancy and childbirth, I am not suggesting that these are the most important, and they are certainly far from being the only phases and processes of the transition to motherhood.[31] They are definitely a very relevant part of this transition—both subjectively experienced and objectively positioned as such, given the importance that culture attaches to them and the attempts at their social regulation. I understand the transition to motherhood, therefore, as "a continuous learning process that began with pregnancy and continued through and after birth" (Juarez, 2015).

1.3 Introducing the Project

The topic introduced in the last section has occupied my attention (to a greater or lesser extent) for the past ten years, so the reconstruction of the empirical basis of this book is far from simple and straightforward. The analysis is mainly based on the comprehensive qualitative study I conducted for my doctoral thesis, but many subsequent insights complement it, as I have continued to explore this topic in different ways over the years. In this section I will try to elaborate on this empirical basis by focusing on the methodological aspects of my study. I understand methodology not as a technical means, as an instrument independent of the phenomenon on the one hand and epistemology/theory on the other, but as a way of articulating and pursuing the phenomenon that is inherent to it, as a product of my own entanglement with the phenomenon and my attempt to grasp and understand it. In this sense, the method is not something that can simply be separated from the specific research as an explicit scheme or procedure and applied in other contexts, but rather a logic of thinking and treating the phenomenon that has more heuristic than algorithmic value. It is precisely in this attunement to the phenomenon that I see the main justification for the use of qualitative

[31] An important aspect of women's postpartum experience and one of the most relevant mothering practices is breastfeeding. I considered including it in my analysis, but I realised that the abundance and complexity of the cultural representations and norms regulating this practice, as well as the richness of its embodied aspects, would require much additional space and certainly go beyond the scope of a single book.

methodology in this research—it is an approach that allows for a holistic analysis of complex and dynamic phenomena in a contextualised manner (Camic et al., 2003). Specific methodological decisions and the interpretative approach are essentially shaped by the theoretical frameworks that I set out in the previous part of the introductory chapter.

The empirical aspects of the book are based on in-depth interviews with pregnant/postpartum women;[32] field research in a maternity hospital in Belgrade and antenatal classes in a healthcare centre, which included participant observation and ethnographic interviews with women and a limited number of medical staff (doctors and midwives);[33] and desk research of official documents and medical textbooks. I will first introduce parts of the study that provided me with rich insights into the local medical and institutional environment as well as medical practices and techniques, although I consider these to be more of a preparatory nature—so they will not take a central place in the analysis in the following chapters, although they provide a significant framework for interpretation.

Finally, it should be noted that the research I conducted for my doctoral thesis has extended and fed into various later projects, which have at least implicitly informed my analysis and conclusions in this book. In these later projects, I focused primarily on the topic of childbirth, as it had the greatest political relevance in the Serbian public sphere. Thus, I continued to explore birth experiences and the role of both medical and institutional aspects, drawing on different methodologies and turning to a more diverse sample of women (Pantović et al., 2024; Stanković et al., 2017). I also took every opportunity to speak publicly about these issues (lectures, roundtables, press conferences, documentaries) aimed at policy makers and the general public, and sometimes even in direct dialogue with medical professionals. All of this has allowed me to continuously engage with the topic of women's reproduction and motherhood over the last ten years and to gain a very comprehensive understanding of the

[32] All participants have given their written consent to participate in the study. To protect their anonymity, I use pseudonyms throughout the book and have changed or omitted any other information that might reveal their identity.

[33] Ethical approval was obtained from the ethics committees of the two medical institutions where I conducted the fieldwork.

various aspects that shape it in the local context. This extensive insight has been both a rich source of knowledge and a challenge in writing this book. As is so often the case, the narrative structure of the text may leave the impression of a linear and uncomplicated (although complex) project, but the actual journey through the research and writing is generally much more intricate, with many wanderings, detours and dead ends. The most difficult thing to handle, both while researching and writing, is the feeling that I am trying to outline a clear, systematic and encompassing account of a complex and elusive subject, but what I end up with is actually a relatively (in)coherent jigsaw, carved out from what I imagine to be a more comprehensive picture.[34]

1.3.1 Fieldwork: Familiarising with the Local Normative and Institutional Context

In order to adequately contextualise the lived experiences of Serbian women going through the early transition to motherhood, I needed to familiarise myself with the normative and medical framework in which pregnancy and childbirth are represented and treated in the local environment, i.e. the specificities of the Serbian maternal healthcare system. First, I assessed the normative framework regulating women's reproduction in Serbia by analysing policy documents and clinical guidelines.[35] These documents show that women's reproductive health is recognised as important at the highest level of national legislation in Serbia: "health of women during pregnancy, childbirth, and motherhood is one of the

---

[34] There were always threads that I could follow, and they would lead to the expansion of certain aspects or the inclusion of completely new ones that would just postpone and further complicate the possibility of closure of this project.

[35] I analysed national laws, strategic and policy documents such as national programs and strategies addressing birth or maternal health, public health statistical indicators, and national clinical guidelines for health care during pregnancy and childbirth (Birth Incentive Strategy, 2018; Guidelines for the implementation of the National program of healthcare for women, children, and youth, 2010; Healthcare for women during pregnancy, 2005; Healthcare Law, 2019; Law on Patients' Rights, 2013; National program of healthcare for women, children, and youth, 2009; National strategy for advancing the status of women and promoting gender equality, 2008; Physiological Childbirth, 2009; Selected health indicators, 2012; Standards of health care adapted to the needs of mothers and children, 2011).

priorities of the healthcare system of the Republic of Serbia" (National Program of Health Care for Women, Children and Youth, 2009).

When it comes to the quality of maternity care, official documents and legislation usually advocate an "emancipatory approach to childbirth" that, in addition to avoiding unnecessary interventions and procedures and providing pain relief, also includes "humanising birth by using new methods and techniques, developing mother- and baby-friendly medical institutions, opening the possibility for the partner's presence during childbirth, and developing alternative childbirth methods such as out-of-hospital and home births" (National Strategy for Advancing the Status of Women and Promoting Gender Equality, 2008, p. 32). There have also been successful attempts to develop guidelines for good clinical practice during pregnancy and childbirth to set standards for the doctors' and midwives' work (Healthcare for Women During Pregnancy, 2005; Physiological Childbirth, 2009), in line with WHO recommendations and international standards.

Before entering the field, I read textbooks on gynaecology and obstetrics written by local doctors and medical professors, from which future obstetricians study (Milošević et al., 1988; Mladenović et al., 2008; Plećaš et al., 2005; Ristić, 2001); I talked to medical students and attended lectures on gynaecology and obstetrics at the Faculty of Medicine in Belgrade. These activities helped me to prepare for fieldwork and conversations with medical staff and to gain insight into the local variants of medical knowledge and practices (known as the Belgrade School of Obstetrics). I also managed to familiarise myself with the organisation of medical care for women's reproductive health and the prescribed examinations and interventions during pregnancy and childbirth, which form the normative framework for actual medical practice. However, I was aware that this normative framework is reflected in practice in very different ways. Therefore, I spent several months collecting information in medical institutions, which constituted the ethnographic part of my study.

A long process of negotiating entry into maternity healthcare facilities—notoriously closed and guarded institutions in Serbia—provided valuable insights into their internal organisation, sometimes opaque but firm hierarchies and a plethora of (implicit) norms and rules. Even finding out who the gatekeepers are was not a straightforward task, let alone convincing the doctors and management to let an outsider (in at least a twofold sense—a person outside the institution, and a non-medical expert) snoop around. Eventually, I managed to gain access first to the birth preparation classes at a healthcare centre and later to the maternity hospital in Belgrade.[36] I spent several days a week there over several months, observing daily practices and taking detailed notes, but also talking to a number of pregnant and birthing women and, less frequently, medical professionals. With few exceptions, the doctors and nurses/midwives were usually too wary or too busy to let me interview them, but I learned a lot from having the opportunity to observe their practices and interactions with the women.

While the ethnographic interviews with women attending the birth preparation classes, sitting in the waiting room of the maternity hospital and lying in the maternity ward were not systematically analysed,[37] they helped me to identify both the typical moments and the specificities in the interviews I conducted outside the institution. All of this facilitated the analysis of the in-depth interviews with the women I subsequently interviewed and boosted the credibility of my interpretations.[38] The whole experience has convinced me that any social science research without at least some ethnographic work must be somewhat limited or short-sighted.

The field research enabled me to gain a closer understanding of the organisation of medical institutions, as well as the norms, standards and

---

[36] The higher the healthcare level, the greater these resistances were and the more rigid the boundaries. So it was much easier for me to get permission to visit a healthcare centre (which is at the primary level of healthcare) than to enter a maternity hospital (which is at the secondary or tertiary level of healthcare).

[37] The conversations I had with the women inside the hospital were very chaotic and frequently interrupted, markedly public and often unfinished. I regularly talked to them in crowded hospital rooms with babies present (sometimes there were six or more women in the same room with their babies), which often made either recording or later transcription of the material unfeasible. The conversations were disturbed not only by the crying and needs of the babies, but also by the interjections of other women and their babies, as well as by the appearance of various medical staff. This circumstance implied a very poorly controlled environment from a methodological point of view, but at the same time it provided ecological validity, as all the features of the real institutional context were directly present in (almost) unaltered form.

[38] The research strategy in this study can be recognised as a kind of data triangulation from various sources that shed light on different aspects of the phenomenon, which is suggested as a way to ensure validity in qualitative research (Flick, 1992).

procedures of reproductive health care provision. It also provided an insight into the considerable discrepancies between the recommendations in policy documents and national guidelines and the situation in medical practice on the ground.[39] In reality, Serbian women are left with few reproductive options—they are required by law to give birth in hospital maternity wards, and until recently, over 99% of women in Serbia gave birth in public health facilities[40] (National program of health care for women, children and youth, 2009), almost exclusively in hospitals and clinical centres.[41] The institutional organisation is rigid and hierarchical, with an extremely unequal distribution of power and privileges between obstetricians, midwives and women. An active and technocratic approach to childbirth is followed, that relies on outdated protocols and practices (e.g., regarding the practice of informed consent, support during labour, birthing position, active management of labour protocols, etc.; Pantović et al., 2024; Stanković, 2013; Stanković et al., 2017).[42]

[39] This is expected for a post-socialist country that is undergoing a (prolonged) process of transition. Researchers of post-socialism have criticised the representation of social and institutional transitions as shifts from one defined state to another (Verdery, 1996). They argue for recognising the unique characteristics of the emerging social orders in post-socialist countries. Thus, when studying changes in post-socialist healthcare and the challenges faced in recent decades, it is crucial to view transition as more than a straightforward shift or top-down reorganisation.

[40] The first private maternity wards have been opened in Belgrade in recent years, but due to limited capacity and very high prices compared to the average economic standard, they are not accessible to the vast majority of Serbian women. There is no available data on the number of women giving birth in private facilities. The obstetricians who work there are mostly the same as those who work in public maternity hospitals. So apart from better conditions and more courteous service, the medical protocols and procedures or standards of care are not significantly different. Since the existing norms of communication and intervention are widely accepted and considered unproblematic by caregivers, women can hardly find a way to avoid them by simply moving to a private sector facility.

[41] Maternal healthcare is publicly financed through mandatory healthcare insurance and provided through a network of medical institutions organised at three levels—university hospitals and clinical centres, maternity departments in general hospitals and small maternity units within primary healthcare facilities (Matejić et al., 2014; Pantović et al., 2024).

[42] Childbirth is treated as an exclusively medical event that is carefully monitored and managed (even in cases considered low-risk), so a number of potentially unnecessary and problematic obstetric procedures are routinely used, especially in first-time mothers—routinised labour stimulation through the administration of hormones, pressing the abdomen during the pushing phase of labour, compulsory enemas, shaving and episiotomies (and suturing the incisions without anaesthesia), lithotomy position with the aid of stirrups, etc. Many of these aspects of treatment are discussed in more detail in the following chapters. They differ significantly from the recommenda-

It should be taken into account that the broader sociocultural setting—specifically in relation to the local politics of reproduction—is a relevant context in which the institutional regulation of childbirth is taking place. As in most European countries, during the last 20 years, a steady decline in birth rate is recorded in Serbian population, which also makes reproductive health an issue of national importance (National Millennium Development Goals, 2006). As a consequence, socio-political context in Serbia is characterised by the dominance of nationalist and patriarchal tendencies that are promoting a pronatalist population policy (Drezgić, 2004; Sekulić, 2014). Under these circumstances women (and their bodies) are seen primarily in instrumental terms—their reproductive potential is treated as an important capital for the state (and the market economy) and it is therefore carefully monitored and managed. "White plague" discourse describing the pattern of a low birth rate that is threatening the survival of Serbian nation is commonly introduced in official documents and public debates surrounding reproduction (Bracewell, 1996; Djoric & Gavrilovic, 2006; Shiffman et al., 2002), in order to present women and their reproductive behaviour as an issue of public interest. Women and their "modern" or "western" way of life, their interests and habits (being selfish, spoiled, career girls) are often blamed for the low fertility rates (Vilenica, 2013). Therefore, current social climate is characterised by great public interest in female reproduction, but also by the tendency to marginalise women's experiences, perspectives and needs, both in institutional settings and in the broader socio-political context.

1.3.2 Interviews: Grasping the Embodied Experiences of Pregnancy and Birth

The main research data consisted of thirty in-depth semi-structured interviews[43] with fifteen women—first at the late stage of pregnancy

tions of the World Health Organization (WHO), which prescribes appropriate standards and protocols for maternity care that are evidence-based (WHO, 1996, 2018).

[43] All interviews were recorded, transcribed and processed in qualitative analysis software (MAXQDA) prior to analysis. This data was supplemented by extensive research notes from the ethnographic part of the study. Since all the material (interview transcripts, ethnographic notes,

(eighth or ninth month) and second shortly after childbirth (up to the third month).[44] The interviews were relatively long, most of them lasting over two hours. They all took place in the women's homes so I was introduced to their life contexts in more detail. This temporary immersion into the lifeworlds of my participants, during which I occasionally witnessed some very intimate moments and practices (especially in post-birth encounters), reminded me of the following quote: "Interviewing is rather like marriage: everybody knows what it is, an awful lot of people do it, and yet behind each closed front door there is a world of secrets" (Oakley, 1981, p. 31). Although the usual genre of methodological reporting leaves the impression that the interviews within the same study were similar to each other, my impression is that they were quite different from each other. This was true not only for different women, but also for the same women, depending on whether the interviews were conducted during pregnancy or after childbirth. The later interviews always included another actor whom I admittedly had not considered sufficiently in advance—the baby. This actor was all the time implicitly and often explicitly present during the interview, and its role was difficult to reduce to just that of the subject of conversation. I also directly witnessed the rhythm of early motherhood, a rhythm still dominated by corporeal or, more precisely, intercorporeal necessities. Postpartum interviews lasted for hours, interrupted by (breast)feedings, pumping sessions, diaper changes, sleeping cycles, etc. It was clear to me that my old methodology professor would definitely not approve of such research conditions. However, what seemed completely unproblematic was that these

---

analysed material for the desk research) was in Serbian, I had to translate it into English while writing this book. I did my best to stick to the original meaning, especially when metaphors, idioms and slang were used.

[44] I decided to interview the women about their pregnancy while they are pregnant and not in the period after birth, because I assumed that a retrospective narrative reconstruction would omit many problematic, elusive or ambivalent aspects of pregnancy experience. This assumption was empirically confirmed, as a comparison of the current and later descriptions of pregnancy shows considerable differences between them (Smith, 1994). The women tended to describe even difficult periods during their pregnancy in positive terms after some time had passed. They reconstructed a series of events as a stable progression, emphasising continuity and neglecting the diversity of experiences and ruptures during this period. However, both interviews I conducted were certainly selective reconstructions, not reproductions of past events (Bruner, 1991), so the choice of topics and the emphasis on some of them depended on the current phase and present concerns.

conversations were extremely ecologically valid. It was hard to sugarcoat the picture or leave out important aspects of the experience when numerous reminders of all the challenges that characterise early motherhood were constantly and intrusively present.

A flexible schedule and content of the topics during the interviews allowed unexpected aspects of the phenomenon to emerge and gave participants the opportunity to shape the narratives about their experiences relatively freely. I opened the interviews with the broad question, "Can you tell me about your experience of pregnancy/childbirth?" and the short instruction, "You can start from the beginning". In this way, participants had the opportunity to articulate their personal meanings and perspectives and narrate their stories in their own chronological order (e.g., some started with how they found out they were pregnant, while others began with when they were trying to conceive). I had prepared a list of questions, but most interviews proceeded in a spontaneous manner, and I tried to follow the narratives of participants with sub-questions and prompts. The women were asked to describe in detail what was happening to them (particularly in relation to their bodily changes and how their altering state was monitored and treated), how they felt about it and how they responded to these changes.

I tend to think of the interviews I conducted as conversations rather than formal meetings in which I assume the role of someone asking questions. This is not to say, of course, that my contribution to the interaction was proportionate to theirs. The women did most of the talking and shared much more with me than I did with them, although the exchange was sometimes mutual. Therefore, the outcome of the interviews is inevitably a co-construction. I consider myself a partial co-author of their verbalised experiences because I did, to some extent, encourage and direct their narrative flow—especially when it came to elaborating on bodily experiences.

All the women were very motivated, committed and generous, both in terms of the time and the experiences they shared with me. These encounters were, at times, very intense—women often experienced strong emotions, both positive and negative, some of them cried. My emotional involvement was unproblematic in these situations and it was not at all difficult for me to connect with them and empathise with what they were going through. Some of the women explicitly commented on how significant it was for them to be given the opportunity to talk about negative experiences without restraint, especially after a traumatic birth, and to try to integrate them into their life narratives.[45] They told me that some (particularly inappropriate and traumatic) details were not shared with people around them and that they had not heard these details from other women who had given birth. As one participant said, "I don't want to scare those who haven't given birth yet, and those who have, they already know, but probably didn't want to scare me either, so they didn't tell me". This tendency to systematically omit certain less desirable and acceptable aspects of the birth experience, both in the literature on childbirth and in the accounts of women who have given birth, is referred to by some authors as a "vow of silence" (Chadwick, 2009, p. 118).

At the time I interviewed the women, I had no experience of pregnancy and childbirth myself, which put me in a specific epistemological position. I agree with Charis Thompson, who says: "I am not a fan of the identity politics idea that you have to experience something before you can write about it" (Thompson, 2005, p. 22).[46] At the same time, I knew that many authors who write about pregnancy and childbirth have themselves experienced the early transition to motherhood and explicitly acknowledge this as the impetus for exploring the topic (Kukla, 2005; Rich, 1986b; Thompson, 2005). What I see as an advantage of my naïve position is that I constantly encouraged my interviewees to describe in detail how they felt and what it was like for them, as I did not know what it was like to be pregnant and give birth. It seems to me that this enabled me to obtain *their* verbalisation and articulation of some aspects of the pregnancy and birth experience that I might not have gotten if I had known "what it was like". Additionally, since I had not made my own choices regarding childbirth or certain practices during pregnancy, I had the impression that they could freely express their positions (on

[45] An open, flexible and sensitive methodological approach is particularly important when exploring sensitive or potentially traumatic topics, as it allows research participants to narrate their experiences in a personal, detailed and emotionally involving way (Stanković, 2020).

[46] At the same time, this does not mean that I am close to the mainstream epistemological approach in psychology that promotes exclusively an external, disinterested scientific view (Haraway, 1991a).

epidurals, caesareans or taking medication during pregnancy) without fear of conflicting with my decisions.

When selecting the participants, the only relevant criterion was that they were pregnant with their first child at the time of the first interview and had medically uncomplicated pregnancies.[47] They were not systematically selected according to any form of representativeness—socioeconomic status, education, place of residence, age, etc.—as I have tried to follow the principles of theoretical sampling (Charmaz, 1995, p. 44–47; Strauss & Corbin, 1998, p. 201–217), which excludes the need for composing a balanced sample based on any (apriori chosen) demographic characteristics. All women gave birth in one of the public healthcare institutions in Belgrade. The average age of the participants was 30 (ranged from 26 to 49 years), almost all of them were well educated,[48] two thirds were employed and almost all of them lived in Belgrade at the time of the interview. All pregnancies were wanted and accepted (although some of them were not planned) and all participants were living with their partner and the father of their child. I recruited almost half of the participants at birth preparation classes in a Belgrade health centre (during fieldwork), and the remaining participants were recruited through a "snowball" sampling strategy. I avoided relying on the help of healthcare providers to recruit participants and emphasised to the women that I was not part of the medical establishment.

Probably the biggest limitation of the present qualitative study is the fact that most of the participants were well educated and residing in the capital city, so their experiences may not be representative of a large

[47] I wanted to explore the role of medical knowledge, practices and technologies in what is considered "normal" pregnancy and childbirth. At the same time, the rationale was to keep the sample homogeneous, as it is relatively small, in order to facilitate the process of generalisation. The sample size was due to the idiographic nature of the research, which involves detailed analysis of individual cases, i.e. attention to the specific characteristics and life contexts of individuals. This impacts the sample size, which rarely exceeds single digits in such studies (Eatough & Smith, 2008, p. 186). There is also an advantage to interviewing a small number of participants multiple times as this provides rich and contextual insights into subjective experience, which is the strategy I adopted. However, I did include negative cases (Strauss & Corbin, 1998)—one participant was pregnant with her second child and one had a very complicated and high-risk pregnancy due to previous health conditions—to increase the credibility of my findings.

[48] Half of the women interviewed had completed a university education, and just one completed only high school education. There were no medical professionals in the sample and only one participant had a background in psychology.

number of women in Serbia. For example, for women outside Belgrade, reproductive options are even more limited (e.g. they cannot choose between different maternity hospitals or opt for an epidural). However, despite this limitation of the sample, it should be noted that the participants in this study do not belong to some privileged class that has the resources to resist or challenge the hegemonic medical model of care and often oppressive institutional treatment.[49] In this sense, they probably had similar experiences to any other Serbian woman, even though their expectations were perhaps different and they were more inclined to evaluate the situation in a negative light.[50] This is corroborated by the fact that the experiences of the women encountered during the fieldwork did not differ significantly, although this sample was not as biased in terms of the educational level and social status of the women. Furthermore, this is also confirmed in a later quantitative study on a large sample (Stanković et al., 2017), and the present findings are consistent with those of other studies in similar settings (and even with highly disadvantaged women, e.g. Arsenijevic et al., 2014; Chadwick et al., 2014; Esposito, 1999). However, the limitations of the study's sample should be borne in mind especially when considering the reproductive experiences of seriously deprivileged and disempowered women—extremely poor, Roma, with very limited cultural capital or access to information—as their voices are not represented in this study. There is previous evidence suggesting that this category of women is very often discriminated against in the healthcare system, that their access to care is restricted and that the quality of care is much more difficult to negotiate for them (Janevic et al., 2011). In addition, women who experienced unwanted pregnancies and did not identify with their condition, as well as those who lacked support from the child's father or their family and close ones, were not included. The fact that the pregnancy was desired, or at least accepted, is emphasised as a

---

[49] Only one interviewee considered an alternative model of birth outside the hospital institution, so she attempted a home birth.

[50] Expectations and the discrepancy between expectations and actual experiences have been shown to be important determinants of birth experience and satisfaction (Ayers & Pickering, 2005; Hauck et al., 2007; Hodnett, 2002). A more representative sample and the inclusion of women from different social classes and cultural backgrounds may explain the positive evaluations of birth experiences and maternal care identified in some studies (Matejić et al., 2014; for a detailed critical evaluation, see Stankovic, 2017).

significant factor in determining how the transition to motherhood is experienced (Young, 2005b, p. 47), since: "Pregnancy and motherhood are experienced in very different ways depending on whether they take place in revolt, resignation, satisfaction, or enthusiasm" (de Beauvoir, 2011, p. 657).

The framework for analysing and interpreting the data was both phenomenological and critical-discursive. My approach to women's embodied experiences is closest to interpretative phenomenological analysis (IPA), which aims to gain an in-depth understanding of individual experiences (Smith, 1995). This approach emphasises the importance of moving beyond the first level of descriptive and emphatic interpretation (Eatough & Smith, 2008) in order to offer "a more overtly interpretative analysis, which positions the initial 'description' in relation to a wider social, cultural, and perhaps even theoretical, context" (Larkin et al., 2006, p. 104). Following this suggestion, I tried to situate the analysis and my understanding of the participants' accounts within the local institutional and sociocultural context and interpret them by drawing on numerous theoretical resources. In contrast to the usual IPA approach, which does not rely significantly on phenomenological literature in its analysis (Zahavi, 2018), concepts and ideas from phenomenology provided an important resource for me during the interpretation of the material, especially concerning the embodied and pre-reflective aspects of the experience. Additionally, the context in which reproductive experiences and the early transition to motherhood take place was analysed through critical discursive lenses, as I paid particular attention to how women are represented, treated and positioned, as well as the material aspects of their environment, to understand what fundamentally shapes their possibilities of experience and agency.

Most of the material I draw on throughout the analysis is in narrative form, which means that the analysis focuses on verbalised experiences that are structured in a specific way.[51] The structure of a narrative involves

[51] The fact that events are not only selected and linked together to form a narrative structure, but that each of them is reconstructed in the light of the whole evolving narrative, imposes specific demands on the analysis. Understanding each individual experience and event thus depends on understanding the whole story, which in turn can only be understood through the interpretation of a series of individual events—a plot traditionally known as the hermeneutic circle (Smit, 2005).

a sequence of events that are interconnected and unfold over time, i.e. the narrative has an "irreducible temporal dimension" (Bruner, 1991, p. 6). This becomes particularly evident when we come across the narration of something like pregnancy, which is a paradigmatic example of a process that unfolds over time, has its phases and duration. However, imposing a coherent and continuous structure that characterises narrative reconstruction of events (Ochs & Capps, 1996) poses a challenge when it comes to certain experiences, especially during childbirth. It was relevant for me to observe what narrative patterns the participants relied on to integrate and organise the occasionally chaotic and overwhelming flow of events. We will also see that they sometimes fail to do so consistently, resulting in a "chaos" narrative (Frank, 1997, p. 97) that depicts the incoherent and disrupted birth experience.

1.3.3 The Outline of the Book

In addition to the introductory and concluding chapters, the book will contain three broad analytical chapters that will attempt to focus on those aspects of the early transition into motherhood that are simultaneously present and closely interwoven in concrete experiences. My thesis is that a woman's subjectivity—her experience and agency—is simultaneously mediated, embodied and distributed. Nevertheless, some aspects of the phenomenon I am examining can be analysed while temporarily ignoring or bracketing this complexity. Therefore, the logic of this book is designed to introduce one layer after another.[52] First, in the next chapter, *Situated Subjects*, I will focus on the sociocultural mediation of the early transition

---

This had practical consequences for the way in which the material was analysed—all narratives were first analysed as case studies in order to understand individual experiences in the context of specific narratives, and only then were such interpreted individual experiences of different participants compared with each other in order to gain insights into similarities and relevant differences between them.

[52] I have tried to find a suitable metaphor for the logic of the book's structure, and it seems that the relationship between figure and background might be the most fitting. Every time we focus on something, it emerges as a figure from the background, but it is essentially shaped by the specifics of the background, which is not in our focus at the moment. Shifting the analytical gaze allows different figures to emerge for closer analysis, taking into account the dynamic relationship with what is currently the background, but which formatively defines them.

to motherhood—the dominant discursive and normative frameworks that shape women's representations, conduct and decisions, without a clear or salient influence of bodily aspects of the phenomenon. In the third chapter, *Embodied Subjects*, I will then focus on the embodied aspects of this experience and how they are shaped as a result of specific sociocultural conditioning and mediated by historically specific tools. Finally, in the fourth chapter, *Distributed Subjects*, I will consider the embeddedness of this phenomenon in (predominantly institutional) contexts that have specific discursive-material aspects and constellations of actors leading to different outcomes for women as subjects. This means that I will try to analyse the phenomenon by gradually introducing layer by layer (if one can put it that way), implying that my theoretical focus will be somewhat different in the three central chapters. While the sociocultural situatedness of subjects is adequately addressed through a sociocultural perspective, understanding their embodiment requires resources from phenomenology, and their embeddedness in specific discursive-material (institutional) environments calls for theoretical resources from contemporary materialist approaches.

Finally, it should be noted that the empirical analysis will follow the temporal progression of the early transition to motherhood, but only to a certain extent. While the prevailing cultural representations and practices, norms and taboos are particularly pronounced at the beginning of pregnancy, when not many bodily changes are yet taking place (which requires a discursive and sociocultural perspective), the pregnant body (and thus also the baby) later increasingly becomes the focus of a woman's attention, calling for a phenomenological perspective. Finally, the institutional environment, material practices and medical technology, although involved from the beginning of pregnancy (often even before that), are crucially and intrusively present at the moment of birth and its immediate aftermath, which is why I draw on materialist approaches. This shifting focus implies that I will add new layers to the analysis in each new chapter, drawing on the theoretical resources and analytical insights introduced in previous chapters.[53]

---

[53] Additionally, some of the topics are dealt with in more than one chapter, but in different ways. For example, the theme of pain appears in all three chapters, but in the "Situated subjects" it is

Pregnancy and childbirth, as crucial aspects of the early transition to motherhood, are the meeting points of nature and culture, biological events in which social beings are the main actors (Oakley, 1979). In the past century or two, there has been a radical transformation of earlier sociocultural representations of pregnancy and childbirth into a dominant articulation of these processes as biological, leading to their becoming objects of medical knowledge, practices and techniques, and turning the pregnant woman into a patient of obstetricians. Various aspects of this relatively new historical situation, as well as the alternative models that have emerged through critical responses to it, will be critically examined in the second chapter. I will attempt to illuminate the various historical, political and sociocultural aspects that together shape the experience of pregnancy and childbirth for contemporary women.

In the third chapter, the woman as subject is not treated as a simple, unproblematic whole, the centre of experience and agency with clear and stable boundaries. A detailed phenomenological analysis will show that for the woman herself, her own body and the baby in her womb appear not only as embodied, but often also as mediated by knowledge and technology, which in contemporary circumstances are primarily medical in origin. A dynamic relationship between embodied and technologically mediated modes of experience throughout pregnancy will be analysed in detail, especially focusing on the complex process of individuation of the baby for the becoming mother. The title of this book is intended to refer to this double process. The baby becomes a new subject for the mother during pregnancy, even before it leaves her body at birth. But the process of gestation and birth of a child is at the same time the process of a "birth" of a mother—radical transformation of her self-understanding, her experiences and her corporeality. The transition to motherhood is thus a process of becoming two subjects, each specific but intertwined with the other.

---

linked to how women represent labour pain and decide on pain relief, drawing on different discourses and norms; in the "Embodied subjects" it is linked to the phenomenological experience and interpretation of pain by women as individual subjects (while also relying on different discourses and norms); and in the "Distributed subjects" pain emerges with a specific quality and intensity as a product of the entire discursive-material network in a constellation of a hospital birth.

This process does not take place in a vacuum, but the relevance of the concrete socio-material aspects of the environment culminates at birth. Starting from theoretical resources and analyses introduced in the previous chapters, and relying on both phenomenological and critical discourse analysis, the fourth chapter focuses on the specific constellation of medical encounters, implicit and explicit norms, relational patterns and material features of the institutional environment that crucially shape women's experiences and sense of agency during childbirth. For many of them, this event represents a very dramatic and personally important rite of passage that significantly shapes how they experience themselves as new mothers, how they handle the care for their babies and how they function in their daily lives in the weeks or even months that follow. The analysis in this chapter, which addresses the importance of a functioning network of different actors in the situation, will also highlight the distributed nature of women's agency.

In the concluding chapter, I summarise and connect the main theoretical issues raised in the previous parts of the book. I revisit the crucial aspects of maternal subjectivity and address the specificities of its embodied, mediated and embedded nature. Finally, I argue for recognising pregnant and birthing subjectivity as a paradigmatic model for subjectivity in general, a model that challenges modernist representations of the subject—as stable, bounded and clearly differentiated from others. The often dramatic process of the early transition into motherhood and the visible ruptures in ordinary functioning and experience reveal the processual, (technologically) mediated and distributed nature of subjectivity that is not so easily recognised in other, more stable and regular circumstances. The analysis in this book therefore calls for a revision of a psychological theory of subjectivity and offers some important resources that might help us move away from modernist accounts.

* * *

Before we turn to the following chapters, in which crucial aspects of the early transition to motherhood are dealt with somewhat separately, I would like to introduce an illustrative example referring to the beginning of pregnancy that showcases the entanglement of these aspects. While this case is quite atypical, it nonetheless contains many typical and interrelated aspects of the phenomenon I am interested in—uncertainty, false starts, difficulties in appropriately integrating and interpreting embodied experiences, the prevailing cultural norms and representations, the broad availability of medical knowledge and the role of medical practices and techniques, as well as the importance of specific institutional circumstances and patterns.

> *"I have an interesting story about how I found out I was pregnant. In March, my period was twelve days late, which is very strange for me because I have regular periods, on time. So I go to the pharmacy and buy a test and it's negative. But it wasn't with the first morning urine. So I wait a few days, buy another test, try with the first morning urine, and it's negative. Okay. I go to the hairdresser and she tells me, 'Oh, I got pregnant, I have nausea.' I ask, 'What kind of nausea?' She says, 'It's not nausea, it's more like heartburn.' And I'm like, 'Aha, okay.' That night I wake up, can't sleep, and I have heartburn. 'Oh my God, I'm pregnant, I'm pregnant!' But then I get my period. A few days later I get my period normally, fully, everything as usual. And I'm like, ok, I don't know what that was. In April, the next month, my period is late again. And I'm like there's no way I'm pregnant now, because if I wasn't pregnant last month, there's no way now, and I don't even feel the heartburn. So I relax, don't think about it, and it's late, I don't know, ten days, fifteen days, twenty days. And I don't think about it at all because there's no way I'm pregnant. And I was even like, I am not buying a test this time, because the other two were negative, this one can't be positive. (…) Finally, I go to the doctor at the health centre and he tells me it's a cyst. Imagine, you go to the doctor and tell him your period is a month late. And he says from the door, 'Ah, you have a cyst'. And he says, 'Come in on Friday for an ultrasound.' (…) So I go on Friday for the ultrasound and I'm lying there. He looks at the ultrasound and turns to the nurse, let's say her name was Jelena—'Jelena, come see, Jelena!' You see, he doesn't turn to me, but to Jelena, come and see Jelena, look Jelena. And they're both looking… 'Look, look, do you see what I see? She's pregnant!' Imagine, the doctor telling me such important news in this way. I'm like 'What!?' and he says, 'You're pregnant.' And this Jelena says to me, 'How did you not know you were pregnant, for heaven's sake?! Every woman knows when she is pregnant!' I say, 'The doctor told me I have a cyst! And last month my period was late and I wasn't pregnant.' And she says, 'God, it's so strange you didn't feel it.'" (Saška)*

This complex case highlights significant aspects of a woman's experience during the early transition to motherhood. Especially at the beginning of pregnancy, but also throughout it, bodily sensations are unclear and ambiguous. Women typically rely on various mediators—(medical) knowledge, technological means such as hormonal tests or ultrasound, the experiences of others—in their attempt to correctly interpret and make sense of their condition so that they can orient themselves practically and plan and carry out further activities. In Saška's case, the realisation that she was pregnant was preceded by an unusually long period of uncertainty. As we will see, this period of uncertainty, during which women are unsure how to interpret their bodily situation, also occurs with other participants, although often not as long and complex. Normative expectations regarding pregnancy symptoms, formed in women under the influence of others' experiences or commonly available medical knowledge, determine which aspects of the bodily experience they pay attention to and how they interpret them. This of course applies throughout the pregnancy, during childbirth, and continues afterwards, when the baby is born. Despite the complex situation women find themselves in during this period, which is only hinted at here, there is a widespread belief and expectation that they quite simply and immediately know what is happening to their bodies. This belief is succinctly expressed in the nurse's reaction—"every woman knows when she is pregnant"—and it is common among some feminist-oriented authors, advocates of natural childbirth, many medical professionals, as well as women themselves and those around them. I hope that through the following chapters it will become clear how unfounded this assumption is and that actual female experience is much more complex, mediated and uncertain.

Very often, medical techniques play an important role in resolving uncertainty and providing the woman with the necessary knowledge and ability to make informed decisions about her actions. But medical technology also plays various other roles during pregnancy and childbirth, leading to different outcomes for the woman's subjectivity. At least two relevant factors determine this: the attitude towards bodily experience that a woman develops during the long process of her body and gender socialisation and the organisation of the practice in which the technology appears, i.e. the specific way in which the technology is institutionally situated. Both aspects will be examined in detail in the following chapters. Already in the above quotation we see a description that is typical of the local institutional situation, in which the woman as subject is mostly ignored, sometimes even actively neglected and endangered. The doctor addresses the medical staff—and not the woman he is examining and whose body parts are projected on the monitor—to communicate something about her condition, something that is very important to the woman herself and that she only learns accidentally and indirectly.

In the analysis that follows, I will attempt to reconstruct the experience of the early transition to motherhood from the perspective of the women themselves, highlighting its bodily and technological aspects both deeply rooted in a broader network of culturally specific representations and practices, as well as the complex dynamics of their mutual relationship.

References

Akrich, M., & Pasveer, B. (2004). Embodiment and disembodiment in childbirth narratives. *Body and Society, 10*(2–3), 63–84. https://doi.org/10.1177/1357034X04042935

Alhusen, J. L. (2008). A literature update on maternal-fetal attachment. *Journal of Obstetric, Gynecologic, and Neonatal Nursing, 37*(3), 315–328.

Arijes, F. (1989). *Eseji o istoriji smrti na Zapadu od srednjeg veka do današnjih dana*. Rad.

Arsenijevic, J., Pavlova, M., & Groot, W. (2014). Shortcomings of maternity care in Serbia. *Birth, 41*(1), 14–25.

Ayers, S., & Pickering, A. D. (2005). Women's expectations and experience of birth. *Psychology and Health, 20*(1), 79–92.

Bailham, D., & Joseph, S. (2003). Post-traumatic stress following childbirth: A review of the emerging literature and directions for research and practice. *Psychology, Health & Medicine, 8*(2), 159–168. https://doi.org/10.1080/1354850031000087537

Baker, S., Choi, P., Henshaw, C., & Tree, J. (2005). "I felt as though I'd been in jail": Women's experiences of maternity care during labour, delivery, and the immediate postpartum. *Feminism & Psychology, 15*(3), 315–342.

Barad, K. (2003). Posthumanist performativity: Toward an understanding of how matter comes to matter. *Signs, 28*(3), 801–831.

Barad, K. (2007). *Meeting the universe halfway: Quantum physics and the entanglement of matter and meaning*. Duke University Press.

Baraitser, L. (2009). *Maternal encounters: The ethics of interruption*. Routledge.

Benson, C. (2001). *The cultural psychology of self: Place, morality and art in human worlds*. Routledge.

Berg, M., & Akrich, M. (2004). Bodies on trial: Performances and politics in medicine and biology. *Body and Society, 10*(2–3), 1–12. https://doi.org/10.1177/1357034X04042929

Berg, M., & Mol, A. (1998). *Differences in medicine: Unraveling practices, techniques, and bodies*. Duke University Press.

Bielinski-Blattmann, D., Gürber, S., Lavallee, K., Grob, A., Surbek, D., & Stadlmayr, W. (2016). Labour experience and postpartum stress and depression: A quantitative and qualitative examination. *Journal of Reproductive and Infant Psychology, 34*(2), 162–174.

Birth Incentive Strategy. (2018). *Official Gazette-Republic of Serbia, 25/2018–16.*

Blagojević, M. (1997). *Roditeljstvo i fertilitet: Srbija devedesetih*. ISIFF.

Boesch, E. E. (2001). Symbolic action theory in cultural psychology. *Culture & Psychology, 7*(4), 479–483.

Bracewell, W. (1996). Women, motherhood, and contemporary Serbian nationalism. *Women's Studies International Forum, 19*(1/2), 25–33.

Bruner, J. (1991). The narrative construction of reality. *Critical Inquiry, 18*(1), 1–21. https://doi.org/10.1086/448619

Buchanan, L. (2013). *Rhetorics of motherhood.* Southern Illinois University Press.

Butler, J. (2004). *Undoing gender.* Routledge.

Cabell, K. R., Marsico, G., Cornejo, C., & Valsiner, J. (Eds.). (2015). *Making meaning, making motherhood.* Information Age Publishing.

Camberis, A. L., McMahon, C. A., Gibson, F. L., & Boivin, J. (2014). Age, psychological maturity, and the transition to motherhood among English-speaking Australian women in a metropolitan area. *Developmental Psychology, 50*(8), 2154–2164. https://doi.org/10.1037/a0037301

Camic, P. M., Rhodes, J. E., & Yardley, L. (2003). Naming the stars: Integrating qualitative methods into psychological research. In P. M. Camic, J. E. Rhodes, & L. Yardley (Eds.), *Qualitative research in psychology: Expanding perspectives in methodology and design* (pp. 3–15). American Psychological Association.

Cannella, B. L. (2005). Maternal-fetal attachment: An integrative review. *Journal of Advanced Nursing, 50*, 60–68.

Chadwick, R. (2006). Pathological wombs and raging hormones: Psychology, reproduction and the female body. In T. Shefer, F. Boonzaaier, & P. Kiguwa (Eds.), *The gender of psychology*. UCT Press.

Chadwick, R. (2009). Between bodies, cultural scripts and power: The reproduction of birthing subjectivities in home-birth narratives. *Subjectivity, 27*, 109–133. https://doi.org/10.1057/sub.2009.1

Chadwick, R. (2018). *Bodies that birth: Vitalizing birth politics*. Routledge.

Chadwick, R., Cooper, D., & Harries, J. (2014). Narratives of distress about birth in South African public maternity settings: A qualitative study. *Midwifery, 30*(7), 862–868.

Charmaz, K. (1995). Grounded theory. In A. J. Smith, R. Harre, & L. van Langenhove (Eds.), *Rethinking methods in psychology* (pp. 27–65). Sage.

Cole, M. (1996). *Cultural psychology: A once and future discipline*. Harvard University Press.

Coole, D., & Frost, S. (2010). Introducing the new materialisms. In D. Coole & S. Frost (Eds.), *New materialisms: Ontology, agency, and politics* (pp. 1–43). Duke University Press.

Creedy, D., Shochet, I., & Horsfall, J. (2000). Childbirth and the development of acute trauma symptoms: Incidence and contributing factors. *Birth, 27*(2), 104–111.

Cunningham, G. F., Leveno, K. J., Bloom, S. L., Hauth, J. C., Rouse, D. J., & Spong, C. Y. (2010). *Williams obstetrics* (23rd ed.). McGraw-Hill Medical.

Czarnocka, J., & Slade, P. (2000). Prevalence and predictors of post-traumatic stress symptoms following childbirth. *British Journal of Clinical Psychology, 39*, 35–51.

Darvill, R., Skirton, H., & Farrand, P. (2010). Psychological factors that impact on women's experiences of first-time motherhood: A qualitative study of the transition. *Midwifery, 26*(3), 357–366. https://doi.org/10.1016/j.midw.2008.07.006

Davis-Floyd, R. (1994). The technocratic body: American childbirth as cultural expression. *Social Science and Medicine, 38*(8), 1125–1140. https://doi.org/10.1016/0277-9536(94)90228-3

de Beauvoir, S. (2011). *The second sex* (C. Borde & S. Malovany-Chevallier, Trans.). Vintage Books. (Original work published 1949).

Denmark, F. L., Klara, M., Baron, E., & Cambareri-Fernandez, L. (2008). Historical development of the psychology of women. In F. L. Denmark & M. A. Paludi (Eds.), *Psychology of women: A handbook of issues and theories* (pp. 3–39). Praeger.

DiPietro, J. A. (2010). Psychological and psychophysiological considerations regarding the maternal-fetal relationship. *Infant and Child Development, 19*(1), 27–38. https://doi.org/10.1002/icd.651

DiQuinzio, P. (1999). *The impossibility of motherhood: Feminism, individualism, and the problem of mothering*. Routledge.

Djoric, G., & Gavrilovic, D. (2006). Between pronatalist population policy and women's reproductive rights: The analysis of exposure of the two discourses in press media after 2000. *Sociologija, 48*(1), 73–95.

Drezgić, R. (2004). *(Re)Producing the nation: The politics of reproduction in Serbia in the 1980s and 1990s* [Unpublished PhD thesis]. University of Pittsburgh.

Duby, G., & Perrot, M. (Eds.). (1992). *A history of women in the west*. Harvard University Press.

Duden, B. (1991). *The woman beneath the skin: A doctor's patients in eighteenth-century Germany*. Harvard University Press.

Duden, B. (1993). *Disembodying women: Perspectives on pregnancy and the unborn*. Harvard University Press.

Eatough, V., & Smith, J. A. (2008). Interpretative phenomenological analysis. In C. Willig & W. Stainton Rogers (Eds.), *The Sage handbook of qualitative research in psychology* (pp. 179–194). Sage.

Edmonds, D., & Warburton, N. (Hosts). (2013, April 2). Ann Oakley on women's experience of childbirth [Audio podcast episode]. In *Social science bites*. Sage. Retrieved from https://www.socialsciencespace.com/2013/04/podcast-ann-oakley-on-womens experience-of-childbirth/

Elmir, R., Schmied, V., Wilkes, L., & Jackson, D. (2010). Women's perceptions and experiences of a traumatic birth: A meta-ethnography. *Journal of Advanced Nursing, 66*(10), 2142–2153.

Endžier, N. (2010). *Žena: Intimna geografija*. NNK Internacional.

Engel, G. L. (1977). The need for a new medical model: A challenge for biomedicine. *Science, 196*(4286), 129–136. https://doi.org/10.1126/science.847460

Engeström, Y. (1987). *Learning by expanding: An activity-theoretical approach to developmental research*. Orienta-Konsultit.

Esposito, N. (1999). Marginalized women's comparisons of their hospital and freestanding birth center experiences: A contrast of inner-city birthing systems. *Health Care for Women International, 20*(2), 111–126.

Flick, U. (1992). Triangulation revisited: Strategy of validation or alternative? *Journal for the Theory of Social Behaviour, 22*(2), 175–197. https://doi.org/10.1111/j.1468-5914.1992.tb00215.x

Foucault, M. (1982). The subject and power. *Critical Inquiry, 8*(4), 777–795. Retrieved from https://www.jstor.org/stable/1343197

Foucault, M. (1988). Technologies of the self. In L. H. Martin, H. Gutman, & P. H. Hutton (Eds.), *Technologies of the self: A seminar with Michel Foucault* (pp. 16–49). University of Massachusetts Press.

Foucault, M. (2003). *The birth of the clinic: An archaeology of medical perception*. Routledge.

Frank, A. W. (1997). *The wounded storyteller: Body, illness, and ethics*. University of Chicago Press.

Frazier, K. E., Jackson, T. E., & Mangione, H. (2015). Commentary: Beyond stigma: Critical approaches to violations of the motherhood narrative. In K. R. Cabell, G. Marsico, C. Cornejo, & J. Valsiner (Eds.), *Making meaning, making motherhood* (pp. 133–150). Information Age Publishing.

Fricker, M. (2007). *Epistemic injustice: Power and the ethics of knowing*. Oxford University Press.

Gergen, K. (2009). *Relational being: Beyond self and community*. Oxford University Press.

Gerson, M., Alpert, J. L., & Richardson, M. S. (1984). Mothering: The view from psychological research. *Signs, 9*(3), 434–453. https://doi.org/10.1086/494070

Gloger-Tippelt, G. (1983). A process model of the pregnancy course. *Human Development, 26*(3), 134–148. https://doi.org/10.1159/000272877

Griffin, S. (2001). Feminism and motherhood. In M. Davey (Ed.), *Mother reader: Essential literature on motherhood* (pp. 33–45). Seven Stories Press. (Original work published 1974).

Gross, H., & Pattison, H. (2007). *Sanctioning pregnancy: A psychological perspective*. Routledge.

Halfon, S. (2010). Encountering birth: Negotiating expertise, networks, and my STS self. *Science as Culture, 19*(1), 61–77. https://doi.org/10.1080/09505430903558062

Hall, G. S. (1904). *Adolescence: Its psychology and its relations to physiology, anthropology, sociology, crime, religion and education* (Vol. 2). Retrieved from https://psychclassics.yorku.ca/Hall/Adolescence/chap17.htm

Haraway, D. (1991b). Situated knowledges: The science question in feminism and the privilege of partial perspective. In *Simians, cyborgs and women: The reinvention of nature* (pp. 183–202). Routledge.

Haraway, D. (1991c). The biopolitics of postmodern bodies: Constitutions of self in immune system discourse. In *Simians, cyborgs and women: The reinvention of nature* (pp. 203–230). Routledge.

Harré, R. (2001). Metaphysics and narrative: Singularities and multiplicities of self. In J. Brockmeier & D. Carbaugh (Eds.), *Narrative and identity: Studies in autobiography, self and culture* (pp. 59–73). John Benjamins Publishing.
Hauck, Y., Fenwick, J., Downie, J., & Butt, J. (2007). The influence of childbirth expectations on Western Australian women's perceptions of their birth experience. *Midwifery, 23*(3), 235–247. https://doi.org/10.1016/j.midw.2006.02.002
Hays, S. (1998). *The cultural contradictions of motherhood.* Yale University Press.
Healthcare for women during pregnancy: National guidelines for doctors. (2005). Serbian Medical Society.
Healthcare Law. (2019). *Official Gazette-Republic of Serbia, 25.*
Hider, N. (1978). *Radikalne perspektive u psihologiji.* Nolit.
Hodnett, E. (2002). Pain and women's satisfaction with the experience of childbirth: A systematic review. *American Journal of Obstetrics & Gynecology, 186*(5), S160–S172.
Institute for Mother and Child Healthcare. (2010). *Guidelines for the implementation of the national program of healthcare for women, children, and youth.*
Institute of Public Health "Dr Milan Jovanović Batut". (2012). *Selected health indicators.*
Janevic, T., Sripad, P., Bradley, E., & Dimitrievska, V. (2011). "There's no kind of respect here". A qualitative study of racism and access to maternal health care among Romani women in the Balkans. *International Journal for Equity in Health, 10*(1), 53. https://doi.org/10.1186/1475-9276-10-53
Jenkinson, C., Coulter, A., Bruster, S., Richards, N., & Chandola, T. (2002). Patients' experiences and satisfaction with health care: Results of a questionnaire study of specific aspects of care. *Quality and Safety in Health Care, 11*(4), 335–339. https://doi.org/10.1136/qhc.11.4.335
Juarez, L. (2015). Motherhood and becoming: The construction of motherhood through pregnancy and birth. In K. R. Cabell, G. Marsico, C. Cornejo, & J. Valsiner (Eds.), *Making meaning, making motherhood* (pp. 21–40). Information Age Publishing.
Kaptelinin, V., & Nardi, B. A. (2006). *Acting with technology: Activity theory and interaction design.* The MIT Press.
King, H. (1998). *Hippocrates' woman: Reading the female body in Ancient Greece.* Routledge.
Kontopodis, M. (2012). How things matter in everyday lives of preschool age children: Material-semiotic investigations in psychology and education. *Journal für Psychologie, 20*(1), 1–14.

Køster, A. (2017). Narrative and embodiment—A scalar approach. *Phenomenology and the Cognitive Sciences, 16*(5), 893–908. https://doi.org/10.1007/s11097-016-9485-8

Køster, A., & Winther-Lindqvist, D. A. (2018). Personal history and historical selfhood: The embodied and pre-reflective dimension. In A. Rosa & J. Valsiner (Eds.), *The Cambridge handbook of sociocultural psychology* (pp. 538–555). Cambridge University Press.

Kristeva, J. (1990). Motherhood according to Giovanni Bellini. In J. M. Thompson (Ed.), *Twentieth century theories of art* (pp. 441–467). Carleton University Press.

Kristeva, J. (2009). *This incredible need to believe.* Columbia University Press.

Kukla, R. (2005). *Mass hysteria: Medicine, culture and mothers' bodies*. Rowman & Littlefield Publishers.

Kuriyama, S. (1999). *The expressiveness of the body and the divergence of Greek and Chinese medicine*. Zone Books.

Laney, E. K., Hall, M. E. L., Anderson, T. L., & Willingham, M. M. (2015). Becoming a mother: The influence of motherhood on women's identity development. *Identity, 15*(2), 126–145. https://doi.org/10.1080/15283488.2015.1023440

Laqueur, T. W. (1990). *Making sex: Body and gender from the Greeks to Freud.* Harvard University Press.

Larkin, M., Watts, S., & Clifton, E. (2006). Giving voice and making sense in interpretative phenomenological analysis. *Qualitative Research in Psychology, 3*(2), 102–120.

Larkin, P., Begley, C. M., & Devane, D. (2012). 'Not enough people to look after you': An exploration of women's experiences of childbirth in the Republic of Ireland. *Midwifery, 28*(1), 98–105. https://doi.org/10.1016/j.midw.2010.11.007

Latour, B. (1993). *We have never been modern*. Harvard University Press.

Latour, B. (1999). On recalling ANT. In J. Law & J. Hassard (Eds.), *Actor-network theory and after* (pp. 15–25). Blackwell Publishing.

Latour, B. (2005). *Reassembling the social: An introduction to actor-network theory*. Oxford University Press.

Law, J. (1992). Notes on the theory of the actor-network: Ordering, strategy and heterogeneity. *Systemic Practice and Action Research, 5*(4), 379–393. https://doi.org/10.1007/BF01059830

Law, J. (1999). After ANT: Complexity, naming and topology. In J. Law & J. Hassard (Eds.), *Actor network theory and after* (pp. 1–14). Blackwell Publishing.

Law, J. (2002). *Aircraft stories: Decentering the object in technoscience.* Duke University Press.

Law on Patients' Rights. (2013). *Official Gazette-Republic of Serbia, 45.*

Lawrence, J. A., & Valsiner, J. (2003). Making personal sense: An account of basic internalization and externalization processes. *Theory & Psychology, 13*(6), 723–752.

Leder, D. (1990). *The absent body.* University of Chicago Press.

Lehoux, P. (2006). *The problem of health technology: Policy implications for modern health care systems.* Routledge.

Leifer, M. (1977). Psychological changes accompanying pregnancy and motherhood. *Genetic Psychology Monographs, 95*, 55–96.

Leifer, M. (1980). Pregnancy. *Signs, 5*(4), 754–765.

Leont'ev, A. N. (1981). *Problems of the development of the mind.* Progress.

Leontyev, A. N. (1978). *Activity, consciousness, and personality.* Marxist Internet Archive. Retrieved from http://www.marxists.org/archive/leontev/works/1978/index.htm

Lyons, S. (1998). A prospective study of post-traumatic stress symptoms 1 month following childbirth in a group of 42 first-time mothers. *Journal of Reproductive and Infant Psychology, 16*(2–3), 91–106. https://doi.org/10.1080/02646839808404562

Mack, A. (2018). Critical approaches to motherhood. In *Oxford research encyclopedia of communication.* Retrieved July 15, 2023, from https://oxfordre.com/communication/view/10.1093/acrefore/9780190228613.001.0001/acrefore-9780190228613-e-579

Marecek, J., Kimmel, E. B., Crawford, M., & Hare-Mustin, R. (2003). Psychology of women and gender. In D. K. Freedheim & I. B. Weiner (Eds.), *Handbook of psychology, vol. 1: History of psychology* (pp. 249–266). Wiley.

Markus, H. R., & Hamedani, M. G. (2007). Sociocultural psychology: The dynamic interdependence among self systems and social systems. In S. Kitayama & D. Cohen (Eds.), *Handbook of cultural psychology* (pp. 3–40). Guilford Press.

Martin, E. (1992). *The woman in the body: A cultural analysis of reproduction.* Beacon Press.

Matejić, B., Milićević, M. S., Vasić, V., & Djikanović, B. (2014). Maternal satisfaction with organized perinatal care in Serbian public hospitals. *BMC Pregnancy and Childbirth, 14*, 14. https://doi.org/10.1186/1471-2393-14-14

McGrath, R. (2002). *Seeing her sex: Medical archives and the female body.* Manchester University Press.

McLaren, A. (1999). *Twentieth-century sexuality: A history*. Blackwell Publishing.

Merleau-Ponty, M. (2005). *Phenomenology of perception* (C. Smith, Trans.). Routledge. (Original work published 1945).

Miettinen, R. (1999). The riddle of things: Activity theory and actor-network theory as approaches to studying innovations. *Mind, Culture, and Activity, 6*(3), 170–195. https://doi.org/10.1080/10749039909524725

Milošević, B., Rajhvajn, B., & Berić, B. (1988). *Porodiljstvo: Udžbenik za studente medicine*. Medicinska knjiga.

Ministry of Health of Republic of Serbia. (2011). *Standards of health care adapted to the needs of mothers and children*.

Ministry of Labour and Social Policy of Republic of Serbia. (2008). *National strategy for advancing the status of women and promoting gender equality*.

Mladenović, D., Mladenović-Bogdanović, Z., & Mladenović-Mihailović, A. (2008). *Ginekologija i akušerstvo*. Zavod za udžbenike.

Mol, A., & Law, J. (2004). Embodied action, enacted bodies: The example of hypoglycaemia. *Body & Society, 10*(2–3), 43–62. https://doi.org/10.1177/1357034X04042932

Moscucci, O. (1990). *The science of woman: Gynaecology and gender in England 1800–1929*. Cambridge University Press.

Mullin, A. (2005). *Reconceiving pregnancy and childcare: Ethics, experience, and reproductive labor*. Cambridge University Press.

National Millennium Development Goals. (2006). Government of Republic of Serbia.

National Program of Health Care for Women, Children and Youth. (2009). *Official Gazette-Republic of Serbia*, 28.

Nicolson, P. (1998). *Post-natal depression: Psychology, science and the transition to motherhood*. Routledge.

Nicolson, P. (2010). What is 'psychological' about 'normal' pregnancy? *The Psychologist, 23*(3), 190–193.

O'Reilly, A. (2004). *From motherhood to mothering: The legacy of Adrienne Rich's "Of Woman Born"*. State University of New York Press.

Oakley, A. (1979). A case of maternity: Paradigms of women as maternity cases. *Signs, 4*(4), 607–631.

Oakley, A. (1981). Interviewing women: A contradiction in terms. In H. Roberts (Ed.), *Doing feminist research* (pp. 30–61). Routledge & Kegan Paul.

Ochs, E., & Capps, L. (1996). Narrating the self. *Annual Review of Anthropology, 25*(1), 19–43. https://doi.org/10.1146/annurev.anthro.25.1.19

Olde, E., van der Hart, O., Kleber, R. J., van Son, M., Wijnen, H., & Pop, V. (2005). Posttraumatic dissociation and emotions as predictors of PTSD symptoms following childbirth. *Journal of Trauma & Dissociation, 6*(3), 125–142.

Pantović, L. (2021). Somebodies or nobody's patient: The importance of social positioning and informal relations during childbirth in Serbia. *Glasnik Etnografskog instituta SANU, 69*(1), 205–225. https://doi.org/10.2298/GEI2101205P

Pantović, L. (2022). Providing a service or seeking a favor? The role of private prenatal care on the continuity of care in Serbian public maternity hospitals. *Birth, 49*(3), 506–513.

Pantović, L., Stanković, B., & Ćeriman, J. (2024). *Iskustva žena u porodilištima u Srbiji tokom i nakon pandemije kovida-19.* UNFPA.

Pelling, M., & Webster, C. (1979). Medical practitioners. In C. Webster (Ed.), *Health, medicine and mortality in the sixteenth century* (pp. 164–235). Cambridge University Press.

Philipp, D. A., & Carr, M. L. (2001). Normal and medically complicated pregnancies. In N. Stotland & D. E. Stewart (Eds.), *Psychological aspects of women's health care: The interface between psychiatry and obstetrics and gynecology* (pp. 13–32). American Psychiatric Press.

Physiological Childbirth: The guide for doctors and midwives. (2009). Ministry of Health of Republic of Serbia.

Pittrof, R., Campbell, O. M. R., & Filippi, V. G. A. (2002). What is quality in maternity care? An international perspective. *Acta Obstetricia et Gynecologica Scandinavica, 81*(4), 277–283.

Platon. (1995). *Timaj.* Eidos.

Plećaš, D., Stanimirović, B., Stanković, A., & Vasiljević, M. (2005). *Ginekologija i akušerstvo: Udžbenik za studente medicine.* Medicinski fakultet Univerziteta u Beogradu.

Porter, R. (2003). *Flesh in the age of reason.* W.W. Norton & Company.

Ratner, C. (1999). Three approaches to cultural psychology: A critique. *Cultural Dynamics, 11*(1), 7–31.

Reis, L. P. C., & Santos, J. E. F. (2015). The experiences of mothers from the railroad suburb of Salvador-Bahia: Conceptualizing a semiotic theory of protection and empowerment in adverse conditions. In K. R. Cabell, G. Marsico, C. Cornejo, & J. Valsiner (Eds.), *Making meaning, making motherhood* (pp. 107–132). Information Age Publishing.

Rich, A. (1986a). Notes toward a politics of location. In *Blood, bread, and poetry: Selected prose 1979–1985* (pp. 210–231). W. W. Norton & Company.

Rich, A. (1986b). *Of woman born: Motherhood as experience and institution*. W. W. Norton & Company.
Riggs, D. W., & Bartholomaeus, C. (2023). *First-time parenting journeys: Expectations and realities*. Cambridge University Press.
Riley, S., Evans, A., & Robson, M. (2019). *Postfeminism and health: Critical psychology and media perspectives*. Routledge.
Ristić, L. (2001). *Praktično porodiljstvo*. Freemental.
Rose, N. (1996). Assembling the modern self. In R. Porter (Ed.), *Rewriting the self: Histories from the Renaissance to the present* (pp. 224–248). Routledge.
Sartre, J. P. (2003). *Being and nothingness: An essay on phenomenological ontology* (H. E. Barnes, Trans.). Routledge. (Original work published 1943).
Sekulić, N. (2014). Social status of motherhood with special reference to Serbia today. *Sociologija, 56*(4), 402–426.
Sekulić, N. (2016). *Kultura rađanja: Istraživanje o seksualnoj i reproduktivnoj socijalizaciji žena*. Institut za sociološka istraživanja Filozofskog fakulteta u Beogradu.
Shaw, J. (2012). The birth of the clinic and the advent of reproduction: Pregnancy, pathology and the medical gaze in modernity. *Body & Society, 18*(2), 110–138. https://doi.org/10.1177/1357034X10394666
Shiffman, J., Skrabalo, M., & Subotic, J. (2002). Reproductive rights and the state in Serbia and Croatia. *Social Science & Medicine, 54*(5), 625–642.
Shweder, R. A., Goodnow, J. J., Hatano, G., LeVine, R. A., Markus, H. R., & Miller, P. J. (2006). The cultural psychology of development: One mind, many mentalities. In R. M. Lerner (Ed.), *Handbook of child psychology* (Vol. 1, pp. 716–793). Wiley.
Sims-Schouten, W., Riley, S. C. E., & Willig, C. (2007). Critical realism in discourse analysis: A presentation of a systematic method of analysis using women's talk of motherhood, childcare and female employment as an example. *Theory & Psychology, 17*(1), 101–124. https://doi.org/10.1177/0959354307073153
Smit, D. K. (2005). Hermeneutika i kvalitativno istraživanje. *Pedagogija, 3*, 315–330.
Smith, J. A. (1994). Reconstructing selves: An analysis of discrepancies between women's contemporaneous and retrospective accounts of the transition to motherhood. *British Journal of Psychology, 85*, 371–392. https://doi.org/10.1111/j.2044-8295.1994.tb02530.x
Smith, J. A. (1995). Semi-structured interviewing and qualitative analysis. In J. A. Smith, R. Harré, & L. van Langenhove (Eds.), *Rethinking methods in psychology* (pp. 9–26). Sage.

Smith, J. A. (1999). Identity development during the transition to motherhood: An interpretative phenomenological analysis. *Journal of Reproductive and Infant Psychology, 17*(3), 281–299. https://doi.org/10.1080/02646839908404595

Soet, J., Brack, G., & Dilorio, C. (2003). Prevalence and predictors of women's experience of psychological trauma during childbirth. *Birth, 30*(1), 36–46. https://doi.org/10.1046/j.1523-536X.2003.00215.x

Spinuzzi, C. (2008). *Network: Theorizing knowledge work in telecommunications*. Cambridge University Press.

Stam, H. J. (2000). Theorizing health and illness: Functionalism, subjectivity and reflexivity. *Journal of Health Psychology, 5*(3), 273–283. https://doi.org/10.1177/135910530000500309

Stanković, B. (2013). Medical practice in transition: The case of Serbian maternity care services and their users. In L. Popovic, M. Vidakovic, & D. Kostic (Eds.), *Resources of Danubian Region: The possibility of cooperation and utilization*. Humboldt-Club Serbien.

Stanković, B. (2014). Woman as a subject of childbirth: Physical, technological and institutional aspects. *Sociologija, 56*(4), 524–544. https://doi.org/10.2298/SOC1404524S

Stankovic, B. (2017a). Women's experiences of childbirth in Serbian public healthcare institutions: A qualitative study. *International Journal of Behavioral Medicine, 24*(6), 803–814. https://doi.org/10.1007/s12529-017-9672-1

Stanković, B. (2020). Qualitative approach to social trauma research. In A. Hamburger, V. D. Volkan, & C. Hancheva (Eds.), *Social trauma—An interdisciplinary textbook* (pp. 335–342). Springer.

Stanković, B., Skočajić, M., & Đorđević, A. (2017). Upravljanje porođajem u Srbiji: Medicinske intervencije i porođajna iskustva. *Limes Plus: Journal of Social Science and Humanities, 14*(2), 197–225.

Stanton, A., Lobel, M., Sears, S., & DeLuca, R. (2002). Psychosocial aspects of selected issues in women's reproductive health: Current status and future directions. *Journal of Consulting and Clinical Psychology, 70*, 751–770.

Stern, D., Bruschweiler-Stern, N., & Freeland, A. (1998). *The birth of a mother: How the motherhood experience changes you forever*. Basic Books.

Strauss, A., & Corbin, J. (1998). *Basics of qualitative research: Techniques and procedures for developing grounded theory*. Sage.

Thompson, C. (2005). *Making parents: The ontological choreography of reproductive technologies*. MIT Press.

Thomson, G., & Downe, S. (2008). Widening the trauma discourse: The link between childbirth and experiences of abuse. *Journal of Psychosomatic Obstetrics & Gynecology, 29*(4), 268–273.

Unger, R. K. (2001). Women as subjects, actors, and agents in the history of psychology. In R. K. Unger (Ed.), *Handbook of the psychology of women and gender* (pp. 3–16). Wiley.

Ussher, J. (1990). Choosing psychology or not throwing the baby out with the bathwater. In E. Burman (Ed.), *Feminists and psychological practice* (pp. 47–61). Sage.

Ussher, J. (2006). *Managing the monstrous feminine: Regulating the reproductive body*. Routledge.

Ussher, J. (2008). Reclaiming embodiment within critical psychology: A material-discursive analysis of the menopausal body. *Social and Personality Psychology Compass, 2*(5), 1781–1798. https://doi.org/10.1111/j.1751-9004.2008.00151.x

Valentine, D. (1982). The experience of pregnancy: A developmental process. *Family Relations, 31*(2), 243–248.

Valsiner, J. (1997). *Čovekov razvoj i kultura*. Zavod za udžbenike i nastavna sredstva.

Valsiner, J. (2002). Forms of dialogical relations and semiotic autoregulation within the self. *Theory & Psychology, 12*(2), 251–265.

Valsiner, J. (2004). Culture in psychology: Between social positioning and producing new knowledge. *Culture & Psychology, 10*(1), 5–27. https://doi.org/10.1177/1354067X04040925

Valsiner, J. (2007). *Culture in minds and societies: Foundations of cultural psychology*. Sage Publications.

Valsiner, J. (2012). Introduction: Culture in psychology: A renewed encounter of inquisitive minds. In J. Valsiner (Ed.), *The Oxford handbook of culture and psychology* (pp. 3–16). Oxford University Press.

van Langenhove, L., & Harré, R. (1999). Introducing positioning theory. In R. Harré & L. van Langenhove (Eds.), *Positioning theory: Moral contexts of international action*. Blackwell Publishers.

Verdery, K. (1996). *What was socialism and what comes next*. Princeton University Press.

Vilenica, A. (2013). Postajanje majkom: Od neoliberalnog režima materinstva ka radikalnoj političkoj subjektivizaciji. In A. Vilenica (Ed.), *Postajanje majkom u vreme neoliberalnog kapitalizma* (pp. 9–31). uz)bu))na))).

Vujadinović, D., & Stanimirović, V. (2017). Rodni odnosi u Srbiji u doba tranzicije—Između emancipacije i retradicionalizacije. In *Studije roda* (pp. 151–177). Pravni fakultet Univerziteta u Beogradu.

Walker, M. B. (1998). *Philosophy and the maternal body: Reading silence*. Routledge.

Wehrle, M. (2017). The normative body and the embodiment of norms: Bridging the gap between phenomenological and Foucauldian approaches. *Yearbook for Eastern and Western Philosophy, 2017*(2), 323–337. https://doi.org/10.1515/yewph-2017-0023

Weisstein, N. (1968). *Kinder, Küche, Kirche as scientific law: Psychology constructs the female.* New England Free Press. Retrieved from http://www.cwluherstory.com/psychology-constructs-the-female.html

Wilson, E. A. (1998). *Neural geographies: Feminism and the microstructure of cognition*. Routledge.

Woollett, A., & Marshall, H. (1997). Discourses of pregnancy and childbirth. In L. Yardley (Ed.), *Material discourses of health and illness* (pp. 176–198). Routledge.

World Health Organization (WHO). (1996). *Care in normal birth: A practical guide.* Department of Reproductive Health & Research, WHO.

World Health Organization (WHO). (2018). *WHO recommendations: Intrapartum care for a positive childbirth experience*. World Health Organization.

Yardley, L. (1996). Reconciling discursive and materialist perspectives on health and illness: A reconstruction of the biopsychosocial approach. *Theory & Psychology, 6*(3), 485–508. https://doi.org/10.1177/0959354396063008

Yardley, L. (1997). Introducing material-discursive approaches to health and illness. In L. Yardley (Ed.), *Material discourses of health and illness* (pp. 1–24). Routledge.

Young, I. M. (2005a). Throwing like a girl: A phenomenology of feminine body comportment, motility, and spatiality. In *On female body experience: 'Throwing like a girl' and other essays* (pp. 27–45). Oxford University Press.

Young, I. M. (2005b). Pregnant embodiment: Subjectivity and alienation. In *On female body experience: 'Throwing like a girl' and other essays* (pp. 46–61). Oxford University Press.

Zahavi, D. (2018). Getting it quite wrong: Van Manen and Smith on phenomenology. *Qualitative Health Research, 28*(6), 854–863. https://doi.org/10.1177/1049732318817547

Zerilli, L. M. G. (1992). A process without a subject: Simone de Beauvoir and Julia Kristeva on maternity. *Signs, 18*(1), 111–135. https://doi.org/10.1086/494781

Zittoun, T. (2006). *Transitions: Development through symbolic resources.* Information Age Publishing.

2

Situated Subjects: Cultural-Historical Contextualisation of Transition into Motherhood

Throughout the history of civilisation, two representations of the female body have persisted that are in many ways contradictory and seemingly exclusive. As Adrienne Rich (1986b, p. 34) describes: "Throughout patriarchal mythology, dream-symbolism, theology, language, two ideas flow side by side: one, that the female body is impure, corrupt, the site of discharges, bleedings, dangerous to masculinity, a source of moral and physical contamination, 'the devil's gateway'. On the other hand, as mother the woman is beneficent, sacred, pure, asexual, nourishing (…)".

This dissociative representation of women and their bodies has been reproduced in culture since at least the beginning of the modern era, although its roots are much older. Rebecca Kukla (2005) points out that since the eighteenth century, a dual image of the pregnant and maternal body has crystallised in public discourse and texts, as well as two sets of opposing practices and regulatory principles that follow from these representations. The first representation entails an idealised image of the future mother who is in perfect natural unity with her child, and whose body spontaneously functions in a perfect manner. It is therefore necessary to protect her from any external intervention—not only from harmful influences, but also from the use of medicine, drugs, artificial

B. Stanković, *Giving Birth To A Subject*, Sociocultural Psychology of the Lifecourse,
https://doi.org/10.1007/978-3-031-77236-8_2

substitutes for breast milk or nipples, etc. In the second representation, the pregnant woman is portrayed as a chaotic, disorderly being, ruled by emotions and whims. She is unpredictable, with permeable bodily boundaries, insufficiently strong to control her desires or fears, and susceptible to many harmful influences. She cannot be trusted to take care of the baby by herself, both while it is inside her belly and after it is born. She, therefore, requires constant monitoring and guidance from external authorities. Kukla refers to these two representations, which lead to the opposing set of practices, as the Fetish and Unruly Mother: "The Fetish Mother is a romantic, idealized character, while the Unruly Mother is an object of distrust and disdain. The first needs protection from external interventions, while the latter needs external interventions for proper discipline and management" (Kukla, 2005, p. 85). It is assumed that both representations of the mother and her pregnant and postpartum body, which have functioned as regulatory ideals up to the present day, emerged simultaneously from a common notion of the maternal body as responsible for "the production of human and social nature, properly governed by normative laws of nature, and easily corrupted and interrupted" (Kukla, 2005, p. 85).

This dissociative representation of the reproductive and maternal body forms the backbone of this chapter, which revolves around the discussion of two prevailing contemporary representational and regulatory models. I will first delve into the dominant medical model of pregnancy and birth, exploring its origins, key features and impact on women's experiences and practices. I will then introduce an alternative natural model that in the local context exists predominantly as a normative ideal. These two models embody specific contemporary cultural-historical expressions of the dissociative representation of the maternal body described above. The remainder of the chapter will attempt to illustrate how the medical and natural models intertwine in concrete practices and experiences and how women navigate the various, sometimes contradictory, discourses and norms associated with these models. Moreover, they will be contextualised in the broader sociocultural landscape characterised by the neoliberal regime of subjectivity, as well as self-sacrifice that serves as both a local and possibly still global ideal of motherhood.

2.1 Medicalisation of the Transition into Motherhood

Entering motherhood, particularly going through pregnancy and childbirth in contemporary Western society, almost inevitably involves contact with health professionals and various forms of medical technology, all within an institutional setting (Lowis & McCaffery, 2004). However, contact with medicine during pregnancy and childbirth is not only a highly probable outcome, but also represents a prevailing social ideal (Lyerly et al., 2007). The medical model is today the predominant way of representing and regulating pregnancy and childbirth, implying the existence of gynaecology and obstetrics as a separate medical specialty responsible for issues related to female reproduction.

The current situation can be seen as the culmination of a long historical process in which female reproduction was placed under the jurisdiction of medicine. Reproduction, traditionally seen as inherently risky and pathological, has been constructed as a purely physical process that can be naturalistically described and regulated accordingly. As indicated earlier, this shift led to the subjective, experiential aspect of these processes being relegated to the private sphere, which simultaneously shaped the way women experienced the early transition to motherhood (and even the preparation for it).

2.1.1 Mechanisation and Pathologisation of the Female Reproductive Body

The so-called *separation principle* is at the centre of the medical approach to phenomena. This is a classic modern principle—Bruno Latour (1993) even calls it the modern Constitution—which finds its paradigmatic expression in Cartesian metaphysics (Leder, 1992). The dualistic separation of mind and body, accompanied by the mechanistic decomposition of the body into a collection of parts, has made it possible to understand the problems of the body as technical issues that require technical solutions. Michel Foucault has pointed out the two levels on which these specifically modern bodies are constituted and shaped: "The great book of Man-the-Machine was written simultaneously on two registers: the anatomico-metaphysical register, of which Descartes wrote the first pages and which the physicians and philosophers continued, and the technico-political register, which was constituted by a whole set of regulations and by empirical and calculated methods relating to the army, the school and the hospital, for controlling or correcting the operations of the body" (Foucault, 1995, p. 136).

This broad historical trend towards the mechanisation of the human body did not spare women's reproductive bodies, which was particularly noticeable in the depiction and treatment of childbirth. In the eighteenth century, Scottish obstetrician William Smellie trained his students on "machines" made from the bones of real women, dressed in women's clothing, from which students delivered foetus-dolls. Less than a century later, James Young Simpson, advocating for the use of anaesthesia in childbirth, suggested that the entire birthing process would be easier for both the obstetrician and the woman if women were sedated. So, a few decades after Smellie constructed an didactic woman-machine from which a foetus-doll was extracted, Simpson, in a way, turned real women into machines from which he extracted real babies (King, 2007, p. 193). Women's reproductive bodies were thus reduced to mechanical devices from which babies, with the assistance of obstetricians and without the mother's involvement, came into the world. Women's consciousness became a contingent part of the birthing process, believed not only to not facilitate but rather to hinder it.

The representation of childbirth in Serbian medical textbooks illustrates this point in a striking manner. Thus, childbirth is defined as "a set of mechanical events, physiologically based, that lead to the expulsion of the foetus from the genital organs" (Ristić, 2001, p. 119) or as "complete expulsion or extraction of the foetus, placenta, umbilical cord, and foetal membranes through the birth canal into the external environment, after the 20th week of gestation" (Momčilov, 2005, p. 342).[1] This representation is fully reflected in the accounts of obstetricians themselves:

[1] In some definitions of childbirth found in medical textbooks, a woman and her body are not even mentioned, and childbirth is presented as exclusively a physiological event, giving the impression that it occurs automatically, similar to other physiological processes such as circulation or secretion: "Normal childbirth is a physiological event that concludes with the birth of the child and the expulsion of the placenta and foetal membranes" (Mladenović et al., 2008, p. 319).

"We say it expertly, to translate, the childbirth object, well, it sounds a bit anonymous. The childbirth object is like a cylinder you know, it is positioned in a certain way, it's physics actually, so it can pass with its smallest diameters through the largest diameters of the birth canal." (from an interview with a doctor)

The commonly held medical conception of a woman giving birth assumes a body composed of a series of parts (uterus, birth canal and vagina) that perform involuntary movements and biologically determined work so that the baby can be born without the woman being involved in any way. Accordingly, the identification of factors influencing the course and outcome of childbirth, referred to in obstetric discourse as obstetric factors, follows this pattern. All potential determinants of childbirth are reduced to three factors: characteristics of the birth pathway or canal (pelvis, cervix, vagina), the birth object (position, posture, presentation and size of the foetus) and the labour forces (which include involuntary contractions of smooth and striated muscles, i.e., labour and pushing contractions) (Čutura, 2005; Mladenović et al., 2008). From a medical point of view, the woman and her actions have no influence on the course and outcome of the birth.[2] These are determined solely by physical processes—the movement of the foetus or birth object and the physical/biological characteristics of a particular part of the woman's body.[3] The representation of the birth process as exclusively mechanical

[2] Since the problem is formulated mechanically, the solution is of the same nature. The obstetrician assesses what is necessary for an object with certain physical properties to pass through an opening with certain physical properties while remaining undamaged, and how much "extra work needs to be invested", meaning how much to enhance contractions by adding medication: *"The art of the obstetrician, as I often tell my students, lies in his ability to assess—and therein lies his greatness and expertise -to assess whether a particular foetus in your uterus can pass through your birth canal undamaged. When this assessment is done well, then you know how much labour force is needed and so on... and that is then a good obstetrician and a good birth"* (from an interview with a doctor). The devaluation of the role of the woman giving birth simultaneously brings the decisive role of the doctor to the fore: "The knowledge and experience of the obstetrician and his ethics are fundamental factors for the successful completion of the childbirth and the birth of a healthy and uninjured baby" (Ristić, 2001, p. 134).

[3] This approach to childbirth has a long tradition and dates back to the first half of the eighteenth century, when one of the first obstetricians, William Smellie, began to view childbirth as a mechanical process. He also introduced cervical measurement and foetal head measurement to predict mechanical factors responsible for a successful delivery (Spencer, 1927). This means that the obstetric representation of childbirth has not fundamentally changed over the last almost three centuries.

and physiological not only determines how the woman and her body are portrayed, but also influences how they are treated. This representation plays a normative and regulatory role and guides certain forms of medical practice, i.e. the actual procedures with women and their babies during childbirth (which is analysed in detail in Chap. 4).[4]

However, while the reduction to the "body-machine" is what all patients actually encounter with the advancement of modern medicine, regardless of their gender specificities, this inherently egalitarian (albeit mechanistic) view of the human body, when it comes to women's reproductive states, becomes distorted due to the predominantly *patriarchal* perspective: "Thus the male body came to be medically viewed as the prototype of the properly functioning body-machine. The female body, as it deviated from the male standard, was regarded as inherently defective and dangerously under the influence of nature, which due to its unpredictability, was itself regarded as in need of constant manipulation by man" (Davis-Floyd, 2001, p. S6). Because the normative ideal is based on the body of the adult male, in which significant physical changes are generally considered an expression of illness or other dysfunction, significant changes in the appearance, processes and functionality of the body that are common in early and late life stages and during the reproductive states of women in adulthood are easily interpreted from the paradigm of "illness", i.e., they are easily pathologised: "Because of their extreme deviation from the male prototype, uniquely female anatomical features such as the uterus, ovaries and breasts, and uniquely female biological processes such as menstruation, pregnancy, birth and menopause are seen as inherently subject to malfunction" (Davis-Floyd, 1994, p. 1126). Thus, the female body is indeed a machine, but a machine that is *inherently and*

[4] Throughout labour, the birthing body is the sole object of medical monitoring and intervention, usually focusing on only one of its parts—the uterus. From the moment a woman enters the delivery room, a number of practices performed on her are directed at the uterus—monitoring the strength and frequency of uterine contractions on CTG, regular examinations to check cervical dilation and performing manual dilatation, influencing uterine contractions by intravenous administration of hormones, and even applying mechanical pressure to the uterus during the second stage of labour (Kristeller manoeuvre). The uterus is thus not only the central, but typically also the exclusive object of medical practice, involving both monitoring and intervention, which results in the woman's role and experience being actively neglected and deemed irrelevant. This approach leads to an objectification and partialisation of the woman as subject.

unpredictably prone to malfunction and disruptions, carrying inevitable consequences for the treatment and regulation of that body (Chadwick, 2006; Kukla, 2005).

Medicine has therefore redefined *normal* physiological experiences (such as menstruation, pregnancy, childbirth, menopause) as medical conditions that need to be monitored and treated (Gannon, 1998; Young, 2005b). Historically, the pathologisation of childbirth was the first to occur.[5] An early American obstetrician, Austin Flint, wondered how a "process that kills thousands of women each year, leaves a quarter of all cases more or less invalided, is attended by severe pain and tearing of tissues, and kills three to seven percent of all babies, can be called a normal or physiological function?" (Flint, 1925; as cited in Caton, 1999, p. 157). His colleague Joseph B. DeLee suggests that everything that commonly happens during childbirth could be labelled "natural to labour and therefore normal, in the same way as the death of the mother salmon and the death of the male bee in copulation, are natural and normal", adding that "labour is pathogenic" since the optimal outcomes for the mother and the baby are "exceedingly rare" (DeLee, 1920; as cited in Caton, 1999, p. 156–7). Following childbirth, pregnancy has also been pathologised and brought under the jurisdiction of medicine, implying "interpreting pregnancy itself as a disruption of health that necessarily requires expert medical intervention, and thinking of pregnancy as primarily about heath and illness" (Mullin, 2005, p. 54).[6]

The evolving trend of medicalisation indicates a tendency to encompass everything related to the reproductive functioning of women, and it has become quite common for medical knowledge and practices to be

[5] As early as the seventeenth century, with the emergence of instruction manuals for midwives (written by male physicians) and the increasing involvement of obstetricians in childbirth, there is a shift towards referring to childbirth as an illness (King, 2007, p. 22).

[6] In Serbian medical textbooks and official documents, pregnancy and childbirth are unequivocally referred to as illnesses, and women who are pregnant or giving birth are referred to as patients (this language is often reproduced by the women themselves). Here is a striking example: "The five most common groups of illnesses in women's healthcare services in the Republic of Serbia include infectious and parasitic diseases, pregnancy, childbirth and puerperium, and tumours. These five most common illness groups together accounted for 98.87% in 2007, and 98.84% in 2011" (Selected Health Indicators, 2012).

involved even in the *preparation* for conception (Tone, 2012).[7] So, it is now generally accepted that "the entire process of pregnancy, childbirth, and child-rearing ought to be *monitored* by a physician, even when there was no indication of a special medical problem" (Kukla, 2005, p. 71).

The preventive involvement of medical expertise "even when there is no indication of a special medical problem" indicates the presence of the *discourse of risk*, under the influence of which natural variations and physiological changes throughout pregnancy and birth are scrutinised as potential complications and disorders. A key role in establishing and maintaining the hegemony of the medical model has been played by the widespread belief that placing pregnancy and childbirth under the jurisdiction of medicine has significantly reduced the riskiness of these processes and increased the overall safety of mothers and infants. A cursory glance at obstetric textbooks thus clearly shows the connection between pathologisation and risk: "The concept of normal childbirth can only be established retroactively, after the fourth stage of labour has been completed. In other words, one must be aware that childbirth can become pathological at any moment" (Momčilov, 2005, p. 345).

If every pregnancy and childbirth are to be treated as risky until proven otherwise, i.e., considered normal only retrospectively, then the preventive use of medical techniques and interventions is justified (Savage, 2003, p. 105). While the obstetric approach in the eighteenth and nineteenth centuries was characterised by an attitude of "watchful waiting" (I will come back to this shortly), the understanding of pregnancy and childbirth as high-risk processes led to the adoption of an "active" approach and the establishment of interventionism as the prevailing norm in the treatment of reproductive processes in the early twentieth century. Accordingly, American obstetrician Joseph B. DeLee promoted

[7] Historically, childbirth first fell under the auspices of medicine. Over the last century, the trend of medicalisation and pathologisation gradually expanded to the entire course of pregnancy, leading to the standardisation of antenatal care, which involves medical monitoring of all pregnancies. However, childbirth remains the most medicalised aspect of women's reproduction. As an illustration, while the percentage of women in Serbia giving birth in hospitals with the presence of medical staff is over 99%, the coverage of antenatal and postnatal care is much lower, standing at just over 50% (National Program of Health Care for Women, Children, and Youth, 2009).

a method that "interferes much with Nature's process"[8] (DeLee, 1920; as cited in Caton, 1999, p. 156), and led women to "experience the birth as an entirely medical event, not unlike any other surgical procedure" (Rothman, 2007b, p. 17). As a result of the pathologisation of female reproduction, an *interventionist approach* has prevailed that remains unchallenged in most contexts, as I will elaborate in detail later.

However, monitoring and intervention are not only reserved for childbirth, as evidenced by regular check-ups, screenings and a variety of medications (hormonal preparations and supplements) during pregnancy aimed at early detection of abnormalities and preventive risk reduction. Women generally adhere to all prescribed procedures, examinations and medications without exception. It is also assumed that they actively work to reduce and avoid potential risks during the planning phase of pregnancy by having regular gynaecological examinations, taking recommended supplements such as folic acid and adjusting their overall lifestyle to the impending condition. The adaptation of everyday practices continues throughout pregnancy and is particularly prominent because modern women have internalised the medical discourse of risk, further reinforced by the prevailing cultural narrative of what a good mother should be.

2.1.2 Medical Discourse of Risk in the Age of Intensive Mothering

There is a very common and widespread conception when a woman becomes pregnant (and later gives birth to a baby) that this is the most important thing that happens to her at this stage of her life and that it should be at the top of her priority list (Riggs & Bartholomaeus, 2023). This is particularly appealing to first-time pregnant women, who often experience pregnancy as a project to which they are fully committed.

[8] DeLee's "active" approach involved administering ether to the woman during the dilation phase to render her unconscious, and then pulling the baby out with forceps, facilitated by a surgical incision in the perineum called an episiotomy. The placenta was then removed manually. Childbirth became a process divided into stages associated with a series of statistical norms and treatment steps that were to be followed (O'Driscoll et al., 1973) and necessarily took place in a hospital setting.

Everything else, from life plans to daily practices, is subordinate to their altered state. As Iris Marion Young (2005b) points out, although their condition actually delays or prevents them from carrying out their projects, women do not perceive this as an obstacle. Pregnancy becomes the "priority" and all other things that were previously perceived as important or crucial temporarily lose importance.

> *"I know what my priority is, what is happening to me right now. But from the moment you become pregnant, at least that's how I see it, everything else absolutely becomes irrelevant, absolutely everything is irrelevant. Since I became pregnant, I no longer think about the bar exam, how I am going to pass it, or how I will find the time to prepare for it. I simply think about the present moment, and things will unfold as they should. I am completely relaxed. So, it's normal for a pregnant woman to only think about that because it's the most important thing to her." (Maja)*

I tend to see this as an expression of the dominant contemporary ideology known as "intensive mothering" (Ennis, 2014), which "declares that mothering is exclusive, wholly child centred, emotionally involving, and time-consuming" (Arendell, 2000, p. 1194). This ideology prescribes what a "real" or "good" mother should be like, and these norms determine how many women feel and act from the day they conceive.

Of course, there are also many women who do not attribute such central importance to pregnancy and continue with what they call "normal functioning". They are also often critical of those *"whose existence is reduced to the role of a pregnant woman and who have no life outside of that"* (Sonja). They recognise that some women fully identify with their altered situation from the outset and adapt their lives to normative expectations, while others adjust their functioning primarily under the influence of their changing embodied experience and emerging needs and constraints.

> *"There are pregnant women who are pregnant right away. I mean, as soon as they realize it, they immediately start holding onto their belly. They wear overalls and act like, 'Now I'm pregnant.' And then there are those who keep working, I mean, they just go on functioning, until it's like, 'Okay, something is happening now, and I can't do that something anymore.'" (Ivana)*

What these two groups of women have in common, however, is a heightened sense of responsibility for the baby—e.g. for its health and well-being. As a consequence, they all alter and adapt various daily practices—their level of physical activity, the way they dress, what they eat, the position they sleep in, but also their emotional regulation (avoiding negative emotions—stress, anxiety, sadness). On the one hand, this responsibility can (and should) be seen as perfectly reasonable, useful and even practically necessary. Responsibility is, after all, essential for caring practices (van Nistelrooij & Visse, 2019)—and babies need to be cared for. On the other hand, we should not forget that this primary or even sole responsibility has been socially ascribed to women throughout history (Kukla, 2005)—making it an important aspect of motherhood as a social (or more precisely patriarchal) institution (Rich, 1986b). And the ideology of intensive mothering is exactly the contemporary form of this institution.

The heightened sense of responsibility towards the unborn child has long gone hand in hand with the deeply rooted notion that everything a mother consumes or experiences, including her thoughts and feelings, can influence and potentially endanger the baby (Kukla, 2005). The discourse of risk, which stems from the medical model, is a contemporary successor to this line of thought and its effects are ubiquitous and widespread. For example, when women are encouraged to reflect on their habits, they may talk at length about their sleeping position, their eating habits or their choice of clothing. The sleeping position in particular can serve as a prime example of the shaping of bodily experiences and habits under the influence of dominant representations and expert (or pseudo-expert) knowledge, right from the beginning of pregnancy when the actual physical changes are either non-existent or minimal.

"I haven't laid on my stomach since I found out I was pregnant. They say you shouldn't sleep on your back because the baby puts pressure on blood vessels. ... Well, I imagine that if such a small baby is putting pressure on me, how must I press her when I'm lying on my stomach. I just didn't want to, from the start..." (Tamara)

"Sometimes, when I wake up from a dream, I might forget for a moment. I don't have that feeling the first second I'm awake. So I make this movement to

turn onto my stomach and then I suddenly realize... I remember. It's like a mechanical movement, but then I'm like - no, you can't do that, turn on your side." (Nevena)

"From the beginning, I somehow sleep on my sides because, like, who knows?... I actually like sleeping on my stomach. But how can I sleep on my stomach now? I can't sleep on my stomach because something might happen. Of course, it's probably a mistake; in the beginning, you can probably sleep on your stomach, but I've been sleeping on the side from the start." (Maja)

In these quotations, one's own body is seen as vulnerable and the process of pregnancy as easily susceptible to risks and negative outcomes. This leads women to adjust their everyday practices and habits for fear of endangering or harming the baby, especially during sleep when they are less conscious. Even if women realise that this concern is probably irrational, it doesn't change the situation. Unconsciously adopting a "risky" position during sleep immediately leads them to seek additional validation from experts—whether by negotiating different "expert" opinions or seeking authoritative confirmation from a doctor while relying on medical technology.

"A few weeks ago, I woke up on my stomach. I woke up and I was like, 'Oh my God, I woke up on my stomach!' Because I've always slept on my stomach my whole life, and it's really hard for me to sleep on my back. ... Then they got me all worried, saying not to sleep on the right side; they even read me some articles. That it's not good on the right side, I don't know why, something with the organs. It's something medical, I don't know. And this one friend, who is a nurse, she says no one recommends sleeping on your back, for example. Yes, because it might press on a nerve. ... Yeah, so then I think, 'Oh God, I turned spontaneously, it didn't hurt, it should be okay.' But when I woke up on my stomach I was like, 'Why did I do something like that?' After that, I had an ultrasound, and when they said everything was okay, I thought, 'Oh, it's fine.'" (Sofija)

As already mentioned, consideration for pregnancy and the baby is also present in many other aspects—physical activity, exercise, choice of clothing, and diet. It seems that there is no aspect of daily life and behaviour that does not need to be adjusted or at least scrutinised as it could pose a potential risk.

"I had this horrible feeling that I have to start paying attention to everything now. I start climbing stairs, then it occurs to me that I shouldn't do it so quickly, so I say to myself, 'Wait, take it slow', This is how you burden yourself with all these things..."" (Maja)

"But then you feel in your conscience, 'Oh, maybe I shouldn't be doing this,' bending down, leaning over, and so on. And then you need to seek help from others." (Saška)

This change in behaviour is not related to their altered physical state or changed embodied experience, but to a consideration that women perceive as "external". They often feel well, "like they could", but refrain from doing so out of a sense of responsibility and following norms that prescribe increased caution because a woman's condition is perceived as risky and easily influenced.

"I was full of energy. I mean, you really feel strength that, I mean, for me, it was a problem, for example, physically. Everyone told me not to carry things, not to carry, but I really feel the strength to do everything. And then I forget that and I start pulling things up very often and then it's like, 'I shouldn't be doing this', not because you feel like you shouldn't be doing it, but just because you've been told from the outside. But you don't feel that..." (Una)

Due to the fear 'of harming the baby,' women change their practices such as dressing, even when they are aware that the baby is only a few centimetres in size in the early months, so this concern is not rationally justified.

"The only thing I was preoccupied with was whether everything would be okay. Right from the start I unbuttoned my pants, bought them two sizes bigger and then started wearing maternity clothes just to make sure I don't squeeze the baby and hurt her. That was and still is my biggest concern." (Tamara)

"All I have in my head is that she's fine, whether I've hurt her somehow. And when I get upset, I think, am I allowed to be upset? These things have bothered me the most throughout the whole pregnancy. Whether I... I mean, my belly is flat, I'm three months pregnant, nothing is showing, you know, but I'm like 'are these jeans too tight now, does it bother her, maybe she can't...?' But she's still so small, she can do whatever she wants." (Sofija)

A similar disproportion between recognising the unfounded or even irrational nature of beliefs and the strength of the norm that is still adhered to is encountered in the area of nutrition. Although the foetus is extremely small in the first weeks of pregnancy, the cultural pattern of "eating for two" to ensure proper development of the baby is strong enough that many pregnant women increase their food intake from the beginning of pregnancy.

> *"And for the first few days all I have in my mind is, 'Give me something to eat, give me some fruit, give something.' It's more like, I want it all to be good, so I better eat something... And if the zygote is like this [showing something the size of a bean] and you still think you should eat for two..." (Mirjana)*
>
> *"And I had nausea because I ate like a pig. I probably thought, now that I'm pregnant, I can eat. I mean, as if I hadn't eaten without restriction before. No, it's not that. It's more like I have to eat for two now. Those are the crazy moments—I go for a check-up, and I have ten kilos more, but the baby weighs 350 grams." (Una)*

Sometimes this cautious attitude and heightened sense of responsibility are only linked to the uncertain beginning of pregnancy and cease afterward. Women sometimes engage in more activities and adopt a more relaxed approach towards the end, compared to the beginning or middle of pregnancy, even though it becomes more physically demanding due to the large belly, increased weight and pressure of the baby. The reason for this is the perception that they cannot endanger their condition too much, and the onset of labour is seen as "the worst that can happen".

> *"Maybe because I have it in my head now, even if it starts now, well, so be it. That's it. I don't have to be so careful anymore. The worst that can happen, I'll give birth." (Anđela)*

It seems that women feel less responsibility for their condition and use their bodies more freely because they believe that they can no longer make serious mistakes, which is consistent with the medical representation of the early stages of pregnancy as particularly risky.

The Loss of the Most Private Space: Emotional Regulation During Pregnancy

Moving from bodily practices and habits into the realm of the psyche, the effects of the internalised discourse of risk, reinforced by the ideology of intensive mothering, become even more pervasive and burdensome. Sharing one's body with the baby implies, in a sense, a loss of the most private sphere. Women often feel that they cannot allow themselves any negative emotions, stress or frustration because it will all affect the baby. Therefore, they should not only refrain from substances and practices that physically affect the body (alcohol, medication, physical exertion), but also make an effort to regulate their mental states and reactions out of responsibility to the baby, because "the baby can feel it all" and could suffer as a result.

> *"I felt responsibility, in the sense that... Stress can't be avoided, really. But the responsibility to minimize it. When you're alone, you can burn yourself out in that stress, in that anger, in everything. Now it's like I am literally aware that I mustn't burn out, that it's not just about me, it's about someone else beside me. And when it comes to me, that feeling was strong, really strong... This being is completely innocent of everything, and there's no reason to burden it along in any way. Whatever troubles me are my struggles, but through me I transfer them onto my child, and that's unfair. It's unfair to this little being who has no problems in her life, and here I am creating them to her. (...) That whole period when I had this conflict with my parents seemed very unfair to me... because I was really stressed at that time, and I felt like, 'Poor baby, what is she going through with me.' 'Poor baby, I'm crying now, why does she have to experience these tears?', that's what I thought." (Nevena)*

The belief that the baby in the womb experiences everything the mother goes through is tied to an ethical demand to approach sources of stress and conflict situations with caution and in a strategic manner, out of consideration for the baby. It implies adapting and controlling one's own reactions to ensure the well-being of the baby.

> *"In that way, I consciously tried to postpone the stress, to go through it as little as possible. For example, before, when there we argued, I would always stay*

until the end, arguing and pushing until the matter was resolved. But the moment I know I'm pregnant... I would give up arguing and do the thing I hate the most—leave and close the door behind me. But I really did it out of responsibility, so I wouldn't experience stress for the baby's sake." (Nevena)

In contrast to the adaptation of everyday practices and habits, the imperative to adjust emotional reactions out of responsibility for the baby is experienced as significantly more challenging and, to a certain extent, even threatening. At the same time, this is also recognised by the women themselves as a very important aspect of becoming a mother and identifying with this new and emerging life role. One participant even emphasised that an expectant father cannot yet feel this kind of responsibility, which makes him still a "fictive parent".

"Yesterday, this whole shit with college and everything hit me. I failed the last exam again, and I would like to grieve. I mean, I'd like to get drunk, that's first. Or if nothing else, I'd like to grieve, cry it out, whatever, to somehow empty myself. And then I said to my boyfriend... this responsibility is so strange, which he still doesn't feel because he is a fictive parent and all that. I can't be sad, I can't take a pill... I can't be too nervous. You know because, yesterday, everything piled up from exams... and my belly started hurting, and I was all... and the discharge, it's madness, it starts immediately, and I got a bit scared, and then I was like, 'Okay, I'm going home to get some sleep, to chill, I don't know.' And I'm thinking I might even go out somewhere, but that's not responsible. And the baby is really quite nervous now because I'm upset. And then I realize how weird that is - it's all luxury now. You can't be sad... Then I remember how my mom never wanted to be sad in front of me and how she hid it and I don't know what. But it seems like it's already started for me. It's been catching up with me over the last few months. I can feel it. And he won't even breastfeed. And I have to do it; my milk depends on how I feel. And the whole story about how I've been acting responsibly towards the baby and how strange it feels. How you are already aware that nothing will ever be the same. Then I just don't have the luxury to sit down and cry. But I need it, it's my release." (Sonja)

Common emotions that could previously be expressed freely (anger, sadness) seem to become a "luxury" for a woman. She then often finds herself in a somewhat hopeless position, because the resources that made her feel better (crying, going out, taking tranquillisers) are also considered harmful. This can lead to an exacerbation of the negative emotions, as she is also aware that they may endanger the baby and therefore represent an additional burden. This vicious circle puts a woman in a somewhat claustrophobic position where she feels she is losing her most private space as she begins to share it with another being. It is important to note, however, that this physiological and phenomenological fact of sharing a body (which I will discuss in detail in Chap. 3) is not itself responsible for her situation since it is a product of the pervasive medical discourse of risk that dominates feelings and imaginations of women in contemporary society.

2.1.3 Interventionism as an Unquestioned Norm and the Rigidity of Medical Practice

The assumption that the application of the medical model reduces risk and enhances safety was so self-evident that for a long time it was not empirically studied and the efficacy or risk of iatrogenic consequences of many obstetric procedures was not known. Robbie Davis-Floyd (2001) presents data indicating that by the late 1970s only 20% of procedures routinely used in obstetric practice were scientifically based, while in the 1990s this percentage still amounted to less than 50%.[9] Practices such as the uncritical use of hormones during childbirth to expedite it or routine episiotomies have been widespread for decades without any proven benefit (Goer, 1995). In fact, many interventions not only persisted but were often interconnected, with the occurrence of some leading to a modification of the entire pattern of childbirth. Thus, since the 1980s, childbirth has become more painful, mainly due to the increasing use of contraction-stimulating hormones (oxytocin), which has led to more frequent use of epidural analgesia, which in turn has resulted in more forceps deliveries and a higher number of caesarean sections (O'Dowd & Philipp, 1994,

[9] Some authors argue, for example, that maternal mortality during childbirth was reduced primarily by the introduction of antiseptic substances and procedures that prevented puerperal fever, which killed a relatively high percentage of women in the eighteenth and nineteenth centuries (Moscucci, 1990), and that this had nothing to do with obstetric practices.

p. 28). This pattern has also been empirically confirmed in local obstetric practice—the occurrence of one intervention significantly increases the likelihood of other interventions (Stanković et al., 2017).

In recent decades, evidence-based medicine has been advocated, which entails a more systematic empirical investigation of the consequences and effectiveness of various procedures. This has led to the formulation of clinical recommendations for appropriate obstetric care (WHO, 1996, 2018), which have also been translated and adapted for use in the local context in the form of national guidelines for good clinical practice (Healthcare for women during pregnancy, 2005; Physiological Childbirth, 2009). And just as Robbie Davis-Floyd (2001, p. S19) claimed prior to the official publication of these guidelines that "if obstetrical care in most hospitals were to become truly evidence-based, then most standard interventions, including routine IVs, routine use of Pitocin, and the lithotomy (flat-on-the-back) position would have to be eliminated; women would eat, drink, and move about freely during labour; and they would give birth in upright sitting or squatting positions". However, she observes that physicians' appreciation of scientific progress is often declarative in nature. In various areas of practice, they are reluctant to change standard procedures, even if they contradict scientific evidence. Local medical practice convincingly confirms this assertion, as there is a significant discrepancy between the recommendations for good clinical practice from the national guidelines (Physiological Childbirth, 2009) and actual practice in maternity wards regarding informed consent, support during labour, birthing position,[10] active management of labour, etc. (Arsenijevic et al., 2014; Stanković et al., 2017).

[10] The supine position (lying on the back) historically became predominant only with the transfer of childbirth to hospitals, as it is convenient for the doctor and allows the easiest access to the woman's reproductive organs. Prior to this, a variety of birthing positions existed, with those that facilitated the baby's progress by utilising gravity (standing, squatting and occasionally kneeling; Shorter, 1991, p. 55–56) being preferred. The practice of giving birth lying down is thus consistent with the delegation of authority over childbirth to doctors. From a physiological perspective, this is an irrational choice—apart from being a common cause of complications, giving birth on the back restricts the opening of the pelvis, hinders effective pushing and reduces the baby's blood and oxygen supply. Accordingly, modern recommendations also support upright positions (Physiological childbirth, 2009; WHO, 2006, 2018). However, despite these recommendations, local maternity hospitals still insist on the lithotomy position (Stanković et al., 2017).

Therefore, various obstetric procedures that may be unnecessary and potentially harmful are frequently used. These include the routine administration of hormones to augment contractions, the application of pressure to the abdomen during the pushing phase of labour, mandatory enemas and shaving and the liberal use of episiotomies (with subsequent suturing of the incisions without anaesthesia). I will analyse in more detail the case of episiotomy, particularly its uncritical and routine use in local maternity wards, as it significantly shapes not only women's birth experiences, but also their experiences and practical possibilities during the first days and weeks with the baby. This case study is not only paradigmatic of the hegemonic status of interventionism in the local institutions, but also demonstrates the broader social embeddedness of medical practices.

Episiotomy is a very common surgical procedure in which an incision is made in the perineum at the end of the second stage of labour to enlarge the vaginal opening. Typically, it is covered in medical textbooks in the chapter on perineal protection. So, the perineum is protected by cutting it. The rationale for this procedure is that it prevents the occurrence of spontaneous tears in the vagina, and with this rationale practitioners have occasionally used the procedure since the early eighteenth century (Spencer, 1927). This controversial surgical intervention became a routine procedure globally from the mid-twentieth century, particularly in primiparous women, and its prevalence has declined significantly in many countries in recent decades[11] (Graham et al., 2005), coinciding with medical guidelines recommending its more selective use (WHO, 1996, 2018; Cunningham et al., 2010; Myers-Helfgott & Helfgott, 1999). However, the prevalence of episiotomy varies widely (from less than 10% to 100%) between and sometimes even within countries,[12] depending on regional medical practices and cultural norms (Graham

[11] In the 1950s, episiotomy was only performed in about 15% of deliveries. In the 1970s, however, it became a common practice and was performed on almost all first-time mothers in the United States, accounting for about 70% of all deliveries (O'Dowd & Philipp, 1994). Although still a relatively common obstetric procedure, this percentage dropped to 40% by 1997 and then decreased to only 18% by 2003, with a tendency to decline further (Cunningham et al., 2010, p. 401).

[12] For example, there are considerable differences between the various maternity hospitals in Serbia when it comes to the frequency of episiotomy, which indicates the importance of institutional factors (Stanković et al., 2017).

et al., 2005). This obstetric procedure serves as a notable example of situated medical practice that is rigid despite the evidence, as it relies on local forms of knowledge, established hierarchies and relationships within institutions, and is influenced by ideological factors outside medicine.

A glance at the local obstetrics textbooks already suggests that episiotomy is a very common and routine intervention. In addition to various medical indications for performing an episiotomy (such as breech presentation, multiple pregnancies, use of instruments at the end of delivery, etc.), it is often added that the woman is a primipara. The episiotomy is therefore recommended as a routine procedure for all primiparous women, with its frequency in practice stated to be around 90%[13] (Plećaš et al., 2005; Mladenović et al., 2008; Milošević et al., 1988; Ristić, 2001).

> *"In modern obstetrics, episiotomy is applied with varying frequency, depending on the school.* ***According to our traditional teachings, often referred to as the Belgrade school of obstetrics,***[14] *episiotomy is quite prevalent as a means of protecting the perineum. For instance, in the case of primiparas, it is performed in approximately 90% of cases."* (Stanojević, 2005, p. 585)

This was confirmed in interviews with women—only one participant did not undergo an episiotomy and was very surprised by this as she, like all the other women I spoke to during the research, had heard that "it is done to all first-time mothers". Women expect to be "cut" because they know it is a routine procedure at the end of labour.

> *"They cut me, which is normal..."*
> *"...yes, like every first-time mother, they have to cut" (Jasna)*
> *"And I asked the doctor: 'How much did you cut me?' and he said: 'Like every woman', and that reassured me" (Saška)*

[13] For comparison: The WHO guidelines (2018) recommend keeping the rate of episiotomy below 10% and only performing it when medically justified. It is also noted that a review study suggests that some of the highest episiotomy rates occur in middle-income countries (Miller et al., 2016), so Serbia fits into this picture.

[14] Occasionally, when I want to emphasise a particular part of the quotation, I use bold formatting. So the highlighting is mine, not the participants'.

Therefore, a practice that is well-known, has a long tradition and is performed in almost all cases has become a practice that is not questioned. The hegemony of local medical knowledge has led to a complete normalisation of the controversial and problematic routine use of this procedure. Its persistence is supported by the fact that it is prescribed in textbooks, but also by the actual practice of doctors who perform it from a position of professional authority.

In such a situation, not only is the question of a woman's consent not raised (Djanogly et al., 2022), but medical practitioners of lower status and authority have no say in the matter. The hierarchical structure privileges the mere preference of the doctor, which takes precedence even when scientific evidence supports an alternative option. The doctor can easily "present an option as *the* answer quite easily, by simply refusing to discuss non-paradigm alternatives" (Davis-Floyd, 2001, p. S8). The following quotation not only illustrates how episiotomy is taken for granted, i.e. how its justification is not assessed in individual cases, but also sheds light on the distribution of power and authority within the medical institution:

"And there's this attending doctor passing by, she says something like 'nothing's happening here'. But the midwife, that midwife there was really nice, very competent... she seemed to know what she was doing. She knows what she's doing, she's clear, directive, well-meaning and says 'we'll do it this way, we won't cut, we'll try this.' Something like that. I mean, it's kind of all right. Then she said, 'Well, you're so dilated that there's really no need to cut.' And then this doctor came along, and that moment was disgusting to me, I mean, that moment in the hospital was really disgusting. Then this doctor passed by, and literally, without exaggeration, um looks and says 'cut.' And the midwife says to her, 'Well, that's not necessary, we don't have to...' and she just takes the scissors herself and cuts. I mean, it doesn't hurt at all, but I felt so awful at that moment. If my leg hadn't been tied,[15] *I think I would have kicked her. She devoted like two minutes to me and said 'Cut!' The midwife said, 'But no!' And the doctor just took the scissors herself and cut. That really sucked, I mean it really sucked because it was the end of the delivery and they could just let me go a bit longer. Luckily it wasn't very busy or crowded. I really don't know." (Una)*

[15] This is another controversial practice still widespread in local maternity wards, where women's legs are tied in the stirrups during the final stage of labour (Stanković et al., 2017).

Although it is assumed that midwives have the knowledge and ability to perform an episiotomy and suture the wound, this is usually the exclusive responsibility of doctors, at least in Serbian hospitals. The midwife is responsible for what is referred to in medical literature as conservative protection of the perineum (as opposed to surgical protection, which is the episiotomy) performed by supporting the baby's head and holding the perineum to prevent tearing. However, to this likely very old, entirely non-technologised (instruments are not involved) and certainly less invasive method is given only one or at most a few paragraphs in the chapters on perineal protection (Stanojević, 2005; Ristić, 2001; Mladenović et al., 2008). It is therefore not a particularly relevant object of obstetric interest and is considered less important than a surgical intervention, not falling within the doctor's remit. Even if they delegate the technical procedure to the midwife, it is clear from Una's case that the decision regarding the episiotomy is the exclusive prerogative of the doctor. Furthermore, the doctor is not obliged to justify his decision or explain why the episiotomy is necessary. It is deemed necessary by default, as stated in medical school textbooks (some of which were published decades ago and are not in line with later evidence-based recommendations), and because their mentors and senior colleagues have done so for at least the last few decades (Davis-Floyd, 1987).

This practice, which is routinely used in local settings and whose incidence has declined significantly in many countries due to a range of potentially harmful consequences, also has dramatic consequences for women's postpartum experiences and functioning:

> *"They cut me a lot, a lot. And after the birth it took at least fifteen days before I could sit normally again. But it's really hard on the side where they cut me. You can't sit, and even when you sleep, you can't sleep on that side. So you have to sleep on one side, which is very uncomfortable. You can't even turn over on that side. You can't do anything."(Maja)*
>
> *"Because the wound, okay, the first day passes somehow, but the second day, when everything has cooled down a bit, the second day is the worst, and it hurts the most. Every movement with your leg is a real effort. You want to put off getting up for as long as possible, and even if you have to go to the toilet... The worst part is getting up and getting back into bed." (Nevena)*

"My wound hurt terribly... The pain from the wound has gotten really bad. And it really hurts. Even when I came home, I couldn't sit. It took a long time, I don't know how many days it took when I returned home from the hospital, it was really really tough." (Jasna)

"In the morning, when I got up, the wound was very sore. Not the wound, but these stitches tighten so much that you can't, I had the feeling that my wound was huge. Huge, even though it wasn't that big, but... All these stitches pull together so much that you can't take a step... My wound was really difficult. I only managed to sit up on the twelfth day." (Saška)

"It was really a disaster for two weeks; I couldn't even sit... And it was really difficult for me because I couldn't stand up by myself. It was, well, it was horrible... I took ibuprofen the whole time I was there and the first couple days when I got home. It was unbearable. And it's really annoying that you can't even sit. You know, I can't, she needs me to hold her. You know, I can only breastfeed her lying down, it's all very uncomfortable. And I can't hold her, I can't sit, and when I stand up I can't walk. It's really been a disaster... And it really feels like an eternity, like you'll never sit again. You can't imagine how it feels...... horrible. But those two weeks felt like five months." (Sofija)

The experiences of women are strikingly similar, and such a large number of quotations have been cited to illustrate how typical this situation is. Something that seems like an almost incidental and insignificant intervention at the end of childbirth significantly determines how a woman feels in the early postpartum period and what activities are available to her. She experiences her body as if she has undergone surgery—she is in a lot of pain, has difficulty getting out of bed, walking, standing or even assuming different positions that she would normally be able to. This means that a woman is barely mobile due to the episiotomy and even the most routine activities, such as going to the toilet or showering, are a great effort or are completely unavailable to her. As a result, she becomes dependent on the help of others, which she often cannot receive in the local maternity wards due to a lack of staff and their lack of interest. The situation is further complicated by the fact that she has to look after the baby, change diapers, hold the baby when it cries, breastfeed or feed it. These practices are often challenging enough and a source of frustration for mothers who have given birth to their first child. Then they are further complicated or hindered because the women are in such a physical state after giving birth. Furthermore, the period they spend in this state until they have recovered is perceived as very long (even like an eternity), because it is not just a week or two of ordinary life and usual functioning, but the first days of adjusting to radically changed circumstances, new responsibilities and a new life role. Unable to perform these tasks independently and adequately, they feel incompetent and helpless, and the poor conditions in the maternity ward and the lack of attention and care are experienced much more intensely. It therefore appears that the first days with the baby are marked by negative emotions such as feeling overwhelmed and powerless.[16]

> *"It's horrible… you know what terribly annoyed me in that maternity ward, and it's quite a traumatic experience for me, I'm still furious about it to this day. They treat you, I mean, they literally make you an invalid. I walked into that maternity ward all on my own, I mean, I knocked, 'Good evening, I'm in labour, I need some help with this.' And when the childbirth was over, I was in such a state that I couldn't move from the bed because the wound was so big (points with her hands). And the maternity ward itself looks like Zombieland; I mean, these women are walking by holding on to the wall." (Una)*

It is obvious that this problematic and controversial practice (at least when applied liberally) persists in local maternity wards because it represents an expression of local medical knowledge (the "Belgrade school of obstetrics") and serves as an indicator of the authority and power of obstetricians. However, it is essential to also consider possible additional influences that support the persistence of this practice, particularly in terms of its ideological roots, i.e. its association with a patriarchal cultural pattern. Some critics have even referred to this procedure as "our western way of female genital mutilation" (Kitzinger, 2006, p. 134).

[16] It is an open question how far-reaching the consequences of this situation are and whether the problems in the first days and weeks significantly shape the woman's relationship with the baby (especially in connection with breastfeeding) and her perception of herself as a mother. However, it can be assumed that women without sufficient social support and resources (e.g. single mothers and women who are marginalised or very poor) are significantly more vulnerable and susceptible to negative consequences.

"The scar I feel is formed by the folding of flesh over flesh. The vagina is tightened. This is called the 'husband stitch'. Doctors often tighten the vaginal opening a bit so that the man can enjoy sex more later. The vagina becomes more pleasing for the man." (Gudović, 2013, p. 252)

The episiotomy therefore not only has a preventive function (it prevents spontaneous perineal tears and replaces them with a surgical incision), but in a certain sense also a therapeutic function—it eradicates the consequences of childbirth and restores the shape and size of the female reproductive organ to what it would look like in a woman who had never given birth. I received a similar explanation in a conversation with one of the obstetricians:

"...with the passage of such a large head, the floor of the small pelvis widens, like any connective tissue, it stretches and never returns to how it was. And it is no longer as elastic as it once was, the elasticity never fully returns. And when we perform that episiotomy, we stitch it up, and when it's stitched well, even I can't see whether it's been stitched (laughter)." (from an interview with a doctor)

Although these potential ideological roots are often concealed and rarely emerge in accounts of women, this is not always the case. The first quote below refers to a period from several decades ago, but the second one pertains to an experience from two years ago, from a central Belgrade maternity hospital. This indicates a long and persistent tradition.

"I don't know, my mom told me that during the prenatal classes the midwife advised them not to resist that cutting and that it's good to have it done. Because when it's cut, they stitch you up to the original size afterward. And it's important for that sexual experience later on. But when it stretches and separates, it never goes back to how it was before." (Sonja)

"I had an episiotomy that was so horrific that my wound couldn't heal for two months without exaggeration. From the very start, I had the feeling that something was not stitched properly and later these stitches got infected. Anyway, so the stitching was hell for me and it lasted about 45 minutes, and they told me that they couldn't give me any anaesthesia for it, that there was no pain relief for the stitching. (...) and they even told me, 'There's no anaesthesia for this, literally - keep quiet and endure!.' The culmination of all that was when

the doctor said, 'Here's a little stitch for your husband, to tighten it a bit better.' And literally, that last stitch, like it was obvious that it was just too tight, and that stitch ended up getting infected. I mean, with the wound, I don't know how it was supposed to be, but with me it literally took weeks, weeks..." (from a recent interview with a woman who gave birth in a central maternity hospital in Belgrade).[17]

The analysis of the case of episiotomy compellingly demonstrates the hegemony of interventionism and the rigidity of medical practices, firmly embedded in the nexus of institutionally bound relationships and additionally supported by patriarchal ideological influences. It also displays the absolute dominance of doctors in local maternity wards. But what happens when women occasionally decide to challenge and question their authority?

The Status of Medical Authority in the Local Context: From Passive Objects to Active Users of Maternity Care (and Back)

While women in previous generations were generally passive recipients of medical treatment, lacking resources to resist or even question the practices imposed upon them, today's women, primarily due to the accessibility of the internet, have access to both medical knowledge and the experiences of women in other countries navigating pregnancy and childbirth in different healthcare contexts. This has led to a situation where, in interactions between women and healthcare professionals, there is no longer a tension and potential conflict between lay and expert knowledge. Instead, two types of *expert* knowledge meet and collide—*local* and *global*, and, in the context of the Serbian healthcare system, *traditional* and *contemporary*. In this constellation, pregnant or birthing women themselves often become primary advocates of global medical

[17] This citation was extracted from an interview conducted as part of the recent research project my colleagues and I carried out on women's childbirth experiences and (dis)respectful maternal care in Serbian maternity hospitals during the Covid-19 pandemic (Pantović et al., 2024, p. 36).

knowledge. The consequence is a desynchronised transformation of reproductive healthcare in the local context, where conventional models of medical knowledge and practice are rigidly applied to transformed service users who are not only well informed but often want to take an active role in the process of care.[18]

The first clear indicator of this transformation of Serbian women from *patients* to *users of healthcare services* in local maternity wards was the emergence of a civic initiative called "Mother Courage" over a decade ago. Initially, it publicised the (mostly traumatic) birth experiences of anonymous women and set itself the goal of changing the situation in Serbian maternity wards[19] (Arsenijevic et al., 2014). It was the first local mobilisation of women that attempted to challenge common and entrenched practices and medical authority. It succeeded in drawing media attention to the questionable and problematic conditions in public maternity hospitals and the questionable medical practices used there. However, the fact that various similar initiatives with the same agenda and goals have emerged in the following years to date shows that conventional medical practices cannot simply be called into question.[20]

---

[18] Recognising the characteristics of today's environment and the broad availability of medical knowledge, one author (who is also a doctor herself) questions the future role of medical practitioners: "Will the health professions survive—or will women with internet printouts come to view the professionals merely as childbirth technicians?" (Savage, 2003, p. 115). The formulation of this question nicely illustrates the fact that women have access to declarative but not procedural knowledge and skills (knowing *that*, but not knowing *how*).

[19] Unfortunately, this initiative, which described itself as "the result of a spontaneous rebellion of women dissatisfied with the treatment in Serbian maternity hospitals: inappropriate behavior of the staff, outdated and inhumane hospital protocols, and corruption", ceased to exist after some time. Their website (http://www.majkahrabrost.com/), which featured hundreds of childbirth experiences submitted by women, is no longer in service.

[20] In fact, while finalising work on this book, one such public mobilisation was triggered by a case of obstetric violence that resulted in the death of a baby during childbirth (for example, https://n1info.rs/vesti/sagovornice-n1-nasilje-u-porodjajnim-salama-zene-trpe-decenijama-tolerisu-ga--sve-strane/). As in previous cases, this leads to the accumulation and public expression of citizens' dissatisfaction (in the form of protests, petitions and initiatives), a media focus on this issue (a series of newspaper articles and television debates) and even reactions from the healthcare system (such as statements by professional associations, announcements of monitoring and control of maternity hospitals and even declarations by the Ministry of Health that the situation will change). However, based on my experience so far, I am sceptical that this will lead to anything more than some declaratory and cosmetic changes.

If organised resistance efforts are not overly effective, what happens when an individual woman tries to challenge a doctor's interpretation or decision and question his authority? The long quote below illustrates this very well.

"Then I happened to search online for something like 'hardening of the stomach' because it started from the fourth month for me. And I find this text that says... there's even on our websites, not just the American ones, these are Braxton Hicks contractions that can occur as early as the fourth or fifth month. These are preparatory contractions. It literally means that the uterus is practicing. So it is practicing from the very beginning and preparing itself. And then there are examples like if you want to run a marathon, you have to prepare for months. Similarly, the uterus prepares for nine months to do its job. So I recognized this is happening to me. And I realized that these are Braxton Hicks contractions. And I said, "Okay," and I just lived with it. (...)

But when I told my doctor what is happening, he prescribed medication. And I didn't want to take it. First, it seemed pointless to take more female hormones during pregnancy when I'm already full of female hormones, but I heard that's how it's done, and that it's no big deal. And after two days of taking it, I was woken up in the middle of the night by menstrual pains. And they were terribly strong. I called him and told him: 'Doctor, after the second pill the pain increased'. He said, 'I've never heard that in my entire practice, and I've been working for thirty-five years. I've never heard of the pain increasing because of the medication. You're a special case.' I say, 'I know it's my fault, but I know how I feel.' And he even teased me when he said that, as if to say, 'You're impossible, I don't know what to give you.' But when I stopped taking it, the pain stopped. It was proof to me that I didn't need that medication at all. It's like my body was protesting, unbelievable. And he even told me it's all psychological, it's in my head. How can something to do with hormones and menstrual pain be psychological, I really can't believe it. (...)

But then, in the 6th month, when he heard that it hadn't stopped for me, he gave me a different medication for the contractions. But it's a very tricky drug, it raises your blood pressure, you tremble, so you have to take another drug to bring it down. And I ask him: 'Why should I take all this when I've been feeling it since the beginning of my pregnancy?' And he tells me: 'But it shouldn't persist; you shouldn't feel it. These are contractions; it could lead to a miscarriage. After all, you are six months pregnant. Don't exert yourself under any circumstances.' (...) So I went and bought these medications and started taking them.

Then I read about them and thought: 'Oh God, this is terrible!' Because the second drug, which eliminates the side effects of the first, is harmful to the foetus. And because I was very scared, I called him again and I was like: 'Doctor, do I really need this medication since I don't tremble much? Only my hands started shaking a little. Do I really have to take this medication?' And he said I had to take it because it relaxes the uterus further. Then I talked to my mother-in-law, talked to my mom, talked to my boyfriend, talked to this one, talked to that one - should I take this medication? And everyone was like 'Listen to the doctor!' And then I thought, okay, if I don't take it, what could happen to me? My blood pressure could spike, oh, that's dangerous for the baby. So how can I decide not to take it on my own? How am I supposed to know how much harm the first drug will do to the baby? So I continued to take it. (…)

And I went for the next check-up. By then, I was already in the seventh month. I told him: 'Doctor, I've taken everything you said, but I have the same symptoms' And he said: 'Oh, that's not good! This is threatening, premature labour. You know that contractions shouldn't start until around 30 weeks; you shouldn't be feeling any of this right now!' I said, 'But doctor, remember that I've been feeling this throughout the entire pregnancy.' But he doesn't listen. He said, 'Now we're going to look at the condition of your cervix'. And he examined me and everything was perfect, the cervix was long, closed, firm. He even wrote 'clinically undocumented contractions' because he couldn't see any contractions on the ultrasound. But he kept the medication. (…) And in the eighth month I said to him, 'Doctor, I'm still on these drugs, but I still feel the same.' And he said: 'So we have to increase the dose' And I said: 'Why?', 'Because you still feel the same.' I was against it, but he insisted: 'It has to be, Saška, we have to get to 38 weeks, then we stop and whatever happens, happens. Until the 38th week you will take this.'" (…)

"You know what's funny, because I take these medications, and every day I have the same symptoms as before I started taking them. I feel like a complete idiot. Now it's even more frequent, but somehow it's normal, in the eighth, ninth month it's normal. They even say that these Braxton Hicks contractions intensify as the pregnancy progresses, the uterus exercises more, prepares itself more. And somehow I'm swallowing this and waking up every four hours; I can't sleep like a normal person because of these medications. And I still have all the same symptoms. Now that he's increased the dose to six a day, the side effects are severe and haven't lessened a bit. So my body is not getting used to the medication at all. About twenty minutes after taking it, my heart starts pounding rapidly, like I don't have enough air. I tremble all over, even when I'm standing;

it's very difficult for me. I have to sit down or lie down as if I'm about to faint. And it lasts, sometimes only half an hour and sometimes until the next dose, which is about four hours. (...)At the last CTG[21] *he told me that the baby's heart is at the upper limit. And he just told me that it's this first drug that goes through the placenta, which means it raised my blood pressure and sped up her heartbeat through the placenta. It seemed horrible to me, but he spoke so casually, like this happens to everyone. And then I kept quiet, I just swallowed it. I mean, it stays here/she points to her chest/and I feel sorry I'm doing this to the baby." (Saška)*

Let us start with a very crucial aspect of this case that we are already familiar with—the woman feels an enormous responsibility, because it is not only her health and well-being that is at stake, but also that of her baby. Such an initial situation already makes it difficult to resist medical authority, because women who refuse to comply with recommended interventions are often labelled irresponsible and as putting their baby at risk (Kukla, 2008; Lyerly et al., 2009). Furthermore, the doctor's interpretation encourages her to perceive her condition as potentially risky, even without any indication based on her own bodily experience, because she feels well and functions normally. However, the discourse of risk also recognises the use of medication (introduced to reduce the potential risk of contractions) as risky. Saška is thus torn between choices that both seem risky and uncertain—to follow the doctor's instructions and take potentially harmful and unnecessary medication, or to follow her own embodied feelings and intuitions and risk a premature birth.

Embracing an alternative *medical* interpretation she found online resolves her conflict—it aligns with her embodied experience and allows her to stop taking medications that are harmful to the baby. Based on this, she attempts to negotiate with the doctor and challenge his interpretation and treatment. However, her repeated attempts at negotiation and

[21] CTG or cardiotocography is a non-invasive diagnostic procedure that enables the simultaneous monitoring of uterine contractions and the frequency and quality of foetal heartbeats (Mladenović et al., 2008, p. 232), and, based on this, the assessment of the foetal condition (Plećaš et al., 2005, p. 340). The practice of listening to foetal heartbeats originated in the mid-nineteenth century, and by the end of the century, it was recognised that fluctuations in heartbeats were related to the condition of the newborn. Since the 1960s, electronic monitoring of heartbeats has become possible (O'Dowd & Philipp, 1994, p. 27).

resistance prove futile. On the one hand, the doctor downplays or ignores her bodily experience—when she informs him that she feels no pain or discomfort during contractions but experiences pain and later very unpleasant side effects such as palpitations and tremors due to the medication. Since her bodily experience does not fit adequately into his interpretation, it seems that the experience itself is problematic and the interpretation remains unquestioned (Saška even says: "I know it's my fault, but I know how I feel"). On the other hand, the doctor rejects the alternative interpretation of her condition that she offers—that these are preparatory contractions that are not only risk-free but also beneficial. The participant herself interprets this as a conflict between two expert knowledges and recognises regional and contextual specificities that determine the medical understanding of certain bodily conditions and processes and the resulting prescribed interventions.

> *"And now that I think about it, I'm really angry to think that I may have been taking these medications for nothing since the sixth month. If I lived in another country, I wouldn't be taking these medications and everything would be the same as it is. My family friend who is a gynaecologist in Canada told me that doctors in Serbia don't recognize Braxton Hicks contractions. Literally, they are informed about it, but they don't acknowledge the existence of these preparatory, false contractions that can start from the fourth month and are not only not dangerous, but even desirable. Imagine if I'm really taking all of this for nothing! I've raised my blood pressure, sped up the baby's heart, so I'm pumping myself with drugs, trembling and feeling uncomfortable because of it. And for what? Maybe my pregnancy would be the same. But, I say it again, it will remain a mystery. If I hadn't taken them, maybe I would have given birth in the seventh month. Because if I hadn't taken them, maybe something would have happened and I would have spent my whole life saying, 'Damn, Saška, you're pretending to be a doctor and you're paying a man to treat you' (...) But that's exactly my biggest struggle during pregnancy; I couldn't follow my instinct. And my instinct was telling me that what I am feeling is normal. Yet, I stuff myself with medications." (Saška)*

However, despite her understanding of the situation and appreciation of her bodily experience, this participant is unable to resist the doctor's authority.[22] The feeling of responsibility is too heavy to be carried alone. The status of medical knowledge and the authority of doctors in the local context are so pronounced that women usually receive no support from their environment or are even exposed to additional pressure, especially from their partners and family. Thus, the doctor remains the primary and sole authority when it comes to the interpretation and treatment of their pregnancy. The norm of interventionism—interfering in the risky process of pregnancy to prevent undesirable outcomes—persists, even in the absence of "objective" symptoms (such as a shortening of the cervix, which would indicate premature birth).[23]

The rigidity of usual medical practice and the unequal distribution of power prevent women from resisting or being recalcitrant to the authority of doctors. This pattern is already firmly established during pregnancy, i.e. before women go into labour and enter the medical institution. It is no wonder then that the hegemony of doctors in maternity wards generally remains unchallenged (as will be demonstrated in Chap. 4). The early transition into motherhood is significantly shaped by the dominance of the medical model, and women do not have sufficient resources to resist and choose alternative practices and contexts. While all of this strongly suggests that this model is dominant and unchallenged during pregnancy,

---

[22] Saška even tries to find an excuse for the doctor and to understand him. She attempts to put herself in his shoes and justifies his actions by saying that he is simply afraid and worried about her condition and that he bears responsibility for the outcome of her pregnancy: *"I have gone through different phases; I have justified him. And then sometimes I think, poor man, imagine, every time you see him, you say, 'Oh, it hurts, oh, I feel contractions.' I mean, even if he sees that the cervix is good* etc., *the man is scared. This girl is paying me, maybe he's even more worried about me than others. This girl comes to my private practice, trusts me, pays me, and I will deliver her. And I'll let her go without medication... And imagine if something happens to her, and everyone will blame him"*. So doctor's responsibility is further emphasised by the fact that she visits him in his private practice, not just at the state hospital, leading to a typical "too much too soon" approach (Miller et al., 2016).

[23] It is important to emphasise that some women manage to defy the doctor's opinion and the prescribed medication, but they usually do so with the support of another doctor's expert opinion: *"I was given that medication because of some invisible contractions. I mean, I didn't see them, the doctor saw them on the ultrasound. And I was given this medication to stop the contractions. And then this one drug affects the heart, like, I think it contracts it also. It affects all the muscles. And then you take another drug that's supposed to bring your heart like back to normal. I was freaked out from that drug, and I was right, because to me, that medication, I mean, your heart starts pounding. Like my heart was really pounding, which wasn't pleasant at all. So I went to another doctor who didn't see these contractions and was like, 'Why are you even taking this?' And then I decided on my own not to take it..." (Ivana)*

birth and the postpartum period, an important alternative is also present—more as an ideal and normative standard than as realised in practice. This is the topic I turn to next.

2.2 Alternative Discourses and Practices: The Naturalness Ideal

The practical and ideological trend of medicalisation, despite its undeniably hegemonic current status, is accompanied by a set of practices and normative standards oriented towards the ideal of naturalness. Although this model is not very common in the local context, as it requires ample resources for women to resist the hegemonic medical model, it nevertheless represents a significant normative ideal.

The early reaction against pathologisation and the interventionist approach to reproductive processes emerged during the eighteenth century, originating from the circles of obstetricians themselves.[24] They believed that interventions only endangered and jeopardised a process that unfolded naturally with the best outcomes for both mother and baby.[25] Unlike the first generation of British obstetricians, represented by William Smellie, who strongly advocated the use of forceps, the second generation overwhelmingly rejected this practice (Moscucci, 1990). William Hunter, a student of Smellie, remarked about forceps: "Where

[24] In some countries, the original position was not interventionism, but there was a strong naturalistic orientation from the beginning. For example, one of the first Dutch obstetricians from the seventeenth century, Hendrik van Deventer, ardently advocated natural childbirth and believed that medicine should only intervene when clear pathology is present (Dunn, 1998). In his practice, he avoided the use of instruments and drugs and emphasised the importance of an upright position during childbirth so that the foetus could use gravity. He highlighted the importance of the woman's activity during the pushing phase. As a physician, he saw his role as assisting in difficult births—while performing certain manual interventions (attempting to dilate the birth canal and rotate the newborn's head), he simultaneously encouraged the woman, recognising that a positive outcome resulted from their combined efforts. Like many obstetricians of the time, he was a firm believer in God and nature.

[25] The early period of the history of obstetrics was thus characterised by disagreement among the doctors themselves—"for the most part this was a debate among gentlemen concerning the proper care and handling of maternal bodies" (Kukla, 2005, p. 86).

they save one, they murder twenty" (as cited in Moscucci, 1990, p. 48).[26] Another renowned physician of his generation, Thomas Denman, was vehemently opposed to the use of instruments in childbirth, believing that, despite their occasionally justified and life-saving use, they did far more harm than good: "But if we compare the general good done with instruments, however cautiously used, with the evils arising from their unnecessary and improper use, we might doubt whether it would not have been happier for the world if no instrument of any kind had ever been contrived for, or recommended in, the practice of midwifery" (as cited in Holland, 1951, p. 916). The naturalistic approach prevailed and almost until the end of the nineteenth century "for the most part the delivery of normal cases was left to the forces of Nature, which is, in Harvey's[27] words, 'a perfect operatrix'" (Spencer, 1927, p. 165).[28]

The contemporary natural childbirth movement, which emerged in the mid-twentieth century and has since exhibited considerable historical and cross-cultural variation (Lowis & McCaffery, 2004), can be seen as a legacy of the naturalistic obstetric tradition. It generally draws on very similar, if not the same, arguments and representations. This movement revolves around embracing inherent and intuitive knowledge and know-how, with a strong emphasis on avoiding or minimising medical interventions and allowing the natural or undisturbed progression of reproductive processes.[29] It developed under the direct influence of the

[26] The emergence of the first maternity wards—specialised hospital departments where women were admitted to give birth—in London in the mid-eighteenth century was actually a reaction to obstetrician circles advocating the use of forceps. As normal childbirths took place in these wards, it could be directly demonstrated that the use of instruments was unnecessary or harmful (Moscucci, 1990).

[27] Dr William Harvey, a famous English physician from the seventeenth century.

[28] In medical circles of later generations, this entire phase was described as extremely conservative, regressive and harmful, which is very well illustrated by the address of one of the doctors to the London Obstetrical Society in 1879: "These illustrious men thought it right to exert all their authority in discouraging the use of instruments, and in inculcating blind faith in nature as the better way. So earnest was their zeal, so commanding their authority, that men were driven into the opposite extreme of supine inaction . . . Rules were laid down, and widely obeyed, which too often allowed parturient women to drift into danger, injury and death" (as cited in, Holland, 1951, p. 916).

[29] Childbirth has historically been the most medicalised part of the early transition to motherhood, which is why the natural model of birth has been the most prominent and articulated. But the

ideas of the English obstetrician from the first half of the twentieth century, Grantly Dick-Read (Caton, 1999), who argued that the unbearable pain and problems faced by "civilised women" during childbirth were completely unknown to "primitive women":[30] "The primitive [woman] knows that she will have little trouble when her child is born. [...] Natural birth is all that she looks for; there are no fears in her mind; no midwives spoiling the natural process; she has no knowledge of the tragedies of sepsis, infection and haemorrhage. [...] Eventually, and probably whilst even yet at her work, labor commences.... There is unquestionably a sense of satisfaction when she feels the first symptoms and receives the impatiently awaited indications that her child is about to arrive . . . [she] isolates herself, and, in a thicket, quietly and undisturbed she patiently waits" (Dick-Read, 1943; as cited in Caton, 1999, p. 175). Similarly, in the description by Sheila Kitzinger, a woman giving birth naturally is "totally absorbed by what she experiences; nothing else counts, nothing can disturb her. It is as if she has withdrawn in her own separate circle. She knows exactly what to do, she does not need instructions, because she is totally tuned to her body and to the energy that waves through her with coming and going urge to push the child out" (Kitzinger, 1984, p. 8; as cited in Akrich & Pasveer, 1998, p. 109). Therefore, going through childbirth need not and should not be a threatening or intimidating experience for a woman, but on the contrary, an empowering experience. As Barbara Katz Rothman (2007a, p. XVI) puts it: "Birth *matters.* (…) Birth matters in shaping a woman's sense of herself, her own body, and her sexuality, but also her relationships with others".

belief that reproductive processes should occur without medical or professional intervention and be as natural and unmediated as possible certainly extends beyond childbirth. It encompasses a variety of practices such as minimally supervised pregnancy, early initiation followed by exclusive, extended and baby-led breastfeeding and parenting practices that encourage responsive care and close physical contact. This model is also closely linked to "natural/attachment parenting", which promotes the idea that parents should trust their instincts in upbringing and avoid unnecessary interference and regulation of their children's sleeping and eating habits, preferences, activities, etc.

[30] Medicine recognises only the pharmacological way to deal with the pain of childbirth, which for decades has exclusively implied that a "civilised woman" cannot go through the process of birth "awake and aware" (Beckett, 2005, p. 253). However, the medical approach only involves treating symptoms and may not address the root cause of the symptoms. All that is needed is to overcome the fear that civilization has instilled in women: "If fear can be eliminated, pain will cease" (Dick-Read, 1944, p. 19, as cited in Rothman, 2007b, p. 22).

For a woman to experience the empowering nature of childbirth, however, she must reclaim autonomy and a central role in her reproductive experience. The crucial prerequisite for this is to break up with obstetric practice and de-hospitalise birth, i.e. to move birth out of the hospital setting. Speaking about the impossibility of implementing her "midwifery model" of childbirth, Rothman (2007a, p. XX) says: "Setting—place, location—counts. The differences between medical and midwifery models of birth are not just about 'attitudes,' and not just a set of guidelines for practice. Different bodies of knowledge are produced in different settings. (…) And hospitals are settings where medicine sets the rules…". In line with this, the movement advocated home births attended by midwives instead of obstetricians. The midwife's role should be to facilitate the woman's childbirth by unobtrusively supporting her and allowing her to rely on her natural abilities. Therefore, the woman, or more specifically her body, is portrayed as having innate and perfectly adequate competencies to navigate through reproductive states and events. On this basis, the woman herself is the only one who has authentic and direct knowledge of the reproductive processes taking place in her body and the intuitive ability to act appropriately during these processes.

Since the local context, as already mentioned, is dominated both ideologically and institutionally by the medical model, we can ask whether and how the natural model is present at all. As expected, it is rarely present in a pure or obvious form—e.g. a negligible number of women in Serbia give birth at home.[31] However, in many situations throughout pregnancy, birth and its aftermath, naturalness figures as an important normative ideal. The fact that this ideal is often in conflict with local practice and its prevailing principles—and sometimes also with the embodied realities of women (Riggs & Bartholomaeus, 2023), as we will discuss in the next chapter—necessitates its context-specific adaptation

[31] Home birth represents a kind of grey area, as it is not mentioned in any of the official documents regulating this area, given that all births should take place in a maternity hospital. Nevertheless, home birth is not explicitly prohibited, but it is actively discouraged by registering newborns exclusively through a medical institution, which poses a practical complication for parents who opt for a home birth (Simić & Jerinić, 2014).

and negotiation in the concrete life circumstances.[32] The following sections will thus try to elaborate on how the two seemingly mutually exclusive models—medical and natural—actually intertwine in practice, and how women attempt to navigate very different discourses and norms in relation to reproduction—firstly in preparing for childbirth and learning pain management techniques, and secondly in deciding on options for pain relief.

2.2.1 Childbirth as a Process That Comes Naturally, but Requires Serious Preparation: The Case of Birth Preparation Classes

While having a limited and dubious role in the childbirth process itself, the natural model was prominent in shaping and envisioning the childbirth preparation program in Serbia. Prenatal classes were introduced in the middle of the last century under the influence of naturalistic theories about childbirth as a natural and spontaneous process that could and should be painless. They were not introduced as an alternative to the prevailing medical model, but rather as a complement to hospital birth, in which doctors still played a central role.

The book "Painless Childbirth" describes in detail the theoretical foundations and concrete methods of psychophysical childbirth preparations carried out in local maternity hospitals (Milošević & Prica, 1968).[33]

---

[32] It is important to keep in mind that these opposing discursive and regulatory frameworks—medical and natural—are not confined to separate and clearly demarcated spaces. Rather, both emerge in the most private spaces and thoughts of women themselves, as well as in a doctor's office. In the example with which we concluded the introductory chapter, we have seen that this perception is prevalent in the local context and sets the expectations for women today, even where we would least expect it. For instance, a nurse expresses surprise that a woman at a gynaecological examination, where pregnancy is detected at a very early stage, did not already know that she was pregnant, because "every woman knows when she is pregnant".

[33] The authors belong to a team of obstetricians who introduced this method of childbirth preparation in 1957 at the Clinic for Gynaecology and Obstetrics in Belgrade. This method is still used relatively unchanged in some health centres in Belgrade, while in others it has been significantly shortened and adapted, as it consists of only a few classes and focuses mainly on theoretical preparation. Women who have undergone this abbreviated version of preparation do not assess it as overly useful: *"The theoretical story is okay, but I did not learn anything special there"* (Sofija). During the fieldwork, I participated in a preparatory program that was very similar to the originally implemented and involved relatively long and frequent attendance at the classes.

These preparations combine the principles of the Dick-Read model of natural childbirth with the Soviet psychoprophylactic method of painless childbirth, which has been developed and widely used in the USSR since the 1950s. Both methods emphasise the significant role of psychological factors in the occurrence of labour pain, which is not considered only as a product of the activity of an isolated organ (the uterus) and does not have an exclusively physiological basis. Rather, its origin lies in the relationships a woman establishes with her environment in the course of her life and the dominant representations she is surrounded by.[34] Alternative representations of childbirth are implemented by educating women about the physiological basis of childbirth, its course, the functioning of their bodies, the origin of labour pains and ways to reduce them. In this way, their folk representations built over the course of their lives are replaced by scientific, i.e. medical, representations of childbirth. These form the basis for establishing a new conditional relationship between contractions and specific breathing and muscle relaxation techniques, which takes the place formerly occupied by pain.

Here we have a peculiar case of the integration of the natural and medical models of birth. Initially, the inherently normal and physiological nature of birth is acknowledged, which does not require any medical intervention. However, this nature does not exist in reality, as actualised, but only as a capacity, as a specific potential of a woman and her reproductive body. In the existing sociocultural environment, this capacity not only remains unrealised, but is also disrupted. Expert and medical interventions are therefore used as a means of restoring it. In a sense, the medicalisation of birth is moved out of the delivery room and incorporated into the woman's preparation for birth—with the aim of helping her to first gain an adequate understanding of her birth (through adopting medical knowledge) and then the competencies to deal with it (through techniques such as breathing and pushing).

[34] Dick-Read's basic idea is that the pain of childbirth is a consequence of certain cultural beliefs that induce fear and muscle tension in women. The Soviet authors explained this by relying on Pavlov's theory of conditioned reflexes. They reinterpreted pain as the result of emotional conditioning. From childhood, women are surrounded by representations of childbirth as an extremely painful event, creating an association between pain and labour contractions. The aim of the preparations is to unravel this conditioned reflex and create new conditioned connections based on positive representations of childbirth.

What do the theoretical principles described above look like in practice? Each prenatal class lasts two and a half hours. Women attend once a week in the seventh month of pregnancy, twice a week in the eighth month and three times a week in the ninth month. Each class is completely identical to facilitate conditioning. It begins with physical exercises, followed by breathing exercises (practising three types of breathing to be used during the different stages of childbirth) and ends with muscle relaxation. The longest and central part of the session is dedicated to theoretical instruction and overlaps with the development of the conditioning reflex. Concretely, this means that the midwife says: "The contraction is starting—react!" and winds up a clock she holds in her hand. The pregnant women lie on their backs and breathe in a certain way while the midwife, using medical terminology, describes relevant aspects of a particular stage of labour during the imaginary contraction that the women are mentally going through at that moment. Then, at a certain point, the clock rings and the midwife says: "The contractions are subsiding!" and the women begin to breathe normally. Therefore, practising breathing techniques and imagining contractions are accompanied by a corresponding medical narrative (e.g. when practising the third type of breathing used in the pushing stage, the theoretical story refers to that stage). The information women receive about childbirth is presented chronologically and ranges from the signs of the onset of labour and appropriate responses (i.e., women should start timing the contractions to recognise when to go to the maternity ward), to descriptions of the types of contractions, all stages of labour, and the postpartum period. This also includes the bodily changes, what a woman is likely to experience as a result of these changes, and everything she will encounter in the maternity ward (e.g. where she will be taken, what procedures she will undergo, what medication might be administered, etc.). This detailed understanding of the childbirth process and expected treatment, as well as instructions on how to behave, is something that women often highlight as the greatest benefit of these preparations:

> *"I'm not afraid of childbirth itself, it doesn't scare me. I just want to know what happens. If it's unknown, I feel insecure. The moment I know that contractions are starting, there are those types of contractions. I'll recognise my contraction,*

I'll know it will hurt here and there, for so long and then there's a pause. I'll cope with this type of breathing; if it doesn't work, I'll switch to the other breathing technique. I know roughly what pushing looks like, what the pain will be like. And somehow the fact that I know what's happening there makes me feel relieved. (...) The most important thing for me is that I prepare myself mentally for what awaits me there. I am only afraid of the unknown, not of the act itself, but of what will happen to me there. Explain to me what it is, what will be done, how it will be done, what might be waiting for me there, how long it will take, and I have no problem with it in that case. I also have no problem with being told that I am going to be in labour for 24 hours or end up with a C-section. What's going to happen is going to happen. But the fact is that I know what it is and that's it. That's why I think these preparations are good, because, practically, for the last two months, every other day, I've been going through the signs to go to the maternity ward, what will happen to me there, how I will give birth, how it will end, what will happen after childbirth, what I need to do all the time, what I need to think about, and what certain signs mean for me. So it makes it a lot easier for me. Since I have known these things, I am practically more relaxed." (Teodora)

"It means so so much to me to be absolutely prepared and to know what could await me at any moment. Unreadiness somehow... I mean, you'd probably panic more. When it starts... from my perspective now, when I know what's coming, which phases, how the childbirth unfolds, I somehow feel that when I recognize this, I'll be calmer. If I had gone into labour not knowing what to expect, I would probably be lost, probably get confused, and I definitely would be... And I assume that as the childbirth progresses, you're like, 'Ah, just this, then this,' because you kind of know what to expect. But when you start and you don't know, you probably think it's going to take 100 years..." (Maja)

Without exception, women embrace this knowledge as something that enables anticipation and reduces uncertainty during a process they perceive as very stressful and precarious. This is even more valuable under local institutional conditions, as the women are not informed about the course of childbirth in any other way, and this knowledge truly helps them to orient themselves and not feel overwhelmed. However, familiarity with childbirth does not only serve to provide information and thus reduce uncertainty. It plays an essential role in the realisation of conditioned responses, as it enables women to recognise and monitor their condition and thus identify the conditioned stimulus that is supposed to trigger the learned response.[35]

In this way, birth preparation, although originating from an approach that promotes spontaneity and non-intervention, actually intricately introduces a medical framework and representation of childbirth into a woman's understanding, simultaneously disciplining her bodily reactions:

> *"This is literally like school. It's like preparing for an exam. One you have to go to and ace with a perfect score, because that's it. And there's a kind of like semi-military atmosphere. I mean, not that someone is yelling at us, but there's an expectation that the story is learned, and you can repeat it word for word, which I'm already doing. And all of this is to create a conditioned reflex for childbirth. That's it."* (Teodora)

The fundamental idea behind birth preparation classes is therefore seemingly paradoxical—while it is suggested that childbirth is something completely natural and that every woman is capable and prepared for it because she has innate competencies, it is simultaneously portrayed as an act that requires extensive preparation in order for a woman to perform it correctly. Despite years of training and preparing expectant mothers for childbirth under a strict regime that emphasises the need for discipline, practice and mastery of breathing techniques and theoretical knowledge about childbirth, the midwife leading the sessions often repeats to the women: *"As soon as a female child is born - a mother is born"*. This is one of the key messages she tries to convey to pregnant women—that being born as women, they have an inherent capacity to give birth.[36] One participant, Teodora, who took part in a birth preparation programme, has internalised this message and describes birth as a *"normal instinct, like*

---

[35] Unlike the usual situation of conditioning, the conditioned stimulus (e.g. a certain type of contraction) is missing here. Women are supposed to imagine it during the prenatal classes and associate a corresponding reaction. However, it is crucial that they learn to recognise it in a situation of birth. Therefore, they are expected to be able to repeat verbatim what the midwife is saying, and each time one of them repeats the story during the class.

[36] The quote from another midwife, who advocates natural childbirth and also runs antenatal classes, illustrates this attitude well: "A woman's body is capable and created to give birth, and knowledge about childbirth is innate in every woman" (taken from http://www.biljeizdravlje.rs/code/navigate.php?Id=331&editionId=36&articleId=; accessed on 15.9.2023).

every other instinct in the body". However, she also believes that extensive and serious preparation is necessary for childbirth to go smoothly. She even expresses surprise after attending the prenatal classes, stating that she was *"simply amazed at how women managed to give birth without these exercises"*.

As we have already mentioned, this paradox is only apparent because, in line with Dick-Read's theory, it is assumed that problematic social influences have led to inadequate conditioning, preventing childbirth from occurring spontaneously. Additional efforts are therefore required to counteract this negative influence. Importantly, the new outcome is not some spontaneous and immediate unfolding of childbirth but a highly mediated and controlled management of the process and adaptation to it[37]—drawing on the representations and techniques derived from medical discourse and implemented through the network of medical authority of doctors and midwives.

It is difficult to reliably ascertain whether childbirth has ever been a spontaneous and immediate experience and process, but it makes sense to assume that cultural mediation of birth has probably been present since the early stages of human society[38] (although specifically technological mediation is a fairly recent phenomenon). This supports the idea that "only now could the birth itself begin—now, that is, that this event of nature had been immersed in culture, in the ordered ritual which made the birth a social and human act" (Wilson, 2003, p. 135). It is therefore

[37] The entire situation is even depicted as a battle for which a woman must be well-prepared, focused, disciplined and resilient—she must be "extremely active, she must fight for a painless childbirth" (Milošević & Prica, 1968, p. 36).

[38] If we ask ourselves at what point in human history the social regulation of female reproduction begins, a surprising answer might emerge that actually points to a period that we cannot unequivocally claim as part of that history. The fact that at one point, quite early on in human history, childbirth became a social act involving at least one other person besides the woman giving birth, can be explained by the specific features of human physiology compared to other primates—a relatively narrow pelvis resulting from walking upright and a relatively large infant head due to an increase in brain size (Rosenberg & Trevathan, 2002). Additionally, human infants are born facing away from the mother, unlike the offspring of other primates. This makes it difficult for a woman giving birth to handle the baby unassisted (without risking neck and spine injuries) or to unwrap the umbilical cord if it's around the baby's neck. These evolutionary facts resulted in human childbirth being significantly more challenging than that of other species. Evolutionary anthropologists use these explanations to clarify why childbirth became a social act very early on in the development of human culture.

all the more surprising that the notion persists that childbirth can be entirely a physiological and spontaneous act that women are naturally capable of and that can take place without any mediation. However, as we have seen in this chapter, this idea aligns smoothly with contemporary medical mediation of birth. But we will return specifically to the analysis of the actual role played during childbirth by the knowledge and skills acquired during the preparations (in Chap. 4), as this depends on the many actors present and their intertwining within a specific discursive-material institutional context.

2.2.2 The Naturalness Ideal Within the Medical Model of Birth: The Case of Epidural

In the local context, there is an almost absolute hegemony of medical understanding and treatment of the early transition to motherhood. As a result, women in Serbia generally take for granted that pregnancy and childbirth entail constant monitoring and numerous interventions, relying on medical authority and technology. This means that women neither believe that they have, nor realistically have, too many opportunities to challenge or resist this model. The discursive-material nature of the model—in the sense that it is firmly grounded in prevailing representations, but also supported by institutional frameworks, practices and technologies, and well integrated into financial flows—makes it resistant to relativisation (Halfon, 2010).[39] However, when it comes to the *only* elective medical intervention in Serbian maternity hospitals, naturalness comes to the fore as an important normative ideal. Epidural anaesthesia used for pain relief during childbirth is the only aspect of medical treatment during childbirth that women opt for.[40] It is therefore possible to observe how they understand their situation and what guides their decisions and actions when it is up to them to choose their own treatment.

[39] This assertion is further elaborated and substantiated in Chap. 4 of this book, which discusses the ways in which agency is both threatened and maintained within the medical institution.

[40] For any other intervention—such as administering hormones during labour to stimulate it, amniotomy, manual dilatation, administering sedatives or episiotomy—women were not asked for their consent, and often they were not even informed (Pantović et al., 2024; Stankovic, 2017a; Stanković et al., 2017).

Pain relief during childbirth has been a recurring topic for centuries, and not without reason, as childbirth pain can be an extremely destabilising and overwhelming experience (as we will see in later parts of the book). Anaesthetics have evolved throughout history, and the latest form of medicated pain relief allows women to remain conscious during childbirth, which was not the case with earlier forms of anaesthesia. The positions taken in the debate on reducing childbirth pain in different historical periods reflect understandings of women and their reproductive bodies specific to those periods.[41] Interestingly, some of the traditional and longstanding discourses can still be heard in the accounts of the doctors themselves, at least in the local setting:

> *"As I would say, because of your sins when you were created, God cursed you to give birth in pain, but we men... I mean, not men, but science has enabled us to reduce it a bit, or rather, to significantly alleviate it." (from an interview with a doctor)*

The decision about epidural anaesthesia was an essential part of the considerations and deliberations in the last months of pregnancy for all participants in the study. The relatively lengthy and complex decision-making process is also related to the fact that the use of epidural is not a standard or default option in local maternity wards.[42] Certainly, the most

---

[41] Interestingly, an early phase of feminist activism in the first half of the twentieth century focused specifically on reproductive issues, including the struggle for the right to pain relief to be achieved through the use of medical technology (Beckett, 2005). The immediate trigger for this reaction was the emergence of a new anaesthetic method known as "Twilight Sleep". It was an informal term for an anaesthetic method that used a combination of scopolamine and morphine. This combination replaced the previously used anaesthetics ether and chloroform, which were known for their harmful effects, leading to considerable criticism of their use in childbirth at the time (Caton, 1999, p. 135). Early American feminists, who had the opportunity to visit Freiburg and familiarise themselves first-hand with the new technology, celebrated Twilight Sleep as something that enabled taking control of the birthing process. Their reaction was provoked by the slow and cautious response of American doctors to the advent of scopolamine. Doctors were accused of rejecting Twilight Sleep due to conservative beliefs and only because patients were advocating for it, not the doctors themselves, and because they were indifferent to the pain women experienced during childbirth (Caton, 1999, p. 132–143).

[42] There are still no official statistics on its implementation. However, the latest Regulation on Healthcare Quality Indicators and Quality Assurance of Professional Work (2021) includes monitoring of the incidence of epidural anaesthesia in the section related to gynaecology and obstetrics. Reports on the implementation of this regulation are still not publicly available. Nevertheless,

significant determinant when deciding on epidural, even among those participants who generally have a positive attitude towards medicine and technology and do not attribute any particular value to the childbirth experience (or even childbirth pain), is the assessment of the potential risks for the baby. This is to be expected given the dominance of the medical discourse of risk throughout the course of pregnancy, which we have already discussed previously.[43]

> *"I was like, before pregnancy, I always thought I would have an epidural when giving birth. I didn't want to even think about it, I mean, why should I endure pain? But then when you get pregnant and start listening to different experiences and opinions, and when you realise that somehow, there are people who are against epidurals and they are like, you know, it's still unexplored, the consequences are not quite clear. And somehow you want everything to be okay and you think all the time only about the baby being well, that she doesn't suffer. But then again, I somehow think that epidural surely slows down childbirth, and if it slows it down, it means the baby is suffering. And then I think* ***it's easier for me to endure that pain and suffering than for the little being that's about to be born****. And you completely change your mind..." (Maja)*

When the care of the baby emerges as a priority, the woman's decision about pain relief during childbirth becomes more complicated, especially when conflicting views and different risk assessments are taken into account. The belief that anaesthesia ultimately has harmful effects on the baby is supported by the fact that pregnant women are constantly advised of the harmfulness of drugs throughout pregnancy and they do not take them—unless there is a clear benefit to the baby.[44] Therefore, over the course of almost nine months, a woman becomes accustomed to

previous research suggests that this practice is still rare and it is questionable how accessible it is outside of large maternity units in clinical centres due to a lack of anaesthesiologists (Pantović et al., 2024; Stanković et al., 2017).

[43] The discourse of risk thus plays a role both in the evaluation of the safety of reproductive processes when left to unfold without intervention and in the evaluation of medical interventions themselves, as we have seen in an earlier example (in the section "The status of medical authority in the local context: from passive objects to active users of maternity care and back").

[44] Therefore, women typically report that they do not take painkillers or medication to relieve cold symptoms during pregnancy, although they have used them frequently before.

subordinating her needs to the well-being of the baby, and the decision to request medication for herself during childbirth seems contradictory.

> *"I will go without epidural. Who knows, it's all medication. I see all drugs as both good and bad for us. (...) So I also see all these anaesthetics and something that kind of immobilizes you so you don't know if you feel your legs anymore, you don't feel anything. That's something that's happening to my baby. Plus, it's being administered into the spine. (...) On the other hand, I expect to be in pain, but it's not such a big deal, not so dramatic that I would have to give myself anaesthesia. (...) That's my main reason. Basically, the less medication the better. They won't let me take drugs, they won't let me take diclofenac for headaches during pregnancy, and suddenly I can give myself anaesthesia when I give birth. I mean, it's good that it's just for that moment, but somehow a drug is a drug. I don't know, I don't think it's as necessary as women make it out to be. (...)* ***So I'm more confident in myself in that sense that I'll endure, than...*** *" (Teodora)*

Therefore, the medical framework that is normalised and considered unproblematic[45] becomes problematic when there is a possibility of deciding on intervention. When given the choice, many women decide against anaesthesia, primarily because they perceive both the medication and the application procedure as potentially risky for the baby.[46] In particular, women who have undergone psychophysical birth preparation think this way—that the childbirth pain is manageable and that they have more confidence in their abilities (and stamina) than in the harmlessness of the medication they can avoid.

[45] It is important to emphasise that local women expect labour to be induced or stimulated by drugs (especially as first-time mothers) and even given some form of pain relief (most commonly sedatives). They are even prepared for this in antenatal classes. However, the other medications that doctors decide on during labour are never discussed or mentioned, since they are taken for granted as part of regular childbirth care.

[46] It should be noted that epidural anaesthesia generally appeared to be a truly situated technology in their dilemmas and considerations. Local women's decision-making regarding epidural depends not only on the risks and benefits of the technique itself, but also on various situational circumstances and institutional particularities regarding the availability of anesthesiologists (as other hospital procedures requiring anaesthesia take precedence over childbirth), their expertise and experience, (informal) payment for the service and so on. Therefore, epidural anaesthesia appears not only as a generic medical technique whose advantages and disadvantages can be weighed, but as an applied technique in specific circumstances.

However, a very significant role in making this decision is also played by the desire to preserve the "naturalness" of childbirth by avoiding intervention. The concept of natural childbirth, in the local hospital context, translates into a refusal to consent to the sole elective intervention. Thus, the highly medicalised and institutionalised childbirth is referred to as "100% natural" solely on the basis of the absence of epidural anaesthesia.

> *But what they first taught us at university is that every drug has side effects and that these side effects can show up not only immediately but also later on. And ok, there are no side effects at the moment, but what will happen in twenty years' time. (...) And even when they asked me from the sixth month,* ***I wasn't sure if I wanted it 100% natural****. And now in the ninth, I think I won't take it. (Angela)*

It is interesting that the idea of risk, which played a key role in the medicalisation of birth, emerges in this context as something that supports natural birth. However, the meaning of "natural birth" is so heavily adapted in the local context that it is reduced to the denial of pain relief, even though the entire childbirth situation remains highly medicalised and institutionalised, i.e. regulated. But this one unregulated aspect is enough to evoke an appeal to nature and the spontaneous regulation of the process in the women's narratives, i.e. the trust that "nature has arranged everything as it should be":

> *"Well, at first I wanted an epidural, but now I'm giving that up. Because I can't bear to think of another ordeal. You know, I have to think about the pain, about breathing, about this and that, about all sorts of things. And then I also have to think about whether the anaesthesiologist is competent, where they'll give it to me,* ***is there a risk****? So I have the feeling that the epidural is just another element that confuses me. And somehow* ***I want everything to go naturally****. And not to be pumped with drugs during childbirth. But I'm really scared of the pain. And I would really like it if I could feel that pain for just a minute, just to see if I can bear it or not. (...) Yet, that pain isn't constant. That's the most positive thing about it, it comforts me. Everything is arranged,* ***nature has arranged everything so that you can take a break****, then this, then that. I wanted an epidural, but now I think I won't so I don't introduce another element to worry about. Plus, to be honest,* ***the first time I'm a bit curious to***

see what it's really like. And if I take the epidural, I'll never really know what it's like. *" (Saška)*

The trust in the natural progression of the birth process among the women I've spoken with is not generally accompanied by some romanticised or New Age image, but is typically articulated within a scientific discourse—as trust in inherited capacity because women refer to their mothers' childbirth experiences and even explicitly to the role of genetics:

"The only thing that comforts me is that in my family, all women have had positive experiences. They all gave birth very easily. Quite quickly. All of them. So, that reassures me, like, it's genetics." (Saška)

"I don't plan to have an epidural, although I'm not against it. But I... I believe in autosuggestion. So I had a mantra during the first pregnancy and also now with the second: 'My mom had an easy birth and I will too. It's genetic and has nothing to do with anything else.'" (Ivana)

It is important to emphasise that the desire for a natural birth is not based solely on the idea of the risks associated with medical interventions. A certain idealisation of natural childbirth plays an important role in the rejection of epidural anaesthesia, since intrinsic value is attributed to the authentic birth experience that is not disturbed by a medical intervention such as an epidural. This is accompanied by an implicit belief that the birth experience will not be altered or compromised in any way by the fact that childbirth takes place in the context of a maternity hospital, where it is carefully monitored and intervened in. Thus, women highlight their desire to feel "what it is like, what it feels like" to give birth, regardless of the negative aspect of the experience associated with pain:

"I don't plan to have an epidural. I want to feel what the experience is like. Maybe I'll only have one child, and I want to know what that feels like. Is it a privilege to give birth or not? I don't know what's so scary about it. And it sort of wraps up the story of pregnancy for me. (...) And there's this woman who had an epidural, and she tells me, 'it's cool, I'm sitting there chatting with the midwife, and she says to me,' 'Hey, shut up, you're giving birth.' I don't think that's cool at all. I didn't want to say that to her, but to me it's messed up, not cool. You don't have to scream, far from it, but the baby needs oxygen, and

you're chatting with the midwife. You're being selfish, I mean, it's just silly to me." (Sonja)[47]

"But look at it from this perspective, imagine this is my first time giving birth and maybe the only time. And imagine someone takes away that feeling from you. Yes, it's probably painful, but... imagine you're bringing a child into this world. To me, that's an incredible act, man, and you give it away so easily. You don't want to feel it. Like, I'll just break down and pull myself back together and that's it. (...) No, I don't want anyone to take that act away from me, period. That's something every woman should feel. We're so soft and we need anaesthesia and drugs for everything, and 'oh, I can't handle that'... That's what bothers me. Come on man, just hold on a little bit." (Mirjana)

Epidural anaesthesia is seen as something that takes away and deprives women of the experience of giving birth and is perceived by many women as a loss. An inherent value is ascribed to the act of childbirth that justifies and necessitates the sacrifice. This shows the influence of a broader normative framework that links motherhood with the need for self-sacrifice:[48] "The definition of motherhood in our culture is one in which the mother sacrifices herself to the child" (Griffin, 2001, p. 37). While this normative ideal is consistent with the prevailing ideology of intensive mothering (Arendell, 2000) or essential motherhood (DiQuinzio, 1999), it also takes on culturally specific forms and positions within local gender regimes, where it is associated with a mother's sense of power or entitlement tied exclusively to the private sphere (Blagojević-Hjuson, 2014).[49]

---

[47] Sonja is so determined not to have an epidural that she chooses a maternity hospital that does not offer the option of an epidural anaesthesia because she fears that she might give in during moments of intense pain: *"I want to make sure I can't get that epidural. I might scream there to make them knock me out. But that can't happen. Then I have to fight not to give in"* (Sonja).

[48] The connection between the role of a mother and her willingness to make sacrifices is also evident in the reactions that women who opt for an epidural anaesthesia receive from those around them: *"And when I say I want an epidural, you get the whole 'What kind of mother are you if you can't do it naturally?' (Nevena)".*

[49] The concept of "self/sacrificing micro-matriarchy" suggests that Serbian women not only internalise self-sacrifice for their children and family, but also emphasise it by "turning necessity into virtue" (Blagojević-Hjuson, 2014, p. 392), thus drawing agency at the micro-level from the private sphere to which they are centrally bound. This tendency was especially pronounced during the prolonged period of social crisis and lack of resources after the dissolution of Yugoslavia and the socialist political regime. While the same author observes a trend towards more equality, primarily in the private sphere, through a more balanced division of roles and responsibilities in relation to children, the link between maternal sacrifice and her power or rights in the family sphere still persists.

> *"You know when I give birth to him tomorrow, and then in about five years when he really misbehaves and annoys me, and I grab him and slap him of course... So you see, if you give birth to him so easily and you didn't even struggle and all that. But when everything really hurts you, you know, and then one day when your kid starts to (misbehave)... 'Oh, just wait until I get my hands on you, you know what you did to me, man! How much I've struggled for you and you treat me like this now!'" (Mirjana)*

To summarise, the arguments stemming from the natural birth model—such as trust in nature, rejection of intervention and appreciation of authentic birth experiences—have been significantly altered to fit the prevailing medical model. Within the constellation of a radically transformed childbirth, opting out of epidural anaesthesia, the only intervention that women are actually consulted about in local maternity hospitals remains the sole guarantee of "naturalness" that has already been severely and inevitably compromised. This often puts women in a position of even greater powerlessness and lack of agency, as I will analyse in detail later. On the other hand, the ideal of naturalness is reinforced by the patriarchal model of self-sacrificing motherhood, which silences and pacifies women.[50] Instead of giving them the opportunity to affirm and strengthen their own capacities, it often leaves them without sufficient resources to deal with the challenges of both their bodily and the local institutional situation, as we will analyse in detail in Chap. 4.

---

[50] The normative expectation of self-sacrificing motherhood also frequently leads to women's (lack of) reaction to the mistreatment and violation of dignity and bodily integrity in the maternity wards. It also influences their assessment of their negative (even traumatic) birth experiences. At the outset of the interview (or during the telephone call when arranging our meeting), most participants asserted that they "can't complain" because "it was fine" or "everything went well". However, their birth narratives, with few exceptions, differed markedly from these brief evaluations that they routinely shared with others. Women avoid lamenting or complaining because they fear appearing selfish and ungrateful for having a healthy baby. This phenomenon is widespread and has been documented in the international literature (Hauck et al., 2007; Soet et al., 2003)—in many contexts, women feel compelled to "be happy with their birth and to put the baby's health and needs before their own" (Soet et al., 2003, p. 43), making it challenging to empirically assess their negative experiences.

2.3 Medical & Natural Models: Mutually Exclusive or Complementary?

The analysis of the contemporary cultural-historical situation and the experiences and conduct of women situated within it has shown that the prevailing discourses, practices and values that represent and regulate female reproduction and motherhood can be grouped into two models—medical and natural—both with a long history, but also with significant contemporary specificities. Both models are not equally relevant, either globally or especially in the local context. However, despite the considerable hegemony of the medical model, both models are present, leading to specific forms of their interaction and adaptation. Moreover, both are entangled with the broader contemporary sociocultural and political context, so their respective roles and implications should be addressed by taking this into account. While analysing their influence, I have attempted to situate both the medicalisation of the transition to motherhood and the alternative ideal of naturalness with respect to culturally specific narrative patterns and internalised social norms (e.g. the self-sacrificing model of motherhood). It is suggested that women often find themselves in a challenging situation when trying to understand their changing position, navigate their lives and prepare future actions during the early transition to motherhood, as they are surrounded by contradictory discourses and practices. On the one hand, local medical institutions adhere to a Cartesian and paternalistic model that reinforces an exclusive focus on the risky body and positions women as passive objects of care. On the other hand, the prevailing ideology of intensive mothering and the neoliberal discourse of choice and personal responsibility position them as accountable for their actions and decisions, and they are expected to play an informed and active role in their pregnancy, birth and taking care of the baby. Therefore, they must grapple with contested representations and norms in order to navigate this complex sociocultural landscape. To conclude this chapter, I will critically reassess both models and then focus on some of their similarities, not just the obvious differences that make them seemingly exclusive.

There exists a long feminist tradition of critically engaging with the medicalisation and technologisation of pregnancy and birth. The introductory chapter mentioned authors belonging to second-wave feminism who affirmed and appropriated pregnancy, birth and motherhood by repositioning women as subjects of these processes and taking the lived female experience as a starting point (O'Reilly, 2004; Rich, 1986b; Young, 2005b; Zerilli, 1992). Building on such a conceptualisation of reproductive capacities, medical science and technology are considered as sites of gender-based discrimination, exercised by the masculine epistemology of science that turns women's bodies into objects of knowledge and experimentation in the name of subordination to the patriarchal system (Cussins, 1996). The medicalisation and technologisation of pregnancy and birth are seen primarily as a means of increasing efficiency and gaining greater control over "the production of babies". It is assumed that such approaches not only contribute to gender inequality but also directly threaten women's health and well-being (Lorentzen, 2008; Oakley, 1979). Feminist critiques concern the nature of medical knowledge, medical practices and institutions (Davis-Floyd, 1993, 2001; Ginsburg & Rapp, 1991; Hubbard, 1997; Stewart, 2004; Treichler, 1990; Turkel, 1995), and especially medical technology.

As one of the main proponents of this line of critique framed it: "The female generative organs, the matrix of human life, have become a prime target of patriarchal technology" (Rich, 1986b, p. 127). Throughout the world, medical technology that has been turned into "a major industry" has become "a means of alienating women from the act of giving birth, hence from their own bodies, their own procreative powers, and of keeping birth itself so far as possible in male control" (Rich, 1995, p. 268). Woman's experience during pregnancy and childbirth is perceived as alienated because medical technologies "objectify internal processes in such a way that they devalue a woman's experience of those processes", and because the organisation of the medical context "reduces her control over her experience" (Young, 2005b, p. 55–56). Medical experts are the ones who take control of the reproductive process from the start, so women are forced to play a passive role in it and their competence to adopt certain choices and decisions is totally devalued (Beckett, 2005,

p. 255). Thus, institutionalised medicine and technology are unambiguously positioned opposite the realm of female subjectivity and agency.[51]

Throughout the book I will argue that the uncritical use of medical technology, sometimes leading to direct obstetric violence, is a serious problem, and that current local institutional contexts lead to many aspects of the alienation that women still experience today. However, in the following chapters, I will also suggest that medical representations, techniques and practices appear as necessary (sometimes even essential) given the specificities of pregnant and birthing embodiment, and thus serve as tools or resources for the women themselves. Considering that women's reproductive experiences and processes have been regulated and mediated throughout much of our known history, medical knowledge/technology represents a historically specific form of mediator that should not be seen as an inherent obstacle to authenticity and agency. In fact, through a contextualised empirical analysis of women's experiences of pregnancy and childbirth, I will show that various forms of technologically mediated and regulated reproductive processes in the contemporary era are not necessarily alienating for women, but can even be potentially empowering. At the same time, I will endeavour to show that the role of medicine and technology is inevitably situated both materially and discursively, and that the particularities of this situation determine the concrete consequences for women and their bodies.

In contrast to the medical model, which has been rightly criticised for decades (even if many arguments need to be and will be re-examined), the natural model appears inherently beneficial for women. It assumes women's experiences and competencies as crucial and positions them as central actors during pregnancy and childbirth. Like the "primitive

[51] It should be noted that earlier feminist authors did not see medicine and technology in this way. In the introductory chapter, the significant critical gesture of Simone de Beauvoir (2011) was mentioned, who conceptualised reproductive processes as inherently oppressive and alienating, at least under existing social conditions. This conceptualisation led to the recognition of medicine and technology as tools that could help women overcome subjugation to their species and avoid the sacrifices that come with it: "With respect to nature, the conflict between the interest of the feminine person and that of the species is so acute it often brings about the death of either the mother or the child: human interventions by doctors and surgeons have considerably reduced—and even almost eliminated—the accidents that were previously so frequent. Anesthetic methods are in the process of giving the lie to the biblical affirmation 'In sorrow thou shalt bring forth children'" (de Beauvoir, 2011, p. 674).

woman" in Dick-Read's descriptions, the contemporary woman who has chosen natural childbirth according to Sheila Kitzinger's and Barbara Rothman's descriptions knows exactly what she is doing, even if she has no specialised knowledge about childbirth. She does not need "knowing-that" because she possesses superior innate "knowing-how". She has no reason to doubt herself or shy away from birth. Her states and experiences are uniquely accessible to her and she does not rely on anything else in her surroundings. She is the sole expert and authority on what is happening to her—the one who instinctively understands this natural process occurring in her body and can respond appropriately and completely spontaneously.

The belief that women have a privileged and immediate insight into their conditions and that any external influence (from other people or technology) is necessarily threatening is also often associated with a nostalgic reminiscence—or rather an idealised projection—of an earlier historical period when pregnancy and childbirth were treated as natural processes left to unfold spontaneously and without outside intervention or regulation, relying solely on the embodied experience of women (Duden, 1993; Ehrenreich & English, 2010; McTavish, 2005). It is thus argued that in the contemporary context, the natural and spontaneous course of pregnancy and childbirth—which earlier generations of women experienced as embodied agents and sole authorities (authority was possibly only shared with other women, midwives, who assisted them)—was hijacked, alienated and associated with the oppressive practices of institutionalised medicine. However, this perception is based on idealised and historically questionable representations of the past. Historians studying medical knowledge and practices in the pre-modern and early modern periods argue that there was hardly a single authoritative type of knowledge concerning pregnancy and childbirth (Green, 2008a, 2008b; McClive, 2002) and that women's embodied experience hardly ever had an unproblematic social status.[52]

[52] The German historian Barbara Duden writes that until the late modern period, confirmation of a woman's pregnancy was based primarily on her ability to feel the foetus moving in her belly (Duden, 1993). Thus, women were able to diagnose and publicly announce their pregnancy based solely on their embodied experience: "This was a time when women quickened; it was taken for granted that women have this experience, make it public, and thereby establish the fact of preg-

However, regardless of these problematic historical arguments, the natural model convincingly promotes spontaneity, intuitive and unmediated knowledge, as well as self-control and self-reliance (without shared or delegated authority),[53] which implies a general focus on individuality (of bodies and persons). It thus prescribes to a particular normative model of subjectivity that is typically modernist—a woman is well bounded and unproblematically differentiated and separated from the rest of the world, a sole possessor of her own capacities and agency (Venn, 1998). In an ontological sense, this model is in many ways problematic, as I will try to show in detail in the next chapters by analysing women as embodied, mediated and distributed subjects.

---

nancy" (Duden, 1993, p. 79). The author concludes that pregnancy was once "a publicly recognized, haptic state of woman known essentially through her own testimony" (Duden, 1993, p. 83). In contrast to this image, the process of confirming a pregnancy today is completely detached from women's agency and experience, as it is linked to a series of objective indicators determined by a doctor using medical procedures and techniques (home pregnancy tests, ultrasound, beta-HCG blood test). However, the historical account offered by Duden is questionable. Long before the modern era, women were not believed because "the female body conceals 'truths' in ways that the male body does not, and pregnancy is one example of this" (McClive, 2002, p. 211). It was therefore highly likely that a woman's narrative would be questioned or met with suspicion. That the picture Duden paints is historically problematic can also be inferred from her own earlier work, in which she cites numerous examples of doctors questioning a woman's interpretation of her own condition and treating her with distrust. She even concludes: "To outsiders—the doctor, the family, the neighbors, the priest—the true thing hidden behind a big belly came to light only with the birth" (Duden, 1991, p. 160).

Even the competence to adequately assess the foetal movements (and thus determine whether it is a pregnancy or not) was not solely a privilege of women, but was also considered an aspect of midwifery expertise. This is evident from the words of Louise Bourgeois, a renowned French midwife from the early seventeenth century: "These movements are easy to judge for those midwives who know what they are doing" (as cited in McClive, 2002, p. 215). This certainly raises questions about the authority over knowledge, which cannot unequivocally and exclusively be attributed to women. Even Hippocrates claimed in his work "On the Diseases of Women" that women's diseases were particularly difficult to recognise because only women had experience of them and they could not be considered reliable witnesses of their bodily condition (King, 2007). Therefore, distrust in women's embodied experience certainly has a much longer history than the beginning of the modern era, let alone the contemporary period.

[53] However, this aspect can also be problematised. Home birth is portrayed as a practice that restores autonomy to women during childbirth, although it often simply implies heteronomy in which the actors are nature or God (even though medical intervention is rejected precisely because of the threat to women's autonomy). Among women who choose home birth and associations that promote such a form of birth (especially in the United States), there is often a fetishisation of nature or some higher power that guides birth and is a source of power independent of human will or agency (Klassen, 2001).

This problematic portrayal of the woman as subject clearly entails a negative image of the role of medical knowledge and technology in female reproduction. In an ethical-political sense, this is problematic, as it assigns to women the (exclusive) responsibility for reproductive outcomes that are both socially relevant and collectively shaped.[54] It might therefore put undue pressure on women to avoid (medical) interventions or assistance, even when these are necessary (or expected to be helpful), or lead to feelings of guilt or failure in those who do not conform to a certain ideal of a "good" mother or "good" birth experience (Ennis, 2014; Kukla, 2005; Locke, 2015). This model can therefore be both empowering and oppressive for women. This is evident when women feel guilty or disappointed in themselves when they ask for an epidural after opting for a "natural birth". A parenthesis is needed here because, as stated earlier, natural birth is planned inside the hospital where there is a plethora of medical interventions performed without consent or even announcement, but women tend to avoid the only elective one. Similarly, when it comes to breastfeeding, women who struggle to establish and maintain exclusive breastfeeding for their babies (without the use of formula or even pumping) often feel unsuccessful and guilty. When breastfeeding is portrayed as a spontaneous and natural practice for which women (i.e. their bodies) are simply (naturally) capable and competent, the important role of other close people, of knowledge and preparation, and of resources that can assist the woman (such as nipple shields and breast pumps) is neglected. In other words, women are left with only one desirable outcome that validates their quality of motherhood and proves whether they can adequately fulfil their nurturing role.[55]

While there are many important and obvious differences in these two approaches to female reproduction, body and health that make them

[54] Pregnancy, childbirth and breastfeeding are usually treated as public health issues and even as issues of national importance and are the target of a plethora of reproductive policies. This is evident in strategic documents at the highest policy level, for example, in national programs and strategies promoting birth or breastfeeding (e.g. Birth Incentive Strategy, 2018; National program of healthcare for women, children, and youth, 2009; Standards of health care adapted to the needs of mothers and children, 2011).

[55] A detailed analysis of the problematic consequences of this situation can be found in the chapter "Separation Anxiety" in a book by Rebecca Kukla (2005), which deals with the cultural regulation of the maternal body.

seem contradictory and mutually exclusive, there are also some underlying shared representations and norms. In both medical and natural discourses, the pregnant/birthing body is represented as a biological body, an object with set boundaries and characteristics, with one important difference: "It is either a biological body prone to breakdown and in need of medical intervention or it is a 'natural' body imbued with instinctive power and innate capacities to birth without medicalization" (Chadwick, 20, p. 26). This partly implicit and shared essentialist understanding of the reproductive (pregnant, birthing and breastfeeding) body actually reproduces a dualistic ontology and prevents imagining alternative understandings by enforcing an either/or logic.

Furthermore, both models often prescribe to the neoliberal "notion of health as an individual responsibility managed through consumption" (Riley et al., 2019, p. i). In the context of the medical model, this is particularly the case when it comes to the patient-centred approach that treats women as consumers or users of care. While the paternalistic approach is still typical in local state hospitals (Ninković et al., 2024), this emerging approach is both advocated by women and evidently present in private practice in Serbia. Turning to private practice and services is a steadily growing trend in a country where maternal healthcare is still publicly funded through the mandatory social health insurance and thus available to all women and free of charge, which is one of the legacies of the country's socialist past. However, the individualisation of responsibility is related to the privatisation of certain aspects of reproductive care, such as pregnancy check-ups in a private practice (Pantović, 2016, 2022)[56] and, more recently, giving birth in private maternity clinics.

[56] A very common and widespread practise by which Serbian women try to ensure continuity and quality of care during childbirth and avoid fragmented and depersonalised care is to choose a doctor from the public maternity hospital to see in their private practice (Pantović, 2016). In this way, women can establish an informal connection with the doctor, which is typical of post-socialist contexts where personal connections represent an important resource for navigating public services (Brković, 2012; Rivkin-Fish, 2005). However, it seems that establishing an informal connection with the medical practitioners within the public healthcare system by officially paying for their services in private practice does not protect women from normalised instances of mistreatment and overmedicalised care (Pantović, 2022), as we will also see through the analysis in later chapters of this book. Although there are some cultural-historical specificities of this situation related to the post-socialist local context, we can still recognise these personal strategies of women as examples of the widespread tendency of privatisation of risk typical of neoliberal societies (Elliott, 2002).

Prescribing to the natural model does not exempt women from using private services since they must regularly hire midwives or doulas and attend private childbirth classes to prepare for home birth. Although the natural approach appears to be less resource demanding when compared to the medical approach, it is actually not easily available to women from less advantaged socio-economic backgrounds as it requires ample resources (financial, educational, social support, etc.) and may not even lead to the same outcomes[57] (Klassen, 2001).

Although there are many positive changes promoted in both patient-centred medical approach and the natural model, they are in complex ways related to neoliberal norms and models of subjectivity. Both promote values such as individualism, self-reliance and personal responsibility since both embrace the idea that individuals should be responsible for their own health and well-being—either by seeking appropriate medical intervention and expertise to achieve a safe and healthy pregnancy/birth or by choosing and preparing for an alternative natural approach. The privatisation and commodification of certain aspects of reproductive care urge individuals to rely on their own resources and capacities rather than collective or public solutions, thus influencing universal access to healthcare and deepening healthcare inequalities.

Recognising some shared premises and not just differences between the medical and natural models is in line with Kukla's (2005) suggestion that both emerged and are maintained on the basis of a shared dissociative representation of the mother and the maternal body, as discussed in the introduction to this chapter. Although these representations appear to be opposed to each other and are associated with a number of contradictory practices that arise from them, pointing out the shared ideological foundations on which these opposing positions are articulated indicates that they are in fact complementary and together form a common discursive and social space. At the same time, it is contested whether

[57] Birth outcomes for home births have been shown to vary by women's race and class. Middle-class white American women generally had better birth outcomes compared to the average for their social group, while lower-class African American women had worse birth outcomes than the average for their social group (Declercq et al., 1995).

either position is inherently beneficial or emancipatory for women, as they are deeply intertwined not only in broader socio-political discourses, but also in the material constellations of women's reproductive bodies and the environments in which these bodies are situated. This will be the focus of the next two chapters, which will first thoroughly analyse the bodily situatedness and then the specific discursive-material situatedness of maternal subjects.

References

Akrich, M., & Pasveer, B. (1998). We deliver our children—In pain? In B. Brenna & J. Law (Eds.), *Machines, agency and desire* (pp. 109–123). TMV Report Series.

Arendell, T. (2000). Conceiving and investigating motherhood: The decade's scholarship. *Journal of Marriage and Family, 62*(4), 1192–1207. Retrieved from http://www.jstor.org/stable/1566731

Arsenijevic, J., Pavlova, M., & Groot, W. (2014). Shortcomings of maternity care in Serbia. *Birth, 41*(1), 14–25.

Beckett, K. (2005). Choosing cesarean: Feminism and the politics of childbirth in the United States. *Feminist Theory, 6*(3), 251–275. https://doi.org/10.1177/1464700105057363

Birth Incentive Strategy. (2018). *Official Gazette-Republic of Serbia, 25/2018–16.*

Blagojević-Hjuson, M. (2014). Transformation of parenthood: The semiperipheral perspective. *Sociologija, 56*(4), 383–402.

Brković, Č. (2012). The pursuit of relations as a constitutive part of biological citizenship in a Bosnian border town. *Antropologija, 12*(2).

Caton, D. (1999). *What a blessing she had chloroform: The medical and social response to the pain of childbirth from 1800 to the present.* Yale University Press.

Chadwick, R. (2006). Pathological wombs and raging hormones: Psychology, reproduction and the female body. In T. Shefer, F. Boonzaaier, & P. Kiguwa (Eds.), *The gender of psychology*. UCT Press.

Cunningham, G. F., Leveno, K. J., Bloom, S. L., Hauth, J. C., Rouse, D. J., & Spong, C. Y. (2010). *Williams obstetrics* (23rd ed.). McGraw-Hill Medical.

Cussins, C. (1996). Ontological choreography: Agency through objectification in infertility clinics. *Social Studies of Science, 26*(3), 575–610. https://doi.org/10.1177/030631296026003004

Čutura, N. (2005). Porođajni faktori. In D. Plećaš, B. Stanimirović, A. Stanković, & M. Vasiljević (Eds.), *Ginekologija i akušerstvo: Udžbenik za studente medicine*. Medicinski fakultet Univerziteta u Beogradu.

Davis-Floyd, R. (1987). Obstetric training as a rite of passage. *Medical Anthropology Quarterly, 1*(3), 288–318. https://doi.org/10.1525/maq.1987.1.3.02a00050

Davis-Floyd, R. (1993). The technocratic model of birth. In S. T. Hollis, L. Pershing, & M. J. Young (Eds.), *Feminist theory and the study of folklore* (pp. 297–326). University of Illinois Press.

Davis-Floyd, R. (1994). The technocratic body: American childbirth as cultural expression. *Social Science and Medicine, 38*(8), 1125–1140. https://doi.org/10.1016/0277-9536(94)90228-3

Davis-Floyd, R. (2001). The technocratic, humanistic, and holistic paradigms of childbirth. *International Journal of Gynecology and Obstetrics, 75*(1), S5–S23. https://doi.org/10.1016/S0020-7292(01)00510-0

de Beauvoir, S. (2011). *The second sex* (C. Borde & S. Malovany-Chevallier, Trans.). Vintage Books. (Original work published 1949).

Declercq, E. R., Paine, L., & Winter, M. R. (1995). Home birth in the United States, 1989–1992: A longitudinal descriptive report of national birth certificate data. *Journal of Nurse-Midwifery, 40*(6), 474–482. https://doi.org/10.1016/0091-2182(95)00061-5

DiQuinzio, P. (1999). *The impossibility of motherhood: Feminism, individualism, and the problem of mothering*. Routledge.

Djanogly, T., Nicholls, J., Whitten, M., & Lanceley, A. (2022). Choice in episiotomy—Fact or fantasy: A qualitative study of women's experiences of the consent process. *BMC Pregnancy and Childbirth, 22*, 139. https://doi.org/10.1186/s12884-022-04475-8

Duden, B. (1991). *The woman beneath the skin: A doctor's patients in eighteenth-century Germany*. Harvard University Press.

Duden, B. (1993). *Disembodying women: Perspectives on pregnancy and the unborn*. Harvard University Press.

Dunn, P. M. (1998). Henrick van Deventer (1651–1724) and the pelvic birth canal. *Archives of Disease in Childhood—Fetal and Neonatal Edition, 79*(2), F157–F158. https://doi.org/10.1136/fn.79.2.F157

Ehrenreich, B., & English, D. (2010). *Witches, midwives and nurses: A history of women healers*. The Feminist Press.

Elliott, A. (2002). Identity politics and privatisation: Modern fantasies, postmodern after-effects. In V. Walkerdine (Ed.), *Challenging subjects: Critical psychology for a new millennium* (pp. 11–22). Palgrave Macmillan.

Ennis, L. R. (Ed.). (2014). *Intensive mothering: The cultural contradictions of modern motherhood.* Demeter Press. Retrieved from http://www.jstor.org/stable/j.ctt1rrd8rb

Foucault, M. (1995). *Discipline and punish: The birth of the prison.* Vintage Books.

Gannon, L. (1998). The impact of medical and sexual politics on women's health. *Feminism & Psychology, 8*(3), 285–302. https://doi.org/10.1177/0959353598083004

Ginsburg, F., & Rapp, R. (1991). The politics of reproduction. *Annual Review of Anthropology, 20*(1), 311–343. https://doi.org/10.1146/annurev.an.20.100191.001523

Goer, H. (1995). *Obstetric myths versus research realities.* Greenwood Publishing Group.

Graham, I. D., Carroli, G., Davies, C., & Medves, J. M. (2005). Episiotomy rates around the world: An update. *Birth, 32*(3), 219–223. https://doi.org/10.1111/j.0730-7659.2005.00373.x

Green, H. M. (2008a). *Making women's medicine masculine: The rise of male authority in pre-modern gynaecology.* Oxford University Press.

Green, H. M. (2008b). Gendering the history of women's healthcare. *Gender & History, 20*(3), 487–518. https://doi.org/10.1111/j.1468-0424.2008.00534.x

Griffin, S. (2001). Feminism and motherhood. In M. Davey (Ed.), *Mother reader: Essential literature on motherhood* (pp. 33–45). Seven Stories Press. (Original work published 1974).

Gudović, M. (2013). Crtica—Epiziotomija. In A. Vilenica (Ed.), *Postajanje majkom u vreme neoliberalnog kapitalizma* (pp. 250–253). uz)bu))na))).

Halfon, S. (2010). Encountering birth: Negotiating expertise, networks, and my STS self. *Science as Culture, 19*(1), 61–77. https://doi.org/10.1080/09505430903558062

Hauck, Y., Fenwick, J., Downie, J., & Butt, J. (2007). The influence of childbirth expectations on Western Australian women's perceptions of their birth experience. *Midwifery, 23*(3), 235–247. https://doi.org/10.1016/j.midw.2006.02.002

Healthcare for women during pregnancy: National guidelines for doctors. (2005). Serbian Medical Society.

Holland, S. E. (1951). The Princess Charlotte of Wales: A triple obstetric tragedy. *BJOG: An International Journal of Obstetrics & Gynaecology, 58*(6), 905–919.

Hubbard, R. (1997). *The politics of women's biology.* Rutgers University Press.

Institute of Public Health "Dr Milan Jovanović Batut". (2012). *Selected health indicators.*

King, H. (2007). *Midwifery, obstetrics and the rise of gynaecology: The uses of sixteenth-century compendium*. Ashgate Publishing.

Kitzinger, S. (2006). *Birth crisis*. Routledge.

Klassen, P. E. (2001). Sacred maternities and postbiomedical bodies: Religion and nature in contemporary home birth. *Signs, 26*(3), 775–809. Retrieved from http://www.jstor.org/stable/3175539

Kukla, R. (2005). *Mass hysteria: Medicine, culture and mothers' bodies*. Rowman & Littlefield Publishers.

Kukla, R. (2008). Measuring mothering. *International Journal of Feminist Approaches to Bioethics, 1*(1), 67–90. https://doi.org/10.2979/FAB.2008.1.1.67

Latour, B. (1993). *We have never been modern*. Harvard University Press.

Leder, D. (1992). A tale of two bodies: The Cartesian corpse and the lived body. In D. Leder (Ed.), *The body in medical thought and practice* (pp. 17–36). Kluwer Academic Publishers.

Locke, A. (2015). Agency, 'good motherhood' and 'a load of mush': Constructions of baby-led weaning in the press. *Women's Studies International Forum, 53*, 139–146. https://doi.org/10.1016/j.wsif.2014.10.018

Lorentzen, J. M. (2008). 'I know my own body': Power and resistance in women's experiences of medical interactions. *Body & Society, 14*(3), 49–79. https://doi.org/10.1177/1357034X08093572

Lowis, G. W., & McCaffery, P. (2004). Sociological factors affecting the medicalization of midwifery. In E. R. Van Teijlingen, G. W. Lowis, P. McCaffery, & M. Porter (Eds.), *Midwifery and the medicalization of childbirth: Comparative perspectives* (pp. 5–42). Nova Science Publishers.

Lyerly, A. D., Armstrong, E. M., Harris, L. H., Kukla, R., Kuppermann, M., Little, M. O., & Mitchell, L. M. (2007). Risks, values, and decision making surrounding pregnancy. *Obstetrics & Gynecology, 109*(4), 979–984. https://doi.org/10.1097/AOG.0b013e3181888fd8

Lyerly, A. D., Mitchell, L. M., Armstrong, E. M., Harris, L. H., Kukla, R., Kuppermann, M., & Little, M. O. (2009). Risk and the pregnant body. *Hastings Center Report, 39*(6), 34–42. https://doi.org/10.1353/hcr.0.0211

McClive, C. (2002). The hidden truths of the belly: The uncertainties of pregnancy in early modern Europe. *Social History of Medicine, 15*(2), 209–227. https://doi.org/10.1093/shm/15.2.209

McTavish, L. (2005). *Childbirth and the display of authority in early modern France*. Ashgate Publishing.

Miller, S., Abalos, E., Chamillard, M., Ciapponi, A., Colaci, D., Comandé, D., Diaz, V., Geller, S., Hanson, C., Langer, A., Manuelli, V., Millar, K., Morhason-Bello, I., Castro, C. P., Pileggi, V. N., Robinson, N., Skaer, M., Souza, J. P., Vogel, J. P., & Althabe, F. (2016). Beyond too little, too late and too much, too soon: A pathway towards evidence-based, respectful maternity care worldwide. *Lancet (London, England), 388*(10056), 2176–2192. https://doi.org/10.1016/S0140-6736(16)31472-6

Milošević, B., & Prica, R. (1968). *Bezbolni porođaj*. Medicinska knjiga.

Milošević, B., Rajhvajn, B., & Berić, B. (1988). *Porodiljstvo: Udžbenik za studente medicine*. Medicinska knjiga.

Ministry of Health of Republic of Serbia. (2011). *Standards of health care adapted to the needs of mothers and children.*

Mladenović, D., Mladenović-Bogdanović, Z., & Mladenović-Mihailović, A. (2008). *Ginekologija i akušerstvo*. Zavod za udžbenike.

Momčilov, P. (2005). Normalni porođaj. In D. Plećaš, B. Stanimirović, A. Stanković, & M. Vasiljević (Eds.), *Ginekologija i akušerstvo: Udžbenik za studente medicine*. Medicinski fakultet Univerziteta u Beogradu.

Moscucci, O. (1990). *The science of woman: Gynaecology and gender in England 1800–1929*. Cambridge University Press.

Mullin, A. (2005). *Reconceiving pregnancy and childcare: Ethics, experience, and reproductive labor*. Cambridge University Press.

Myers-Helfgott, M. G., & Helfgott, A. W. (1999). Routine use of episiotomy in modern obstetrics. Should it be performed? *Obstetrics and Gynecology Clinics of North America, 26*(2), 305–325. https://doi.org/10.1016/s0889-8545(05)70077-2

National Program of Health Care for Women, Children and Youth. (2009). *Official Gazette-Republic of Serbia*, 28.

Ninković, M., Ilić, S., & Damnjanović, K. (2024). Women's trust in the healthcare system in Serbia: Validation of the Women's Trust and Confidence in Healthcare System scale. *Women's Health, 20*. https://doi.org/10.1177/1745505724124986

O'Dowd, M. J., & Philipp, E. E. (1994). *The history of obstetrics & gynaecology*. The Parthenon Publishing Group.

O'Driscoll, K., Stronge, J. M., & Minogue, M. (1973). Active management of labour. *British Medical Journal, 3*(5872), 135–137. https://doi.org/10.1136/bmj.3.5872.135

O'Reilly, A. (2004). *From motherhood to mothering: The legacy of Adrienne Rich's "Of Woman Born"*. State University of New York Press.

Oakley, A. (1979). A case of maternity: Paradigms of women as maternity cases. *Signs, 4*(4), 607–631.

Pantović, L. (2016). Buying a connection: Private practice in public health care—The case of a Serbian maternity hospital. *Anthropology of East Europe Review, 34*(1).

Pantović, L. (2022). Providing a service or seeking a favor? The role of private prenatal care on the continuity of care in Serbian public maternity hospitals. *Birth, 49*(3), 506–513.

Pantović, L., Stanković, B., & Ćeriman, J. (2024). *Iskustva žena u porodilištima u Srbiji tokom i nakon pandemije kovida-19*. UNFPA.

Physiological Childbirth: The guide for doctors and midwives. (2009). Ministry of Health of Republic of Serbia.

Plećaš, D., Stanimirović, B., Stanković, A., & Vasiljević, M. (2005). *Ginekologija i akušerstvo: Udžbenik za studente medicine*. Medicinski fakultet Univerziteta u Beogradu.

Regulation on Healthcare Quality Indicators and Quality Assurance of Professional Work. (2021). *Official Gazette-Republic of Serbia, 123/2021.*

Rich, A. (1986b). *Of woman born: Motherhood as experience and institution*. W. W. Norton & Company.

Rich, A. (1995). Motherhood: The contemporary emergency and the quantum leap. In *On lies, secrets, and silence: Selected prose 1966–1978* (pp. 259–273). W. W. Norton & Company. (Original work published 1978).

Riggs, D. W., & Bartholomaeus, C. (2023). *First-time parenting journeys: Expectations and realities*. Cambridge University Press.

Riley, S., Evans, A., & Robson, M. (2019). *Postfeminism and health: Critical psychology and media perspectives*. Routledge.

Ristić, L. (2001). *Praktično porodiljstvo*. Freemental.

Rivkin-Fish, M. (2005). *Women's health in post-Soviet Russia: The politics of intervention*. Indiana University Press.

Rosenberg, K., & Trevathan, W. (2002). Birth, obstetrics and human evolution. *BJOG: An International Journal of Obstetrics & Gynaecology, 109*(11), 1199–1206. https://doi.org/10.1046/j.1471-0528.2002.00010.x

Rothman, B. K. (2007a). Introduction: A lifetime's labor: Women and power in the birthplace. In W. Simonds, B. K. Rothman, & B. M. Norman (Eds.), *Laboring on: Birth in transition in the United States* (pp. xi–xxii). Routledge.

Rothman, B. K. (2007b). Laboring then: The political history of maternity care in the United States. In W. Simonds, B. K. Rothman, & B. M. Norman (Eds.), *Laboring on: Birth in transition in the United States* (pp. 3–28). Routledge.

Savage, W. (2003). Professional control or women's choice in childbirth? Is either possible? In G. Boswell & F. Poland (Eds.), *Women's minds, women's bodies: Interdisciplinary approaches to women's health* (pp. 103–115). Palgrave Macmillan.

Shorter, E. (1991). *Women's bodies: A social history of women's encounter with health, ill-health and medicine*. Transaction Publishers.

Simić, J., & Jerinić, J. (2014). Pravo na porođaj kod kuće—Izbor, a ne slučajnost i neke pravne posledice. *Pravni zapisi, 5*(1), 120–161. https://doi.org/10.5937/pravzap0-6103

Soet, J., Brack, G., & Dilorio, C. (2003). Prevalence and predictors of women's experience of psychological trauma during childbirth. *Birth, 30*(1), 36–46. https://doi.org/10.1046/j.1523-536X.2003.00215.x

Spencer, H. R. (1927). *The history of British midwifery from 1650 to 1800*. John Bale, Sons & Danielsson.

Stankovic, B. (2017a). Women's experiences of childbirth in Serbian public healthcare institutions: A qualitative study. *International Journal of Behavioral Medicine, 24*(6), 803–814. https://doi.org/10.1007/s12529-017-9672-1

Stanković, B., Skočajić, M., & Đorđević, A. (2017). Upravljanje porođajem u Srbiji: Medicinske intervencije i porođajna iskustva. *Limes Plus: Journal of Social Science and Humanities, 14*(2), 197–225.

Stanojević, D. (2005). Epiziotomija. In D. Plećaš, B. Stanimirović, A. Stanković, & M. Vasiljević (Eds.), *Ginekologija i akušerstvo: Udžbenik za studente medicine*. Medicinski fakultet Univerziteta u Beogradu.

Stewart, M. (2004). *Pregnancy, birth, and maternity care: Feminist perspectives*. Elsevier Science.

Tone, A. (2012). Medicalizing reproduction: The pill and home pregnancy tests. *Journal of Sex Research, 49*(4), 319–327. https://doi.org/10.1080/00224499.2012.688226

Treichler, P. (1990). Feminism, medicine and the meaning of childbirth. In M. Jacobus, E. F. Keller, & S. Shuttleworth (Eds.), *Body/politics: Women and the discourses of science* (pp. 113–138). Routledge.

Turkel, K. D. (1995). *Women, power, and childbirth: A case study of a free-standing birth center*. Greenwood Publishing Group.

van Nistelrooij, I., & Visse, M. (2019). Me? The invisible call of responsibility and its promise for care ethics: A phenomenological view. *Medicine, Health Care, and Philosophy, 22*(2), 275–285. https://doi.org/10.1007/s11019-018-9873-7

Venn, C. (1998). The subject of psychology. In J. Henriques, W. Hollway, C. Urwin, C. Venn, & V. Walkerdine (Eds.), *Changing the subject: Psychology, social regulation and subjectivity* (pp. 115–147).

Wilson, A. (2003). Participant or patient? Seventeenth century childbirth from the mother's point of view. In R. Porter (Ed.), *Patients and practitioners: Lay perceptions of medicine in pre-industrial society* (pp. 129–144). Cambridge University Press.

World Health Organization (WHO). (1996). *Care in normal birth: A practical guide*. Department of Reproductive Health & Research, WHO.

World Health Organization (WHO). (2018). *WHO recommendations: Intrapartum care for a positive childbirth experience*. World Health Organization.

Young, I. M. (2005b). Pregnant embodiment: Subjectivity and alienation. In *On female body experience: 'Throwing like a girl' and other essays* (pp. 46–61). Oxford University Press.

Zerilli, L. M. G. (1992). A process without a subject: Simone de Beauvoir and Julia Kristeva on maternity. *Signs, 18*(1), 111–135. https://doi.org/10.1086/494781

3

Embodied Subjects: Phenomenological Reconstruction of the Process of Becoming a Mother

Maternal—and especially pregnant and birthing—subjectivity is approached in this book from the first-person perspective and as bodily situated. In this chapter, a phenomenological theoretical framework is introduced to enable a nuanced conceptual reconstruction of embodied experience during the early transition to motherhood. This process is phenomenologically specific and challenging for women's subjectivity for various reasons. By discussing specific lived experiences, it will be shown that embodied experience during this period tends to be vague and ambiguous and that women generally draw on various mediators—medical knowledge (e.g. about the stages of pregnancy), technological means (such as pregnancy tests or ultrasounds), as well as the experiences of others—in an attempt to correctly interpret and even integrate their experiences, and to orient themselves practically in their everyday lives.

The changing shape and functionality of their pregnant body means much more than an altered reflection in the mirror—it entails a different experience of its limits, a modified mobility and an altered perspective from which the world is perceived and acted upon. An essential aspect of pregnant embodiment is also the fact that there is another being growing inside a woman's body that gradually becomes more and more

B. Stanković, *Giving Birth To A Subject*, Sociocultural Psychology of the Lifecourse,
https://doi.org/10.1007/978-3-031-77236-8_3

differentiated and autonomous for her, a process that is closely interwoven with the psychological transition to motherhood. After introducing some relevant theoretical resources for mapping and understanding maternal embodiment, the analysis in this chapter will follow a unique temporality of the embodied experience of pregnancy by focusing on a dynamic interplay of embodied and technologically mediated aspects of this experience as central to both the identification with pregnancy and the individuation of the baby for the mother.

3.1 Phenomenology of the Reproductive Body: Hermeneutic and Practical Challenges

The focus on the body and embodiment pervades social theory and research in recent decades. But while it is easy to define embodiment negatively, as "reducible neither to representations of the body, to the body as an objectification of power, to the body as a physical entity or biological organisms, nor to the body as an inalienable centre of individual consciousness" (Csordas, 1994, p. XI), its positive definition requires us to engage with phenomenological theory in more detail.

The basic phenomenological assumption is that we perceive the world and act towards it through our body, that is—as embodied subjects. Contrary to other things and other people's bodies that can be the objects of my experience, my body, as the focal point of my experience of and action in the world, is a condition of possibility for me to be able to experience any other object and act upon it. It is a medium through which the world presents itself to me. In other words, "the body is considered a constitutive or transcendental principle, precisely because it is involved in the very possibility of experience. It is deeply implicated in our relation to the world, in our relation to others, and in our self-relation" (Gallagher & Zahavi, 2008, p. 135).[1]

[1] The body that forms my perspective on the world must not be confused with "a certain living object composed of a nervous system, a brain, glands, digestive, respiratory, and circulatory organs whose very matter is capable of being analyzed chemically into atoms of hydrogen, carbon, nitro-

Although it functions as the basis of our entire experience, the body is usually absent for us. During normal functioning, it is "given only implicitly" (Sartre, 2003, p. 355) and participates pre-reflexively in our experience. As Merleau-Ponty (2005, p. 104) describes: "(...) I observe external objects with my body, I handle them, examine them, walk around them, but my body itself is a thing which I do not observe". Our bodily experience is thus normally characterised by sheer immediacy and a sense of givenness, so that the body disappears as an explicit object of self-reflection or action.[2] As Drew Leder (1990) argues, it is not only the surface or *ecstatic* body through which we engage with the world (e.g. our sense organs) that recedes into the background of our experience, but also the *visceral* body, which consists of our corporal depths—vegetative organs and processes that have a vital function and are mainly hidden beneath the surface of our bodies.[3] The organs and processes that belong to these systems are largely beyond our control and we are largely unaware of them, so that they are most often outside our phenomenological field (Leder, 1990, p. 36). They are of particular interest to us here because many female reproductive organs and processes are characterised by similar phenomenological features, affordances and limitations. Although

gen, phosphorus, etc." (Sartre, 2003, p. 327). My body could not be the subject of natural science if it could not be regarded as one of the objects in the world, but insofar as it is *mine*, this body is never merely an object in the world, but the medium through which my world begins to exist. In this sense, the objective body that the scientist examines is never *my* body as it is *for me*.

[2] There are multiple ways in which the body is absent from experience. Even the possibility of my experience depends on the withdrawal of my body into the background—its very tacitness is constitutive of my experience of the external world, for the bodily process that disappears constitutes the fundamental source of the corresponding field of experience. Or, as Drew Leder notes: "If I were to apprehend all perceptual events simply as modifications of my body located within the perceiving organ, I would have no experience of the outer world" (1990, p. 15). In contrast to this focal disappearance, so-called *background* disappearance is characterised by the fact that certain "bodily regions can disappear because they are *not* the focal origin of our sensorimotor engagements" in the sense that they are either "relegated to a supportive role, involved in irrelevant movement, or simply out of play" (Leder, 1990, p. 26).

[3] According to Leder, visceral functions have remained largely neglected, in contrast to ecstatic functions, which have been an indispensable topic of most phenomenological studies. He believes that the focus of phenomenological analysis on ecstatic functions in the history of phenomenology is quite understandable, given the role they play in shaping the field of experience. However, the visceral body also exhibits a certain pattern of withdrawal from the field of personal experience and control (Leder, 1990, p. 30) and therefore deserves due attention within the framework of phenomenological analysis.

their biological function is not the preservation of the individual but of the species, they too are largely hidden beneath the surface of the body, which makes them phenomenologically isomorphic to what Leder calls the visceral body.

Under certain circumstances, however, the body itself emerges from the background and becomes the centre of our attention and our actions. For instance, when a part of our body fails us, as in the case of injury or illness, but also when we try to master a new skill. At that moment, our attention is directed towards a specific part of the body or a bodily process, which then becomes one of the objects in the world that we focus on in order to understand or influence it—whether to correctly interpret our health condition so we can improve it, or to apply a different exercise or learning technique in an attempt to master a musical instrument or learn a dance or sports movement.[4] The most common way to refer to this existential duality is to distinguish between the *body as subject* and the *body as object*. This implies that the body can be experienced and understood from two different perspectives—from the third-person perspective, that of the observer, and from the first-person perspective, that of the subject who inhibits this body, and in that sense: "The objective body is [...] the objectification of a body which is also, nonetheless, lived" (Gallagher & Zahavi, p. 136).[5]

Very often throughout pregnancy and birth, the reproductive body emerges from its visceral background and becomes an important object of interest and attention.[6] Women increasingly focus on their bodily

[4] It should be noted that, phenomenologically speaking, there is no fundamental difference between the part of the body we use and the tools we use. Mastering a part of the body is no less demanding than mastering a tool. And if we have already mastered the use of a tool, it "falls into oblivion" just like the body parts we use, and only becomes an explicit topic for us when it is broken. As long as it works properly, we focus on what we are doing and not on what we are doing it with.

[5] This is the anti-Cartesian attitude that has been advocated throughout the history of phenomenology. My relationship to my own body is primarily existential, not objective. Neither *res extensa* nor *res cogitans* can be the result of an ontological analysis, but only the result of an epistemological analysis. Consequently, the distinction between the *objective* and the *lived* body is not *ontological*, but *phenomenological*. The embodied subject herself can thus treat her own body as an object, and of course this does not make her any less embodied. On the contrary, just as our embodiment is a condition of possibility of having the experience of other bodies, it is a condition of possibility of having the experience of our own body (as object).

[6] In many cases, this happens even before conception, especially if conception is not easy and uncomplicated.

processes and changes, thus diverting their attention from the environment to which their attention is directed in ordinary life. Self-focus is only further emphasised by the fact that the inner space of a woman's body is inhabited during this period by a new body that gains more and more autonomy over time. This is not to say that the woman is now simply focused on the baby, but rather that she is aware of her body as the environment in which the baby is kept alive and developing. Women listen to various signals from their bodies, not just the unpleasant ones, and wonder whether these signs are related to the process of pregnancy. Every sensation of the body, even something completely harmless and barely perceptible, is a potential indicator of a process that is inaccessible to them, but which may be important for the health and well-being of the baby.[7] Women often express this epistemic problem when they say: "I am pregnant for the first time, I don't know if this is something significant or not, next time I will know". Especially in the first pregnancy, their body appears to them as something unknown and very often explicitly present and thematised in their experience:

> *"Most of the time there's always something to remind you, it's not the first state, it's the second state (Serb. drugo stanje) and there's always something... different things. Sometimes it's this, sometimes it's that, but it's never been like 'Oh, everything's fine with me now'. There's always something, it's never all great." (Anđela)*

The fact that the reproductive body emerges from the visceral background during pregnancy and birth does not mean that what happens to it becomes clearer. The covertness of many reproductive processes means that even when a woman is aware of these processes and has certain perceptual capabilities to access them, her insight is often limited. This is a result of the fact that the visceral processes are accessible to us through our *interoception*.[8] This perceptual modality is phenomenologically

[7] Bodily symptoms in pregnancy, while often uncomfortable, are generally not a problem for the woman per se—because they are painful or unpleasant—but are relevant as potential indicators of a pathological condition or as signs that they are doing something that could harm the baby.

[8] According to the classical physiological classification, interoceptive perception differs from exteroceptive and proprioceptive perception. Exteroceptive perception pertains to objects in the environment in which the body is situated, while proprioceptive perception relates to balance, position and muscle tension within the body itself.

specific due to three characteristics: qualitative reduction, spatial ambiguity and spatio-temporal discontinuity (Leder, 1990, p. 39–45). Sensations from inside our body have a reduced qualitative range compared to the variety of sensations we receive from the surface of our body.[9] Experience is thus given as a unique perceptual dimension—unlike information from different sensory registers that we clearly distinguish, although they are interwoven and given simultaneously. The fact that interoceptive field is characterised by spatial ambiguity means that we are generally unable to accurately determine the spatial location of the stimuli that trigger our sensory response.[10] Moreover, most of the experiences that emanate from our body (hunger, thirst, fatigue, illness) involve multiple and dispersed localisation.[11] Finally, the information we receive about the external world when we are awake flows continuously, without gaps or leaps. While exteroception maintains the continuity of the world, information from inside the body is received only occasionally and sporadically, making it difficult to recognise causal relationships. This spatio-temporal discontinuity complicates the process of gaining insight and understanding of one's own condition.[12]

It is this phenomenological peculiarity of interoception that makes reproductive experiences vague, undifferentiated and difficult to grasp and considerably complicates any reliable interpretation of women's inner

[9] Even in comparison to a single sensory modality, such as the sense of touch, because we can distinguish between touching, tickling, pain, heat, cold, itching and pressure.

[10] While the differential threshold for tactile sensations on the skin is measured in millimetres, visceral experiences have unclear boundaries and an imprecise place of origin.

[11] In fact, these states or signals from the visceral body have a very generalised effect on embodied experience: "Hunger is not just in my stomach but pervades my mouth, my muscles, my mood. It is everywhere, manifesting as exhaustion and craving, irritability and impatience" (Leder, 1990, p. 51). And not only that, the effects of what happens in my visceral body also spill over into my environment. Fatigue or drowsiness can cause things around me to become overly intense—the colours can be too bright, the sounds too loud, the movements of people and car traffic too fast, and so on. When we are hungry or tired, we not only feel it in our whole body, but it actually colours our experience of the world and affects our projects. In this sense, the difference between the visceral and the ecstatic body, between depth and surface, is only relative and elusive.

[12] The lack of differentiation and clarity of experience is also accompanied by an underdeveloped vocabulary—we do not find it easy to verbally express feelings from within the body and often rely on lengthy descriptions and metaphors. This presents a specific methodological and analytical challenge when researching embodied reproductive experiences.

states. The hermeneutic challenge is paired with the practical one—as much as our visceral body is inaccessible to direct insight, it is also inaccessible to voluntary control: "my corporeal depths disappear not only from perception but relative to my structure of will and action" (Leder, 1990, p. 45).[13] And yet we often want and need to both understand and influence what is going on inside our bodies. Therefore, in order to gain both insight into what is happening to us and control over our bodily processes, we must rely on various means and strategies, and often also on the knowledge and assistance of others. Medical representations/procedures/technologies, as well as medical practitioners, play an indispensable role in this regard, which is important to consider when addressing the embodied experience of becoming a mother in today's medicalised world.

3.1.1 Mediated Relationship with Our Reproductive Body: The Role of Medical Knowledge and Technology

The combination of the vagueness of reproductive experiences and their personal significance is the source of the anxiety that women often feel when going through reproductive processes. For example, when pain of unknown origin occurs, women begin to monitor their bodies excessively, re-evaluate their behaviour immediately prior to the new sensation, and consult various sources. To reduce their anxiety, they often turn to close women around them who may have had similar experiences. Finally, if the issue seems serious enough, they usually consult a doctor who, as the holder of medical knowledge, regularly plays the main role in resolving the epistemic problem they encounter:[14]

[13] We have control, or more precisely, we can intervene in our inner bodily processes to a certain extent, but only indirectly. This is because the unfolding of bodily processes depends on exchanges with the environment, so that certain phases take place via the surface of the body. For example, we can influence our digestion by choosing a specific diet or increasing the level of physical activity after eating. In the same manner, women try to influence the processes that are under their direct control (diet, exercise, sleeping positions, daily practices and habits) in order to indirectly influence the processes that are not under their direct control, so they could affect the health and well-being of the baby.

[14] Although not all participants had such an uncritical attitude towards doctors and medicine as described in the following quote, none of them questioned the authority of medical knowledge.

"My pelvic area hurts a little. But again, it's from the pressure of the baby, especially when I sit for a long time or when I walk for a long time. The pressure is probably greater then, so it hurts a bit, but it's not unbearable pain. ***It was only a problem for me at the beginning when I didn't know why I had this pain.*** *So I asked the doctor about it. Although even before I went to the doctor, I talked to, I don't know, my mum, my mother-in-law, my friends, and everyone said it was from that, and then the doctor also said it's the pressure from the baby. (...) So I relaxed a bit about that. That's been my biggest problem since the beginning of pregnancy, not making a mistake or doing something that could harm the baby. I mean, that's my only problem." (Tamara)*

The unclear origin of bodily events and changes combined with their potential consequences (especially for the baby) leads women to engage in a hermeneutic process—a search for an adequate interpretation in order to eliminate possible risks for the pregnancy and the baby and to establish a regime in which things progress as they should.

While the fact that the female reproductive body is today the subject of detailed medical knowledge and widespread application of medical technology owes much to the portrayal of reproductive processes as fundamentally pathological and risky (as discussed in detail in the previous chapter), it also has an important foundation in its phenomenological quality of being hidden from experience. For the most part, a woman's reproductive body is only indirectly accessible to her, so that she must resort to various means and strategies to gain both insight into what is happening to her and control over her bodily processes. This is why other people, especially those who have a certain level of expertise and are equipped with certain technical means, are often in a better position when it comes to understanding and influencing our own internal bodily processes: e.g. "To those who could hear its message, the pulse spoke truths about a person that the person himself or herself would not or could not say" (Kuriyama, 1999, p. 18). So, by relying on medical knowledge and various medical procedures and technologies, a medical practitioner plays the role of "a hermeneut, reading the text of the surface body for what it has to say about corporeal depths" (Leder, 1990, p. 51).

It's not necessary, however, for a contemporary woman to actually visit a doctor to obtain her own piece of hermeneutics since medical knowledge and expertise is broadly available today. The participant below explicitly refers to medical information from the internet (i.e. stages of pregnancy and the hormonal changes that accompany them) as an interpretive framework for monitoring bodily changes. Although the changes take place in and on their own bodies, they are "tracked online". In other words, women seek information that allows them to recognise, connect, integrate and explain their experiences, even without any negative symptoms as triggers.

> *"And then comes that magical part of pregnancy, where your hair gets thick. For me, the second trimester is like the Belle Époque. I mean, your hair becomes thick and grows, and the body hair disappears. It's brilliant. But then it comes back when you enter the third trimester. I mean, there are these phases, and I track it all online neatly. And hormonally, it makes sense and depends in which direction it goes from that baseline." (Una)*

In the next sections, we will see how the opacity of reproductive processes and the epistemic and practical challenges associated with them come to the fore right from the beginning of pregnancy, which is characterised by the uncertainty as to whether conception has taken place at all. Ambiguity during pregnancy is typical for various events and phases (e.g. how to properly attribute sensations from the abdomen to foetal movements) and accompanies the pregnant woman all the way to the not-so-easy task of recognising the onset of labour. It will be shown that while medical techniques and representations very often play an important role in resolving uncertainties and giving women both the knowledge and the ability to make informed choices about their actions, they also sometimes lead to inducing or deepening their anxiety.

3.2 Uncertain Beginnings

During pregnancy, women undergo significant physical changes and accompanying psychological adjustments (Leifer, 1980). This experience brings growth and transformation, but also uncertainties and challenges. Women often feel anxious during this life phase (Barber, 2012; Heron et al., 2004), which is exacerbated by the pressure to 'get it right' (Slade & Cree, 2010). The beginning of pregnancy in particular is often characterised by uncertainty and challenges (Smith, 1999), as women are unsure how to interpret the bodily changes or whether they are normal or indicative of a potential health problem. The uncertainty is compounded by the fact that some "signs" of pregnancy coincide with bodily experiences that are characteristic of other conditions, such as the onset of the menstrual cycle or that of an illness. The feeling of uncertainty is not only related to an adequate understanding of their body, but also to the physiological process itself—will the pregnancy last and develop properly, or will it result in miscarriage or early labour? All of these questions women face are both hermeneutical and practical, and they come with a demand—women need to address them in order to act and feel like agents during this transitory period.

3.2.1 Epistemological Uncertainties: Am I or Am I Not?

The body does not often speak up in our everyday functioning. Even when it does—as with a sudden cramp in the leg, a sharp pain in the stomach or a warm, pleasant sensation on the skin when we sit in the sun—these feelings remain isolated islands in the sea of our daily experiences focused on the external environment or internal (primarily mental) content. However, during our lives, we begin to treat some of these bodily displays as signs and we start to see connections between them. We link them to a certain condition and realise that our body is communicating with us in a more understandable and stable way—that is how we can recognise the first symptoms of a cold, an impending migraine or an attack of rheumatism.

Premenstrual symptoms are one such phenomenon of relatively stable signalling of the body in most women's lives. Pulsating mild pain in the lower abdomen, headaches, breast tenderness, increased appetite, irritability are usually related and the premenstrual body takes over the stage—often with unwavering regularity.

"I know my body. So I knew that I would get my period then for sure, because when my breasts start to hurt, it means that I will get my period a week later, as by the clock. And it comes almost exactly on the day. So I know it's not going to be late. And since I felt that pain in my breasts, I associated it with my period. So that's it, I should be getting it now. And I was just preparing myself for that, not for pregnancy..." (Teodora)

Premenstrual symptoms almost invariably occur as the first, misinterpreted sign of pregnancy. How and when does a woman's premenstrual body become a pregnant body? A delayed cycle is a sign that calls into question the previous interpretation, although other mediators may also be involved in this process of reinterpreting one's condition—often in the form of significant others.

"I was expecting to get my period any moment. Normally my stomach doesn't hurt. Just back pain and my breasts are a size larger, and I'm nervous. PMS hits me mentally, I get a little depressed and bloated. So I'm a bit bloated, I'm even more irritable because I'm bigger and my boobs are all over the place, and nothing is happening, so I'm already starting to doubt... but I'm expecting something different from PMS. I asked my mom what it was like for her when she was pregnant and she told me 'the same', which made me a little worried... And then I took the test." (Sonja)

While *experiencing* one's own body seems like an unmediated process (although we have already problematised that claim), *understanding* and *interpreting* bodily sensations could be a difficult task with an uncertain outcome. And this is a task that must be solved in order to act in any way. The realisation that she is pregnant prompts a woman to take a series of actions, from changing her diet and taking supplements to prenatal testing, while at the same time making some behaviours undesirable or forbidden for her, for example, the consumption of alcohol or intense physical activity. These are certainly social (and medical) norms that prescribe a responsible and cautious approach to pregnancy for women. However, in the case of a wanted pregnancy, women's goal is to care for the well-being of the developing foetus, and as such they identify with normative societal expectations. Therefore, they feel the inherent need to properly understand their situation in order to be able to act accordingly.

Regardless of whether they interpret the body's communication correctly or incorrectly or, as we shall see shortly, ignore it altogether, what offers most women in modern Western society a final resolution of uncertainty and thus the opportunity to be agents is a relatively simple example of medical technology—a pregnancy test. Hormonal pregnancy tests[15] are not only the most commonly used reproductive technology next to the birth control pill, but also the most commonly used diagnostic technique after the thermometer in the modern world (Tone, 2012). A large number of healthy, sexually active heterosexual women of reproductive age have relied on them at least at some point in their lives, especially in the West.[16] So, for most women, a home pregnancy test is a culturally and historically specific tool that provides an interpretation of bodily condition and resolves a situation of uncertainty. Almost all participants respond to a delay in their cycle and the onset of physical symptoms by purchasing a test to check if they are pregnant.[17] The use of this simple and accessible medical technology allows women to clarify the situation by providing a valid interpretation of unclear and ambiguous physical symptoms and guiding them towards a specific set of future activities.

However, it is important to bear in mind that pregnancy must appear as a possible interpretation of the emerging symptoms for the test to be recognised as a suitable tool at all. One participant was diagnosed with a condition several years before she became pregnant, implying that she would not be able to conceive naturally. Therefore, pregnancy did not appear as a possible explanation for the onset of her symptoms, and there

[15] Over-the-counter pregnancy tests detect hCG, which stands for human chorionic gonadotropin, a hormone whose concentration rises significantly in the early stages of pregnancy (Cunningham et al., 2010, p. 37).

[16] The tests were first sold in American pharmacies in the late 1970s, but their price was relatively high until the mid-1990s. After that, they became very affordable, and the number of women using them increased steadily (Tone, 2012).

[17] Home tests usually eliminate the need for laboratory diagnosis of pregnancy, which is based on the use of immunological tests and is carried out in a medical facility through blood analysis. With these laboratory tests, pregnancy can be diagnosed very early, as early as one week after fertilisation, and they are therefore regularly used only in women who have undergone some form of assisted reproduction (Kastratović-Kotlica, 2005; Mladenović et al., 2008). Accordingly, the only participants who did not independently confirm their pregnancy with a home test but relied on laboratory diagnostics were those who conceived through in vitro fertilisation or started an assisted reproduction procedure.

was never a need to purchase a pregnancy test. In her case, other intermediaries, such as the experiences and involvement of other people, were necessary for her to gain insight into her own condition.

> *"And then when I got pregnant, I was completely shocked. I was... actually, first my friend found out I was pregnant, and then I did. She had been pregnant for a month longer than me. And she calls me to come over... But when I saw this friend some two weeks before that she asked me if my belly was swollen or something like that. And I said, yeah, my boobs are swollen too, like I don't know, I must be getting my period soon, it makes me crazy. And then she started bugging me, 'maybe you're pregnant, maybe you're pregnant!' And I put it down to her—well, she got pregnant a month ago and now she sees pregnant women everywhere. And she calls me and says, 'You know what, we both have a cold and if you're knocked up, please don't come over because pregnant women shouldn't be exposed to viruses.' I said, 'What are you talking about?' 'No, no, just check.'" (Una)*

So here the bodily changes are not noticed and correctly interpreted by the woman herself, but by someone else, and the test only appears to be an adequate means of resolving the situation in this context—it is not intended to show a woman what is happening to her, but to prove it to someone else. What is also interesting is that only when the information conveyed by the test becomes available does the woman begin to recognise and integrate bodily experiences, as it provides a suitable framework for interpretation.

> *"When I realised I was pregnant, my first thought was like yeah, all my clothes feel tight. That's how I felt...* ***my body had really been my safe zone my whole life****, unlike all the other things,* ***but I hadn't really been reading it somehow****. (...) That was an interesting insight for me. The moment I found out I was pregnant, I had the proof, then I started paying attention to my body. And then I noticed a ton of things.* ***I mean, the body sends interesting signals, it's just a question of what you pick up on****. They didn't just show up, I didn't trigger them the day I got the evidence. Then I rewound the tape and it was there all along and completely... First of all, my skin was terribly sensitive. To the touch and like those tiny cuts you get during the day doing the dishes or wiping, that need five days to heal. It had been happening for about a month and a half, but you don't pay attention to it. That was the first thing. And I was*

> *really sleepy. And my breasts were swollen. And my belly was very noticeable from the start. I later got a medical explanation for all that." (Una)*

Not only did she not pay attention to the numerous bodily changes that occurred, nor did she connect them (weight gain, swollen breasts, sleepiness, sensitive skin), but she also ignored very indicative symptoms such as a delayed menstrual cycle, which she noticed but attributed to various causes unrelated to pregnancy (stress, irregular lifestyle, "cycle synchronisation").

> *"This is the first time in my life that I didn't pay attention to my period. I complained to my roommate, for three weeks I was like 'Now I really have to get it finally, I can't take it anymore.' And she insisted that our cycles were now synchronising, so mine was late and hers was coming earlier. It all made sense. I also changed jobs at that time and changed my apartment... and I lived an incredibly disorganised life." (Una)*

Una claims that all her life her body has been a "safe zone" in which she felt comfortable, but still she "did not read it". She believes that the reason she did not notice or pay attention to her bodily experiences and conditions was because she was not properly "tuned in". The realisation that she was pregnant allowed her to retroactively acknowledge and interpret her entire embodied experience. So it's not just about interpreting and understanding her own body, but in a sense also about experiencing and registering its signals. She began to "pay attention" and recognise many symptoms that had escaped her notice in the previous period, only when they could appear relevant as indicators of a particular condition. This case shows that for an adequate interpretation of embodied experience, it is not enough for a person to know that certain physical signs are indicators of certain states; rather, that state must emerge as a possible interpretation.

Finally, in some cases, the resolution of epistemic uncertainty not only changes the women's mere interpretation of their bodily experiences or even their awareness of them, but intervenes even more directly in how they feel. One of the participants, after confirming pregnancy with a home test, suffered from severe, all-day nausea throughout the entire period leading up to the first ultrasound to confirm the presence of the foetus. She easily interpreted this symptom as a sign of pregnancy, but it was only after a medical examination that this interpretation was not only questioned, but the symptom ceased to exist.

> *"And then I went in for that first ultrasound and literally as soon as I walked out of the doctor's office, the feeling was gone, as if by magic. When I went in, the doctor confirmed the pregnancy and it was a huge relief. At that moment, the sickness I was feeling for days literally disappeared as if by magic. And then I went out and came home and had my first normal meal in a week. So then the nausea stopped. And so I connected it in a way that maybe it was not connected to the pregnancy itself. That it was my nerves... this uncertainty of whether I am or whether I'm not, whether everything is ok, and waiting for that ultrasound to confirm that it is. That's exactly what I thought, just for that reason, that impression that the feeling had magically disappeared. If it was something physical related to the pregnancy, it would keep occurring afterwards. Because after that I did not have any of these symptoms. Not even once." (Nevena)*

Only the sudden cessation of the unpleasant symptoms that coincided with the resolution of the uncertainty by medical confirmation of pregnancy enabled this participant to attribute these symptoms to her psychological situation and her reaction to stress rather than to the bodily manifestation of pregnancy. What is interesting in this case is that she believes this situation arose because she had read too much information about pregnancy online as soon as she found out she was pregnant ("I probably stressed myself out then"). The medical knowledge that led her to view her pregnancy as an extremely risky project with an uncertain outcome thus put her in a state that could only be resolved and alleviated by additional (more reliable) medical knowledge—which is also regularly acquired through medical technology. We will see that a similar pattern of the role of medical knowledge/technology both triggering and resolving uncertainty is frequently observed during pregnancy, childbirth and postpartum period.

3.2.2 Ontological Uncertainties: Will It Stick?

In addition to the uncertainty about the adequate interpretation of one's own condition, I have already indicated another source of anxiety that significantly determines how a woman experiences the onset of pregnancy and how she deals with it—namely the uncertainty about whether the pregnancy will be maintained. Medical literature suggests that approximately 15–20% of all documented pregnancies end in miscarriage, with the highest rate (over 80%) occurring before the twelfth week of pregnancy (Cunningham et al., 2010, p. 215; Gracia et al., 2005). Consequently, the first few months are often seen as precarious and risky by healthcare professionals as well as women and their families. As one interviewee put it: "It's all in your head, you just pray for that twelfth week to pass" (Maja). The fear of miscarriage is also linked to cultural customs that dictate not to "spread the news" about the pregnancy before the end of the risky period to avoid "jinxing it": "I'm pregnant but I'm not talking about it, I want to tell everyone but I can't. And we only announced it after the third month..." (Sonja). Therefore, in order for the pregnancy to become socially recognised, a woman not only waits for confirmation that she is pregnant, but also for confirmation that the pregnancy will last.

The availability of early pregnancy detection tests has shifted the confirmation of pregnancy to a much earlier time than was the case a few decades ago, making women aware of the uncertain beginning, when it is still questionable whether the pregnancy will be maintained or not (Tone, 2012). Although uncertainty about the onset of pregnancy also existed in earlier historical epochs, when it was not certain until birth whether the absence of menstruation and the growth of the belly indicated pregnancy or the development of an illness (Duden, 1991, p. 157–170), this uncertainty for the woman herself seems to have been primarily epistemic—"am I identifying my condition correctly?"—and not of an ontological nature—"the condition has been correctly identified as pregnancy, but will it last?" The advent of hormonal tests for the early detection of pregnancy has thus created a completely new situation for the modern woman—both in terms of how she perceives and experiences her body at the beginning of pregnancy and in terms of how she relates to it. She no longer sees her body as maybe pregnant or maybe not, but begins to see it as an environment that might "accept" the pregnancy, or might "reject" it. The woman often tries to take an active stance in this situation and influence the sustainability of the pregnancy—by taking hormones, avoiding exertion and reducing activity, getting more rest—rather than simply waiting for the situation to resolve itself.

A good illustration of this point is the case of a participant who experienced bleeding immediately after a positive pregnancy test, which is commonly considered the greatest indicator of risk of miscarriage (Everett, 1997; Gracia et al., 2005). Although she would have interpreted the same bleeding as a delayed onset of menstruation if she had not taken the test that morning, the fact that the test was positive completely changed the interpretation of the situation and her attitude towards it.

> *"And then we went to my parents' to share the news, and there I went to the bathroom and got my period! And you know what a drama that was! I hadn't thought about having a baby until that morning, but then it all fell apart! I wasn't pregnant, bro! But these tests are really quite reliable, they react to a tiny hormone and can't go wrong. And it says it can be slightly pink and pink, but mine was super pink within three seconds and it was clear I was already pregnant, no doubt about it, and then we were all devastated." (Sonja)*

The fact that Sonja had sufficient medical knowledge to recognise the test as a reliable assessment tool, as well as the realisation that the immediate positive result (she waited only briefly until the red line appeared) indicated a high concentration of hormones in the urine, led Sonja to interpret the onset of bleeding as a miscarriage without any doubt. She vividly describes how the mere realisation that she was pregnant, even though she had not felt ready for a child just a few hours earlier and felt that it was not the right time given the practical circumstances, drastically changed her attitude towards the whole situation. A pregnancy that was not even wholeheartedly wanted becomes something extremely precious, so a spontaneous termination would be a huge loss for her.

"Then I rushed to some private lab to get a blood pregnancy test, and it was late and everything was closed, and then I waited in front of the computer for the test results until they emailed them to me. And I was crying my heart out like I had lost five children, I completely fell apart, no one could calm me down." (Sonja)

It should be noted that such early identification with the pregnancy in the initial phase is atypical and actually only occurred in participants who had a markedly uncertain and problematic start to their pregnancy. Sonja was in a state of anticipation during these first weeks and experienced her body all the time as something that was supposed to retain the foetus and feared that it would reject it. This is evident from her unconscious bodily reaction—she clenched her legs and pressed them together to physically prevent the foetus from "leaking out". This very vivid example makes it clear that it is not just about a different understanding or imagining of one's own body, but that the changed embodiment implies something more than that.

"And I was unconsciously clenching the whole time. My mom told me not to clench, if it's going to leak, it will leak. And I sat there the whole time with legs tightly squeezed, as if to plug it up. And how she figured me out, that was fascinating to me. But she had a miscarriage before she got pregnant with me, so maybe she remembers. But she just told me 'don't, I used to do that too.' But I kept clenching." (Sonja)

Sonja believes that the doctor "played an important role" for her, precisely by affirming this uncertain status of the pregnancy and interpreting the situation in a way that Sonja could not influence it with her actions:

"The doctor was like 'I can't tell you anything, nothing is known until the third month. You are pregnant, but whether it sticks or not, there's literally nothing that can be done except to hit you with these hormones. If your body keeps it... if it doesn't, it doesn't. Get over it.'"

Paradoxically, this interpretation did not seem to take away her sense of agency; instead, it supported her in waiting and accepting the situation.[18] He did not give her "false hope" so that she would identify with the pregnancy too soon, which would increase her sense of loss if the pregnancy did not last. But he also did not completely "crush her spirit" either, so she did not immediately start grieving or become anxious because this condition could harm the pregnancy that had a chance to hold.

For some women, the beginning of pregnancy is perceived as risky, and regardless of the presence of indicative physical signs such as bleeding, they approach their situation very cautiously. This is especially true for those who have conceived through in vitro fertilisation or who have had problems with reproduction in the past. In such cases, reliance on expert knowledge, medical techniques and procedures is very much present, as blood beta-hCG levels are monitored every few days, frequent check-ups are scheduled and hormones are taken as a preventative measure. However, this type of approach to pregnancy is also seen in women who have not yet experienced health problems, which is to be expected given the dominance of the discourse of risk discussed earlier.

The uncertain onset of pregnancy and the absence or unclear and ambiguous presence of bodily signals place a woman in a specific situation at the beginning of pregnancy and allow medical technology to play a very important role for her. This applies in particular to ultrasound examinations, which promise a more "direct" and "immediate" access to her bodily situation, so that women often wait eagerly and anxiously for the results of the first ultrasound examination. However, we will see that the question of the role of ultrasound in the experience of pregnancy is considerably more complex and ambivalent—even when it offers insight and resolution, this often comes at a price.

[18] I am grateful to Jan Valsiner for drawing my attention to this specific and seemingly paradoxical type of agency, which consists in maintaining an unclear and uncertain situation, i.e. not taking action or adopting a definitive stance towards something (personal communication, May 2014).

3.2.3 Can Uncertainty Be Resolved? The Ambivalent Role of Medical Technology

Women regularly seek further technologically mediated confirmation of pregnancy and consult their doctor because hormonal tests (both home and laboratory ones) have one major limitation: they cannot detect ectopic pregnancy, which is a major health risk and can have fatal consequences. This technological shortcoming leads to increased anxiety, which can only be remedied by using a different, more sophisticated technology. Unlike hormone testing, ultrasound offers a more direct (and seemingly unmediated) view of the foetus implantation in the uterus and the ability to hear its heartbeat, which provides reassurance and comfort and reduces uncertainty.

> *"You can't take the test and be like 'Now I'm pregnant.' Because that test really doesn't mean anything. Because, in fact, you know you're pregnant, but you don't know if it's ectopic pregnancy or whether everything is okay." (Ivana).*
>
> *"I believed in that pregnancy test plus ultrasound. I'm of the opinion - what's certain is certain, I'm more in favour of them seeing on the ultrasound that everything is okay. And I thought, how do I know, you do these blood tests and it could be, God forbid, an ectopic pregnancy... It could happen to you... I was really, well, I was very informed. In fact, I used to read a lot. So I was really well informed. And so it was a very normal next step for me to have the ultrasound." (Maja)*

Some authors recognise that the very early detection of pregnancy made possible by home testing has actually led to pregnant women being placed under the authority of medicine even earlier (Tone, 2012). On the one hand, women are sufficiently medically informed about the pregnancy and possible risks, so the need for further verification is quite rational as it can prevent unfavourable outcomes. On the other hand, one can recognise in women's narratives an excess of uncertainty and the need to have what they have detected themselves confirmed by an expert using more sophisticated technology and in a more direct manner. The importance of *seeing* something and not just checking the test result that indicates it is often emphasised. Because of this need, women sometimes put themselves in a situation of even greater uncertainty because they expect something from medical technology that it cannot deliver.

Maja had been trying to get pregnant for over two years and was, as she puts it, "really preoccupied with it". It seems that she transferred the anxiety regarding conception to the beginning of her pregnancy. That is why she needed external confirmation that "everything was fine", and as direct and reliable confirmation as possible. So as soon as she found out, she tried to find a clinic that was willing to perform an ultrasound scan, even though it was a very early pregnancy that could not yet be detected by ultrasound.

> *"I was like, 'Okay, I'm not going yet, it's still too early, nothing will show up on the ultrasound anyway'. But the impatience was so overwhelming, it's just that need to hear that everything is okay. Just to hear that everything is fine. Because you want it so much and then something can happen. Because lately you hear so often that women got pregnant and then it doesn't work out... So I call the clinic and they say it's still too early, that I should wait another week or two. And I'm like, 'Who's gonna wait, I'll look for another one'. I looked for a clinic until I found one that would take me. (...) And the doctor confirmed it was a pregnancy, but it was a small pregnancy. Nothing, the foetus wasn't even visible on the ultrasound. Only that sac was visible." (Maja)*

But even this direct confirmation from the doctor is not enough to completely eliminate the uncertainty, because the image from the ultrasound, which was hoped to provide an immediate insight and unproblematic confirmation, is still ambiguous. Maja does not see what she at least implicitly expected to see—her baby.

> *"She gave me the ultrasound picture and there's only a circle there. No baby in it. And then you start to think, 'Well it is alright, she said everything is alright... but how can it be okay when you can't see the baby?' You're totally...it's all in your head and you're just waiting for that twelfth week to pass." (Maja)*

Maja's case shows that technology, or at least the way it is commonly represented, offers a promise that often cannot be fulfilled—the promise of *objective and unambiguous insight*, a straightforward *proof* of a certain condition. In reality, however, people are confronted with unclear images, figures that can be interpreted in multiple ways and incomprehensible graphics. It is also interesting to consider how the doctor's voice relates to this ambiguity of technology. Doctors are generally seen as authorities and it is very important that they "say that everything is fine". But in situations like Maja's, where there is considerable uncertainty associated with a condition, the lack of absolute consistency between the doctor's words and the technological image introduces additional uncertainty.

"He didn't show me anything on the ultrasound and that was terrible, because he told me: 'I see the gestational sac, like a membrane where the space for the baby is forming, but I don't see the embryo'. (...) And I asked, 'What does that mean?' He said, 'Well, nothing, it's still early pregnancy, I can't see it yet.' I asked him if that was normal, if that happens, and he said: 'Yes, yes, but come back next week for confirmation'." (Saška)

One way to resolve this situation is to seek additional confirmation and the opinion of another doctor, which would provide an additional source of validation. In local circumstances, this very often involves seeking a second opinion in a private practice after an initial consultation in a public healthcare institution.[19]

"This doctor performed a transvaginal ultrasound for me, and she turned the screen and showed me: 'Look, this is the embryo.' She even let me hear the heartbeat and said: 'Here, you can hear the heartbeat, the embryo is vital'. And then I felt relieved, and that was the official confirmation of my pregnancy. But later I heard stories that in Western Europe transvaginal ultrasounds are forbidden in the first three months. So then I started to worry about that, 'why did she do it for me?' Probably because we told her that my gynaecologist hadn't seen the embryo. So she did it so we wouldn't leave without seeing it again." (Saška)

Although this examination was the "official confirmation" of Saška's pregnancy, it created the basis for a new uncertainty due to the potential harmfulness of transvaginal ultrasound in early pregnancy, which can compromise the competence of the cervix and thus increase the risk of

[19] As already discussed at the end of the previous chapter—local women often rely on private healthcare practice to maintain or establish both the quality and continuity of care (Pantović, 2022).

miscarriage. For this woman the technology thus appeared as a means of resolving *epistemic* uncertainty ("am I really pregnant?"), but at the same time it triggered *ontological* uncertainty ("will everything be okay with the pregnancy after this checkup?"). This is not an uncommon situation when it comes to the involvement of medical technology, and we encounter it in other situations during pregnancy and childbirth.[20] Therefore, medical technology plays an ambivalent role for women during the transition to motherhood, and we will return to this topic and the question of what this role depends on at the end of this chapter. One of the key factors is certainly the availability of women's embodied experience of pregnancy, which is constantly changing during pregnancy, especially as the most prominent aspect of this experience becomes present—first through technological mediation and later through the embodied experience of baby's movements, which we turn to next.

3.3 Identification with Pregnancy and Individuation of the Baby: Pregnant Embodiment and the Role of Medical Knowledge/Technology

This subchapter is the longest one in the book, and for good reason. I will attempt to trace a complex process of women's identification with a radically altered state, which I consider both an important aspect of the early transition to motherhood and a precondition for further change and

[20] Prenatal genetic testing is a paradigmatic example because it resolves the uncertainty inherent in the results of a less reliable but entirely safe *screening* test by means of a completely reliable but also risky *diagnostic* test that brings new uncertainties for women. Both types of tests enable the detection of foetal chromosomal abnormalities, but differ in the reliability of the results and the invasiveness of the procedure. In Serbia, all women undergo a screening test, which is a mandatory part of prenatal care (the so-called double test includes an ultrasound examination and the analysis of biochemical markers in serum). This test is completely non-invasive, but is not considered reliable due to a high number of false-positive results (Benn et al., 2001). The diagnostic test (usually amniocentesis), on the other hand, is an invasive procedure and carries a certain risk of miscarriage, but it is absolutely reliable (Mujezinovic & Alfirevic, 2007). When women undergo amniocentesis, they eliminate all uncertainties about the possible presence of genetic abnormalities in the foetus. However, this solution triggers or deepens a new uncertainty—the more reliable genetic testing procedure potentially threatens the pregnancy itself.

adaptation. Pregnancy is a paradigmatic developmental process and follows a unique temporality. And while it is a distinctly embodied process, different medical knowledge and techniques play a significant, albeit changing, role in it, depending on the specificity of the stage women find themselves in.

The pregnant embodiment is a highly specific and exclusively female experience that poses various challenges to a woman's subjectivity and her everyday life. As mentioned at the beginning of the book, the expression "drugo stanje" (the other state) describes very well the changes and deviations from the usual bodily experiences and functioning that characterise the period of pregnancy. Pregnancy seems to heighten women's awareness of their bodies because in many situations, sometimes even all the time, women are aware of their weight, their protruding belly, their swollen breasts and the baby inside them, which leads to altered patterns of movement and new habits. Throughout this process, medical representations and technologies play an important role in a woman's sense of self, her conduct and the process of identification with the pregnancy. This is especially the case in the initial phase characterised by the absence or ambiguous presence of embodied experiences.

In the later part of the chapter I will turn to the most specific and central aspect of the pregnancy experience—the fact that there is another being developing inside a woman's body that becomes increasingly differentiated and autonomous for her, which is why pregnant subject is characterised as being: "*decentered, split, or doubled* in several ways. She experiences her body as herself and not herself. Its inner movements belong to another being, yet they are not other (...)" (Young, 2005b, p. 46). It is said that a woman lives in a body that is "simultaneously dual and alien space" (Kristeva, 1990, p. 441). Various phenomenologically oriented authors have attempted to articulate this liminal situation that a pregnant woman goes through as she experiences both herself and her developing baby as "me/not-me and of-me/separate-from-me that places her in the unique position of getting to know herself-with-another and another-within-herself" (Sandelowski & Black, 1994, p. 607).

The aim of this chapter, then, is to explore various aspects of embodied experience during pregnancy, with a particular focus on the individuation of the baby for the mother, which draws on both embodied and technologically mediated inputs. Ultrasound has a particularly important role in this regard, and I will attempt to analyse its varying and manifold influences. The literature often emphasises the psychological importance of prenatal diagnostics[21] for women, especially ultrasound, which enables them to *see* the baby (Clement et al., 1998). It is noted that the images and information about the foetus provided by medical technology are associated with reducing anxiety (Zlotogorski et al., 1997), but also with promoting attachment to the foetus (DiPietro, 2010; Taylor, 2008). However, I will attempt to show that the impact of technology can be much broader—that it can significantly alter the way a woman experiences pregnancy and her pregnant body, as well as the way she practically addresses various challenges of her altered state.

3.3.1 "Baby on the Screen" and Early Identification with Pregnancy

I have already argued that the beginning of pregnancy is characterised by numerous uncertainties and that medical technology plays a somewhat ambivalent role during this period. At the same time, the fact that it offers women the opportunity to gain an insight into the baby's condition and progress is often significant for early identification with the pregnancy, which has many practical consequences. For many women, being able to see the baby on an ultrasound image in the early months, before the characteristic aspects of the embodied pregnant experience emerge, such as the growth of the belly or experiencing the baby's movements,

[21] Prenatal diagnostics has a long history. Midwives have been palpating the bellies of pregnant women for centuries to feel the movements of the foetus and monitor its growth, while the practice of a male doctor performing this examination did not begin until the late eighteenth century (Kukla, 2005, p. 71). The hands of doctors were replaced by technology in the early twentieth century, when the use of x-rays during pregnancy began. Although there were warnings that x-rays could be harmful to the newborn, it was not until the 1950s that x-rays during pregnancy were shown to be associated with the development of cancer in children, leading to the abandonment of the practice (O'Dowd & Philipp, 1994). Since the 1960s, x-rays have been replaced by ultrasonography, which has become a widely and routinely used technology for monitoring the foetus throughout pregnancy. In Serbia, women with uncomplicated pregnancies undergo four mandatory ultrasound examinations during pregnancy, while this number may be higher for women with suspected risks (Health Care for Pregnant Women, 2005).

makes the pregnancy "real" for them and helps them to "become more aware" of it.

> *"So that first ultrasound was strange. I mean, kind of weird. I didn't actually realise it at the time. (...) So it allowed me to have a little awareness, to see that it's a baby, you know." (Sofia)*

This often serves as an incentive to organise everyday life and practical activities according to the basic principle that guides most women during pregnancy—concern for the unborn child and its well-being.

> *"And I turn to the screen and you see a baby like this, everything is miniature. You see his little spine and everything. Well then, that feeling ... that's my child. Then you do everything just to protect him as best you can. Then you get this urge to take care of yourself. That you have to fight. Whatever you have to do, because you have another life inside you. You are not alone." (Mirjana)*

Mirjana says that she knew she was pregnant, that she was "aware of it", but she experienced it very intimately for the first time when she saw the baby on the ultrasound. For her, the ultrasound played an important role in her early identification with pregnancy and taking care of her body and behaviour. At that moment, she immediately realised that it was no longer just her health and her body at stake, but that she was responsible for another being. This had a very concrete practical consequence—Mirjana stopped smoking almost completely after this ultrasound scan. However, from the fact that the ultrasound played an important role for Mirjana at this *early* stage of pregnancy, we should not prematurely conclude that medical technology was crucial for her identification with the pregnancy and the bonding process with the baby. We will soon see that she actually cites the experience of movement as decisive for her perceiving the foetus as "her baby" and the pregnancy becoming truly "real" for her.

It seems that diagnostic techniques often lead primarily to an easier "cognitive" realisation and appropriation of the pregnancy and the resulting regulation of behaviour, but not to an intimate and substantial identification with the pregnancy, attachment to the future baby and the altered sense of self (as a mother).

"I am mentally prepared for the fact that I am pregnant, and I know more in my head that I am pregnant than I feel it physically in any way. And then when I see that dot or that something, you just kind of visualise it. (...) That's how you start to think, to take more care, to look after yourself. And the moment you see it on the ultrasound ... it's there and it's fine and that's about it. (...) And this is what it means to me, I stop there. It's not like it's triggered that maternal instinct now... No, I really didn't have that feeling. I just know it's there now, so I take care of it, that's important to me." (Teodora)

So, it seems that without diagnostic technology, it may have been more difficult for women to become aware of pregnancy, which is significant for the adaptation of practical measures to changing conditions. At the same time, technologically mediated insight does not seem to suffice when it comes to developing a deeper connection with the baby and identifying with the role of a mother. Many women point out that although they can see the baby on an ultrasound image, they actually get to know it through the embodied experience of its movements and the embodied recognition of the baby's interactions and rhythms, which we will soon focus on.

The gap between the realisation of pregnancy on the basis of the first ultrasound and identification with the pregnancy is particularly evident in women whose condition is complicated by medical problems. Tanja became pregnant in her late 40s after numerous unsuccessful IVF attempts and three previous miscarriages. Aware of all the risks her pregnancy faces (her age, autoimmune syndrome, hormonal problems), what she sees on the ultrasound is just a foretaste of what, if all goes well, will one day be her baby. It's more something that reminds her of "how much she still has ahead of her" and how uncertain it all is.

"And on that first image from the ultrasound, you just can't see anything. Something like white in the middle and everything else black. And then it's like...now this is my child. Especially when you know how much you still have ahead of you and what awaits you. Then you know that this is only the first,

first step. (...) And even later, when I first saw that little, let's say, human-like figure. Something had formed there, now I can't remember what, of those organs. But it's all so strange. I don't know, it's all still to you... I don't know how to describe it. You know you're pregnant, you know it's your baby and everything, but it all still, at least that's how it seemed to me, felt somewhat unreal. And I don't know, there is a kind of emotional connection and all, like you love that child, but it just seemed to me like it was happening to someone else." (Tanja)

In this case, identification with pregnancy is a particularly uncertain and slow process. Although there is a cognitive acceptance ("you know you're are pregnant, you know it's is your baby") and there is also an indication of feelings ("like you love that child"), it is still evident that this woman is far from identifying herself with the pregnancy ("felt unreal", "like it was happening to someone else").

Finally, there are women who privilege their embodied experience of pregnancy and baby so much that what the ultrasound shows is of no consequence to them, even in the earliest stages of pregnancy, when it is the only insight they have. For them, identification with pregnancy only becomes possible through a change in their embodied experience, and before that they feel frustration at the lack of some specific bodily manifestations. As a result, the expected change in behaviour (abstaining from alcohol, medication, physical activity) is perceived as oppressive and external.

"And the motivation for the whole abstinence thing starts at that moment because of the idea that you're pregnant and then you're like, 'No way I'm drinking.' But then from one moment everyone knows I'm pregnant, and it doesn't show at all, nothing's happening. And this baby isn't moving yet, I don't feel anything! And I start getting pissed off. How am I pregnant now, is someone messing with me? Nothing is happening with me, and all these other women are throwing up, moaning, I have nothing. And I can't drink, damn it. Just negatives, no positives. When am I going to get something out of this? But, the baby started moving very early, and that was something different..." (Sonja)

What enables these women to truly identify with the pregnancy are the physical symptoms, the growth of the belly and the experience of the baby's movements, rather than the medical confirmation or technologically mediated knowledge about the baby.

"B: How did you feel when you first saw the baby on the ultrasound?
S: Well, at times I thought they were lying to me. You give up so much, I mean, it's no big deal, but... and everyone treats you differently, and you're the same. And it's supposed to be different, and I don't know how to act. So now what? I shouldn't be lifting things, huh? And everyone around me is urging me to lie down. But I don't want to lie down! What should we do now? And then I'm irresponsible, I'm going to kill my child. I mean, you get the idea... So it meant more to me when I started gaining weight. A lot more. And when it started kicking." (Sonja)

Sometimes it is hard for a woman to "act like a pregnant woman" when she does not "feel like a pregnant woman". She experiences a mismatch between the fact that others treat her differently and expect her to behave accordingly, and the fact that she does not experience this change first hand—"and you're the same". Until pregnancy becomes a lived reality for her, she perceives changing her habits and making sacrifices as a consequence of social pressure.

"Well, that ultrasound scan was nothing special for me. Basically, I didn't even experience pregnancy until my belly started to grow. Ever since we started looking on websites, forums, comments... and someone is like 'oh, my angel' and... I really didn't feel like I was pregnant, and if no one had told me that, especially when the nausea stopped, you feel completely normal, only you're like pregnant. And I didn't have that feeling, like you'd say the maternal instinct was kicking in. No. It was completely... I had nothing, nothing at all. It was weird for us at first, and at first we had all forgotten that I was pregnant. It didn't feel like anything had changed for us. ... It starts to change when the belly starts, for me, when my belly started to grow, then I kind of became aware and when the movements started." (Anđela)

In Anđela's case, too, medical technology neither contributed to the reality of the pregnancy nor helped her to visualise the baby. However, it is important to bear in mind that both participants had their ultrasound examinations performed in a state clinic and never had the opportunity to observe the monitor or receive an ultrasound image of the baby. Women whose pregnancies are monitored in public practice in Serbia usually do not have the opportunity to observe the baby on the monitor during the examinations, which puts them in a very different situation compared to pregnant women in many other countries. This fact may partly explain the peculiarity of the findings in this study that are in discordance with many reports from other institutional settings. How a woman perceives the ultrasound examination and the impact it has on how she experiences the pregnancy, her body and the baby she is carrying depends on how medical technology is institutionally embedded. This issue will be extensively addressed at the end of this chapter, as well as throughout the next one. Now we will focus on what women have already recognised in this section as central to the process of identifying with pregnancy and the transition to motherhood—various aspects of specifically pregnant embodiment.

3.3.2 An Altered Body: Alienation & Identification

During pregnancy, a woman's body changes considerably in shape and weight in a relatively short period of time, and these changes involve far more than just an altered appearance. The very fact that body size changes rapidly and constantly during pregnancy makes its boundaries become blurred. A woman begins to lose a precise sense of how much space her body occupies and where its limits lie, which has profound consequences. As Kristina Lemieux describes in her touching autobiographical essay (2006, p. 77): "I have been told the body is not who you are. And I believed it. But I have watched my body grow, I have watched the stretch marks appear, and it changed how I felt about myself".

The most noticeable physical change, both for the women themselves and for those around them during pregnancy, is the weight gain and the change in the size and shape of the body. Although women accept this change relatively easily as they associate it with pregnancy,[22] the relatively

[22] This change is normalised in women's narratives and seen as "natural", even though it runs counter to the prevailing norm of thinness. This is partly due to the influence of a more significant norm, namely that women should be primarily concerned with the well-being of their baby rather

rapid change in body size can also have a somewhat alienating effect—it often takes a while for them to get used to it, to "embrace" their altered body, and until then they feel strange and cannot fully identify with it.

"I wasn't too worried. I didn't fall into depression because of the weight gain. Of course, it's not like you don't care when you start gaining weight, you stand in front of the mirror sometimes and, ugh, it's not like you don't care. But I also wasn't standing in front of the mirror for hours on end to traumatise myself. I avoided looking at myself too much. (...) I understand that I'm pregnant, that it's normal to gain weight during pregnancy and that I'll lose it after pregnancy. (...) Yet, you just feel bothered by that weight. And then I thought: 'Oh God, how do fat people live? How do fat people live?' Oh, I just want to give birth to get back to my weight and feel normal. But over time, for example now in my ninth month, near the end of my pregnancy, I've gotten used to this weight so it's not as strange to me as it was in the beginning when my body was just starting to transform. So I guess you get used to it, you learn to live with it." (Maja)

Crucial to this adaptation process is not only the passage of time, but also the fact that the woman's body begins to look like a pregnant body. Previously defined body boundaries have changed and this is sometimes experienced dramatically. This situation of uncertainty can be resolved by the growth of the belly and the specific change in body shape, which undoubtedly indicates pregnancy and the presence of the baby—both for others and for the woman herself:[23]

than their physical appearance. Furthermore, during pregnancy they cease to be sexual objects for others, and excessive concern for their appearance could be interpreted as a subversion of the representation of a pregnant woman as a non-erotic object.

[23] Although this is usually the case, for some women the noticeable growth of the belly alone leads them to perceive the body change as too significant and destabilising for their sense of identity, accompanied by a feeling of alienation. But even for them, the process ends with identification with their "new" body: *"And already, towards the end of the fourth or fifth month, the belly suddenly starts to grow, you suddenly start to change, and it's really a trip where you don't recognize your body. It was a trip. I stand in front of the mirror and it's not like some bad feeling, oh I've gained weight... no, not at all. Somehow you know what that stomach is for and then you start to feel the movements and all that, but it's still weird. You look in the mirror and suddenly it's like it's not your stomach anymore. ... But that feeling is kind of over for me, that trip, and then when you get used to it, then it's all ... And now I'm thinking to myself, like what will I do without this bump? Really, it's a feeling, oh, now suddenly this is my body." (Nevena)*

"In the beginning, I found it hard to accept my belly, in the sense that I looked deformed to myself somehow. I struggled to accept my appearance in the mirror. It was a bit uncomfortable and awkward for me. However, the bigger it got, the easier it was for me, that's interesting. Somehow you see that it's a big baby and that's how it should be. But when it was something in between, it felt weird." (Saška)

"So, the biggest crisis I had with my body image was in the beginning... Actually, I started freaking out when I lost my waist. In the third or fourth month. And when I started to gain weight. And when my clothes got visibly smaller and my belly still was not there. Then I moaned: 'I want my belly to show!', not because others would know, but so that I would know what the hell is happening with me. ... Later on, I somehow got some pregnant form, but a metamorphosis into a pregnant woman, it wasn't really. ... You lose your waistline, you lose definition. I had psychological issues and most of my body image... where are my measurements, where is my end? And where's my shape? The first month I had no shape, it was a total drama." (Sonja)

Our bodies have a public dimension, and this public dimension is not only relevant to other people, but also to ourselves—our embodied experience changes as this dimension changes (Clark et al., 2009). As Judith Butler (2004, p. 21) suggests, our bodies "are not quite ever only our own" but have an "invariably public dimension; constituted as a social phenomenon in the public sphere, my body is and is not mine".[24] Bodily changes that unproblematically indicate pregnancy carry positive connotations. Unlike other reproductive phases such as menstruation and menopause, where the uncontrollability and unpredictability of the body (its odour, sweat, bleeding) are often a source of discomfort and shame because the environment reacts negatively to either showing or failed concealment (Ussher, 2008), the physical symptoms of pregnancy are "forgiven".

[24] The fact that information about a pregnancy becomes publicly available due to physical symptoms changes a woman's social status. In this study, the public dimension of the pregnant body, i.e. a woman's experience of her own body as it is *for others*, was not explored in detail, so this relevant and interesting topic remains insufficiently addressed. However, in the narratives, women often talked about their privileged status in public as they became visibly pregnant because people around them treated them with extra care and consideration. Many also expressed a sense of longing in advance for this stage of life, as they are aware that this will change as soon as they give birth, as the baby will then be the centre of attention.

It is important to understand that the new, pregnant embodiment entails much more than just a changed reflection in the mirror. It brings with it a different experience of boundaries, altered patterns of movement, a shifted perspective from which the world is observed and acted upon. Although the process of adapting to the new body is primarily the result of a series of spontaneous transformations, it also involves active adjustments. Adapting to the changed physical situation is not only a passive process, but also a form of learning and practising, similar to acquiring new skills, as women need to master their bodies in order to accomplish some everyday tasks that they performed automatically before pregnancy.

"You find your own technique on how to get up, how to squat, kneel, not kneel, lean to one side, the other side, it's important to have a way to get up." (Ivana)

"Somehow you learn to make it easier for yourself. Because, you find a position, and that's exactly what I said earlier, that it's easier for me to squat, easier to stand up, because it seems like I learned how to do it. And now, at the end of pregnancy, it seems to me that I will never be able to go back to how it was before, I will never be able to bend normally again. It seems like I'll stay like this forever. Now it has become so normal to me that it seems like I will have these movements forever." (Anđela)

After some time women manage to get used to their altered body, its capabilities, limitations and movement patterns. Although they "come to terms with their body schema" and identify with the pregnant form, to the point of wondering what they will do without their belly, they often continue to act as if they have their "old body", which is not pregnant. This is consistent with Iris Marion Young's suggestion (2005b, p. 50) that "in pregnancy my prepregnant body image does not entirely leave my movements and expectations, yet it is with the pregnant body that I must move". Women often inadequately estimate how much space their body takes up and where its limits lie:

"I wasn't aware of my stomach at all, not even now. It always seem to me that I'll go through and then I get stuck. I mean, you can't get through. Or I don't know, there's a coat rack here in our apartment, and there's the light switch, and

I hang up my jacket and turn off the light a hundred times with my belly. ***I don't have the feeling that it's part of my body at all.*** *I haven't gotten used to it at all. Also, when someone is sitting there and I want to pass by, I'm sure I can do it, but I can't. I don't have that sense in my head of how big I actually am and how much space my body takes up." (Anđela)*

"I don't have that sense, I go and I bump into something still. Or now I want to squeeze through something because you're just used to being able to pass through it, you don't think that you're much bigger now. And then you're trying to squeeze through and bump a little bit. Or I bump into the corner of a table, it's a regular thing... ***you don't have the feeling that there's something so big in front of you.*** *" (Jasna)*

What women report when they talk about "getting used to" their bodies actually corresponds to aspects of both body image and body schema—changes in their attitudes and perception of their body as well as changes in the experience of body movement and posture. Both systems are complex and interact closely and intricately during intentional actions (Gallagher, 2005), so that some aspects are adapted more successfully, while others less so. What makes this situation additionally interesting is that it involves not only objective physical changes and their phenomenological aspect. Embodiment in pregnancy, as in other life situations, is mediated by representations and norms that shape our specific experiences and conduct. In the case of pregnancy, the dominant representations and norms relate to the developing baby in the womb and the desire to protect it.

"I've noticed that when it's a tighter space that I put my hand on my belly, but I still estimate that I can get through. So if I'm asking my brain now - I can pass through there. I couldn't figure myself out at all." (Sonja)

"But now, for example, I'm aware that I have a belly because I find myself unconsciously holding my belly when I walk past people. So no one bumps into me." (Sofija)

Consideration for the baby and the need to protect it have thus led to the belly being constantly present, albeit in an implicit way. The fact that women typically identify with their condition during pregnancy implies that they begin to perceive and experience their body as the space in which the baby is developing and as something that sustains its life:

> *"The woman turns into a kind of small cocoon for the baby." (Una)*
>
> *"I feel it, I'm aware of everything every second. I never forget. I was even afraid that I might turn onto my stomach at night, because I like to sleep on my stomach. That's what I was afraid of, but it never happened. I feel like my brain is constantly focused on that. And I've read that pregnant women start forgetting things and they should write them down. And then there's no medical explanation, they're just thinking about the baby. And I'm the perfect example of that. Because I really don't think about anything else, I only think about the baby. I don't know how I passed my exams, how I was able to concentrate. Because I'm constantly thinking about the baby and I can't let anything slip by to make a mistake. ...* ***At every moment I'm aware of my belly and her presence.*** *It never happens to me to forget that I'm pregnant and about her. I'm really focused only on her. Even when I sleep, I don't end up lying on my stomach." (Saška)*

In the next part of the analysis, we will focus on the process during which the baby becomes more and more concrete and autonomous for the woman, even though it is still part of her body. However, it is important to keep in mind that the baby is not only explicitly present in the woman's experience during pregnancy. It is also implicitly present, almost all the time. This implicit presence involves an intensified focus on her own body, which constantly appears in her experience as something that needs to be protected and treated with care. Nevertheless, its explicit presence—experiencing the baby's movements and recognising its activity patterns—significantly changes the phenomenological and existential situation of women and plays a crucial role in the process of becoming a mother.

3.3.3 Birth of Intersubjectivity: From Quickening to the Individuation of the Baby

During pregnancy, women face a specific challenge—how can they experience and imagine a being that is simultaneously present and absent and that changes rapidly and constantly? This section will attempt to identify a process by which a woman begins to experience and imagine the baby as a separate being, possessing a certain degree of autonomy, personal characteristics and patterns of behaviour. A crucial aspect of this process is related to the embodied feeling of the baby's movements being experienced as "truly real", but medical knowledge/technology continues to play an important role, particularly in the early stages. Based on the changing patterns and quality of these bodily sensations, which inform women about the other being's inner movements, women typically construct an increasingly differentiated and complex picture of the presence, activities and characteristics of their future child. This process of individuation of the baby for the mother enables the beginning of a real relationship and a sense of belonging. The gradual emergence of the baby as a relatively autonomous subject is a prerequisite for the expectant mother's personal transition to a new identity, but also announces the beginning of their mutual interaction and communication as "pregnancy is about the making of new individuals, about processes of individuation, about two bodies becoming one, one body becoming two" (van der Ploeg, 2004, p. 155).

Embodied Experience of Baby's Movement: Quickening as "The Real Deal"

The pregnant woman has a privileged epistemic access to the foetus that is in a phenomenological sense very peculiar. Pregnancy is the only life situation in which the sensations coming from the interior of our bodies not only say something about ourselves—our body parts and their functioning—but also about an object in the world, i.e. the Other. This determines the specific quality of this experience, but also the uncertainty that accompanies its appropriate interpretation. It is quite common for us to experience and interpret the coldness we feel on our palm while holding an ice cube as indicating the coldness of the object we are holding, rather than the coldness of the hand itself, even though we actually feel the coldness of the hand. But the hand does not appear to us as an object—it is only implicitly present as a "means" of experiencing the world. If, on the other hand, we feel a cramp or a vibration in our stomach, we usually experience and interpret this as an indicator of processes in the visceral organs themselves, which always appear to us as objects, never as a point of view on the world. In the case of the baby's movements, this is precisely where the peculiarity lies—the woman relies on sensations from inside her body, not to learn something about the body itself, but to perceive the characteristics and activity of another being.

The phenomenological specificities of interoception, as discussed at the beginning of this chapter, determine the possibilities and limitations of the embodied experience of the baby. Albeit vague and often uncertain, a woman's insight is embodied and concrete, and from a certain point in pregnancy she is clearly aware of the baby's touch and movements. Before the advent of technology that allowed very early detection of pregnancy, quickening was considered the first reliable sign of pregnancy. It announced that the process a woman's body was going through, which manifested itself in many other ways, would (probably) end with childbirth and not with a miscarriage or the onset of illness (Duden, 1991).[25] The experience of foetal movement thus had not only a personal but also a social significance, although its authoritative status is debatable, as we discussed in Chap. 2.

The medical literature points out that women who are pregnant for the first time feel the foetal movements exactly halfway through pregnancy—at four and a half months or 20 weeks—which doctors used to rely on when assessing gestational age (Mladenović et al., 2008, p. 289). As a rule, women have an acquired expectation of when they should feel the baby's movements. As that period approaches, they become particularly focused on bodily experiences that can be indicators of movements—experiences that would probably not be noticed at all in any other life situation or would be interpreted completely differently and would have no relevance. Moreover, they are usually familiar with *what it feels like* and then try to recognise it in themselves.

[25] For centuries, quickening had legal significance as one of the criteria by which a foetus was declared alive, and accordingly abortion was considered murder (Duden, 1991, p. 82).

"At the beginning you're not sure at all, with everything you think 'aha, here it comes, it's starting now', because you somehow expect it. And then like you think even from the gut, if your bowels rumble, you think 'aha, baby, baby'. So you're a little bit obsessed with it, just to feel it a little bit. But all the movements feel very, very funny, like something is twinkling in your belly. ... And I think that was it. But I don't know for sure." (Maja)

"They say from the sixteenth to the twentieth week, it all depends on whether it's your first, second, third baby. The first baby announces itself later, but since I'm slimmer, I should feel it earlier. Now, there are different stories about how it feels. Like if you squeeze a chick in your fist and then it moves, to stories like when you have gas in your stomach, it feels like something is tickling you. So these are different stories but in the end it didn't seem like any of that to me... but oh well. And then people start asking you, not intentionally, from about sixteen weeks, did you feel the movements, did you feel the movements? I didn't feel them. That does cause a bit of panic. I didn't feel it, so what now? But it's also normal until the twentieth week. Until the nineteenth week, I was calm. But from the nineteenth to the twentieth I started to wonder if I'll feel it already now, so it wasn't easy for me anymore, I was coming to an end and I was like maybe I did feel it, but I didn't recognize it." (Tamara)

Both the time frame and the quality of the experience are therefore largely regulated—partly by the widely available medical knowledge and expectations, and partly by the experiences of other women. This normative context actually determines when, to what extent and on which physical signals women concentrate and tune in at all. And since it is not so easy to fit one's own—specific, unclear, ambivalent—experiences into the expected normative framework, this process is uncertain and often leads to anxiety and concern. This is another example of how bodily experience, at least until she learns to "read" it, is not a straightforward matter for the individual.

"I wasn't at all sure if that was it. Because I was thinking I should have felt it by now, why haven't I, how, where, what is it, why isn't it. And then I thought, when I did start to feel something, I thought if this was it, but I wasn't sure. And then I read on the internet that some women wrote they started feeling it in the twelfth or thirteenth week, especially if it's the second pregnancy, then you're more aware so you can feel it. But I also asked the doctor and she said,

'No, not until the twentieth week, don't think about it yet'. And afterwards it was like some bubbles were popping in my belly, so I wondered whether it was it, or not. But I could only feel it when I concentrated." (Anđela)

"And then, when you feel the movements for the first time, then you're not sure about these movements. Because I receive text messages from the city of Belgrade, because they send these messages.[26] *So I knew roughly when the movements should be felt and what they should look like, but you're not sure. You're not sure if it's your bowels working or if you're really feeling something or if you're imagining it." (Tanja)*

The first movements are often not at all different from the sensations the women have experienced before, but they have associated them with other conditions, and now they must learn to recognise them as indicators of the baby's activity. They often rely on the experiences of other women around them and try to find out details about the quality of these experiences to recognise them more easily. Sometimes they seek the opinion of a doctor or technologically mediated information, especially if they are going through a long period of uncertainty.

"One day in the twentieth week I went to the doctor for an ultrasound and he told me that the baby seemed restless and constantly moving, that everything was fine. That night I could feel the baby moving. Whether it had something to do with what he told me or maybe I had felt it before but didn't recognise it, I don't know. (...) Of course, I was overjoyed to have felt it at all, but I was calm because I had been to the doctor that day so I knew everything was fine and that I would feel it eventually." (Tamara)

[26] Similar to the numerous pregnancy tracking apps available, a public service was established at one point that sent pregnant women messages to their cell phones with information about their pregnancy—providing week to week insights into what is happening in their bodies, how their pregnancy is progressing and what medical check-ups should be scheduled: *"They send me this two or three times a week. They track your pregnancy and tell you what's happening that particular week, what tests you need to do that week or what might be critical during that period. The messages are very specific and offer explanations if you have any doubts. They also guide you by suggesting, for example, that it's is time for an amniocentesis, a double test, an expert ultrasound or checking antibodies if you are Rh negative. They might remind you that it's time to check smears and blood work, or inform you that the baby is now a certain size and you should start to feel movements. They usually focus on what's characteristic of that week and keep you informed, even if your doctor doesn't"* (Tanja)- This service functions as a kind of monitoring and disciplining technology that introduces medical discourse into the pregnant woman's everyday life and sets norms for her imagination and behavior.

Medical technology freed Tamara from the anxiety caused by the absence of embodied information that was expected due to the assumed norms. This interviewee is specific in that she tends to prioritise medical information and the authority of doctors in various situations, but this role of ultrasound also occurs among women who are inclined to rely heavily on their embodied experience. We will return to Mirjana's case later when we analyse how the process of individuation of the baby takes place, based mainly on her experience of the baby's movements. Initially, however, the ultrasound also allowed her to reduce anxieties and fears arising from the fact that her bodily experience did not fit adequately into the established normative framework.

> *"The first time I felt the movements was around the fifth month. But it was something very gentle. I was even scared, I said 'Oh God what is this, do all women feel like this?' Cause I read on the internet and for me it was... I felt almost nothing. And I got a bit scared, everyone around me was talking about their babies moving back and forth and my baby was not moving. You know, I feel like some little scratching, but it's not... And then like 'Oh God, is everything okay?' You read about how other women feel, but you don't see yourself in that story. And then I went to the doctor and told her all this and she said, 'Do not worry, we'll take a look'. And then she looked at the ultrasound and said 'Everything is fine, it has a normal cardiac response, but it's a quiet baby'." (Mirjana)*

Although it usually takes some time and practise for a woman to begin to distinguish and register different sensations as indicators of the baby's activity, this very specific phenomenological situation often leads her to describe this experience as something very special, sometimes even as a "unique" female experience.

> *"That's a really special feeling, and I told my husband that I'm sorry that men can't experience it and that I'm really... really sorry for them, that they're handicapped for that one feeling. Like, everything in life we can both feel, but that feeling of something moving inside you, we just won't be able to depict it to them, it's just... what does it remind us of, what does it resemble? It doesn't resemble anything, it's just unique. I mean, it's really a special feeling and you can't compare it, at least I can't compare it to anything." (Nevena)*

Given that this kind of experience is relatively rare, and even more so considering the fact that it's not accessible to men, women have no conceptual apparatus readily available to them when they want to describe how they feel. Instead, they have to resort to metaphors and analogies.

"Like when you're swimming in a pool and you pass by someone's body, it's kind of that feeling, but from the inside. And then, you know, more and more, you feel it more and more often because it's bigger and then... So you can clearly see when it moves here, you feel how it shifts, there, back and forth, it's really strange. ***Indescribable****. You have something alive inside you. And that's exactly like that... strange." (Mirjana)*

The quality of the experience of the baby's movements changes over the course of the pregnancy as the baby grows and takes up more space. While the movements are barely noticeable and difficult to differentiate at the beginning, by the sixth month onwards the baby's kicks are clearly felt. Towards the end of pregnancy, the woman is almost always aware of the baby's presence and activity and perceives its movements differently (such as pushing or stretching).

"Maybe in the third or fourth month I started feeling like I had some little fish swimming in my stomach, flipping around. Those were the first sensations. Then in the fifth month, when I saw her and her sex and everything, maybe it started a bit stronger. I felt it regularly, little by little. And I could feel exactly how she was gaining strength and growing. So from these little fish to slightly stronger kicks, like she was slapping me with her little hand. And now it's great because there's no room, so she just wriggles and pushes, not kicking but pushing you because there's no space. I've really felt her grow. It is great." (Saška)

"Well, I don't know, it's something you could mistake for gas in your stomach. It feels like a flickering. Later on, it's just, you really tactilely feel it, it really thumps... earlier she used to thump me here when she was positioned differently, thump, thump, thump, and then she calms down again. But generally, I felt her the most when I was sitting down, when I was lying on my back, that's when I felt her the most, in the seventh, eighth month. No matter what I was doing, or if I was walking, I felt her less then. But as soon as I sat down and adjust a bit, there she goes. It's different than now, for example. Now it's maybe not so much thumping, more like nudging. Maybe there's not so much space now, so she's

nudging more, and you can see it now. The whole belly ripples. And now it doesn't matter whether I'm standing or lying on my side, on my back. Now you simply feel her every move. It's no longer kicks, it's more like nudging, like she's or stretching. Sometimes I really get the impression that she stretches her legs and then pushes off with her foot on my stomach." (Teodora)

While in the middle of pregnancy it is necessary for a woman to calm down and interrupt her activities in order to feel the movements and presence of the baby, as time passes that presence becomes more obvious and continuous. As the baby takes up a significantly larger part of the woman's pregnant body, it becomes constantly present in her experiences and interactions with the world. This implies that it is not so easy for a woman to focus on her life projects (such as work) because there is a parallel occurrence from which she cannot isolate herself so easily. In fact, this is a situation in which, in usual circumstances, the body recedes into the background so that the woman, as an embodied subject, can be directed towards the external world undisturbed. However, due to the activity of the baby, which she feels almost all the time, the woman's body is very often in the foreground at the end of pregnancy and the world withdraws into the background.

"Now in the end, the problem is to keep focus, your brain is bye bye. Because this baby of mine is very restless, pushing and shoving, even at work I can't sit still for that long. Your, let's say, focus of thought, simply shifts." (Ivana)

Over time, the woman becomes "bodily aware" of the baby's presence, and this awareness becomes more frequent and longer as the pregnancy progresses. For most women, this plays the most important role in identifying with the pregnancy and bonding with the baby—initiating a transition from *knowing* to *feeling* that they are pregnant.

"I think with that first movement comes the feeling that you are pregnant. Although, these movements are not like that in the beginning and then somehow ... it always surprises you. You know, you are like 'aha, here she is!' In the very beginning, when my stomach was still flat, it was more like, I don't know, maybe more knowledge than the feeling itself. ***I knew I was pregnant, but now I really feel it****. Any way I turn, there is no way I can avoid it." (Nevena)*

"So I don't know now... for me, apart from these movements that connect me to her, that she pushes me, so now I know 'aha, there she is'. It's just that these are first signs where the two of us get to know each other, and that's something that connects me to her. But if she was very still in my belly, I would feel like I'd put on weight." (Teodora)

We have already seen that, at least initially, quickening is not a completely immediate process, but that medical knowledge plays an important role in shaping expectations and interpretative frameworks. In addition, medical techniques, particularly ultrasound, play a role in how the baby is experienced and how this embodied experience is interpreted. Throughout pregnancy, women adjust their expectations and interpretations based on the evolving patterns of baby's activity. Obvious changes or deviations are then the cue for needing and requesting some kind of external confirmation that all is well.

"With the first baby, the fact that it wasn't moving was normal. But it's a matter of habit. Now when this one doesn't move all the time, then you start to think like he is quiet, maybe childbirth starts, maybe something's wrong? Because you come to understand those movements as the norm, you reach the point where that's how it should be. At first, I didn't feel anything. Then everything was like zoom, zoom, I was like 'What's happening to me now?' And now he moves all the time, and when he doesn't move, then it's not normal for me. (...) I guess you get so used to your child, you learn together with him." (Ivana)

"These last few days I see that she's calmer, and I'm like, 'Is everything okay, man?' And I sit and say to her, 'Come on, give me a little nudge, kick me, do this, do that.' And I see that it's noticeably less. So I went online and did a little searching. And it exactly says like, 'Your baby will become calmer in the 36th week, you might feel it occasionally, but stronger kicks.' And that's just how it is for me right now." (Sofija)

In the later stages of pregnancy, then, technologically mediated experiences or medical knowledge play a significant role for women when they cannot rely on their embodied experience or are unsure how to interpret it. Thus, not only are these two modes of experience not mutually exclusive, but they often interact with each other and appear in a coordinated way in women's experiences during pregnancy. This conclusion is revisited at the end of the chapter.

Evolving Individuation of the Baby for the Mother-to-Be

There is a gradually changing embodied experience of being pregnant and having a baby inside the body. While the evolving of this experience undeniably leads to an increasing identification with pregnancy, it also leads to the individuation of the baby for the mother. Adrienne Rich (1986b, p. 63) expresses this twofold, interdependent and only seemingly contradictory process as follows: "(...) I experience the embryo (…) as something inside and of me, yet becoming hourly and daily more separate, on its way to becoming separate and of–itself. In early pregnancy the stirring of the fetus felt like ghostly tremors of my own body, later like the movements of a being imprisoned in me; but both sensations were my sensations, contributing to my own sense of physical and psychic space".

In the previous sections, the role of ultrasound in early identification with pregnancy was discussed in detail. It was mentioned that the embodied experience of pregnancy, particularly in relation to the baby's movements, plays a much more significant role later on, enabling the woman to experience her altered state as a new reality. This process of appropriation of pregnancy is essentially linked to the fact that the baby becomes more specific for the pregnant woman and begins to be perceived as a separate being. Both medical knowledge/technology and the woman's embodied experience play a significant role in the individualisation of the baby for the (expectant) mother, and we will try to trace the dynamics of their relative contributions and their mutual interaction.

We can reasonably ask ourselves whether there is ever a moment in pregnancy in which a woman experiences a new state without the baby being (at least phantasmatically) present. It is clear from the pregnancy narratives that the baby is present for the woman from the very beginning, even if the modality of its presence changes considerably over the course of pregnancy. It has already been mentioned that all participants adopt a cautious and protective attitude from the beginning, not only towards their condition in general, but specifically towards the fact that another being is developing in their womb. This is reflected in the fact that they often no longer wear tight pants so as not to squeeze the baby, or no longer sleep on their stomachs for the same reason. In the beginning, however, the baby is present in a completely undefined way—it has neither an independent existence nor specific characteristics.

It seems that in the early stages of pregnancy, the images and information provided by ultrasound allow the process of individuation of the baby to begin before the woman begins to feel its movements, because medical technology is then the only source of information. However, the technologically mediated knowledge only provides women with *a generic and unspecified representation of the baby*, which is still far removed from the concrete idea of an autonomous being that they perceive as their own. The first examinations can even trigger the fear that "something is wrong" because women have no fixed normative expectations of what the foetus should look like and how its heartbeat should sound.

> *"B: How did you feel when you saw the foetus for the first time?"*
>
> *"Well, it's as if I have an alien inside me. The heart beats very fast then, something over 150–160 beats per minute, and it goes like 'thump thump thump' (very fast). And while she (the doctor) explains to you that it's normal for it to beat so fast, and you get the feeling ... it's even a bit scary ... it's so small and so out of human shape and you somehow get the impression that something is wrong. (...) You can see that everything is undefined, like a head is springing up here ... I didn't like to look at these first ultrasounds in detail." (Saška)*

Often the strongest impression is the fact that what is seen on the screen (or on the picture the woman can take home) looks too different from the baby after birth, i.e. from the "real baby" Tanja, for example, relies on information from the internet to create a normative context for the assimilation of what she can see during the ultrasound scan.

> *"I didn't really ask them to show me anything, but on several occasions they themselves were like 'look, here are the hands, the legs, look how beautiful he is'. Sometimes they give you that little picture. Although, so to say, in these pictures these babies look like aliens. Like my child looks more like some... I don't even know what, than like a baby, but okay. Afterwards, you look a bit on the internet and stuff, because there are these websites, I leave my email address, and*

> *then they send you something like, 'This is happening in this week, this is how your baby looks like', and then you get a bit used to it...'"* (Tanja)

It seems that many couples, faced with the anxiety of imagining an unfinished, sexless and undifferentiated being, try to alleviate it by giving the foetus a nickname when they see it for the first time.

> *"And then my boyfriend and I called it 'Lizzy', because it seemed to us in the picture, she gave us that picture, it looked like some kind of lizard. And since we didn't know if it was a boy or a girl, then like 'little lizard'. And until about the fourth or fifth month, we called the baby 'little Lizzy'."* (Saška)

The nickname is usually humorous and does not refer to a human being nor does it serve as a personal name—for example, Nevena called the foetus "pasuljče" (because it looks like a small bean), Sonja, "smoki" (because it looks like Flipsy, a type of snack), Saška, "gmiza" (because it reminded her of a little lizard). This name is simultaneously idiosyncratic and in a sense represents endearment, so it seems to enable the beginning of attachment to the foetus, its appropriation and an initial step in the process of the baby's individuation. This way of referring to the foetus is something that future parents share and that is unique to them, causing the not-yet-formed foetus to lose some of its generic character and enter the symbolic universe of the expectant family as a more specific being. Typically, this nickname is retained for the first few months until the woman experiences the first movements, which are an important prerequisite for the further individualisation of the baby for her.

The ultrasound also enables a woman to find out an important characteristic of the baby that is not accessible in any other way—the sex. Then the process of gendering the baby begins as it becomes a boy or a girl for the future parents, which provides different frameworks for attributing characteristics, imagining the future life with the child, and even making practical decisions such as buying baby items or choosing names. Therefore, information about the baby's sex plays a significant role in experiencing the baby as a being with certain characteristics.

"Like when he told me the sex, even though I didn't explicitly say I wanted to know. When he said, 'Oh, it's a boy', I smiled as if it was... And then he asked me, 'Why are you grinning?' and I said, 'I don't know?' I mean, I really don't know, because if he had said it was a girl, it would've been the same for me. The idea that this something has a sex. It's like a little living being, completely incredible. And every time you get an input like that, you feel great." (Una)

In the previous section on the role of ultrasound in identification with pregnancy, it was emphasised that this role primarily pertains to the first few months, when the woman does not yet feel any movements and her belly does not grow noticeably. During this period, the ultrasound confirmation of pregnancy, which makes it possible to see "something"—which is not yet a developed image of the baby and requires a certain amount of anticipation and imagination—makes the pregnancy "more real" for the woman herself. In this way, medical technology relieves the woman from some of the uncertainty that often accompanies the onset of pregnancy and worries about whether the pregnancy will continue. Later ultrasound examinations bring something more than just confirm the health of the baby—they allow her to see something on the screen that closely resembles the shape and features of a baby, enabling a further step of identification with the pregnancy.

"Well, you know, when he's so small, you're like afraid that everything is as it should be. You're in fear, just that everything is as it should be. And then when I saw him looking like a little baby at six weeks, like you know, he has fingers, man, you can see the fingers, it's something incredible. It was like 'Whoa!', you know 'Wow!' Then you truly realise it's a beautiful feeling. You realise that, you know, everything is like alright now. You like breathe a sigh of relief. Okay, it has everything it should have. Somehow, now that it's a bigger baby, you're more connected to it and you really consider it as a being." (Mirjana)

Although the entire narrative is still coloured by concern for the baby's health, the fact that a woman can see that the foetus she is carrying in her womb has fully taken on the form and characteristics of a baby enables a further step in the process of baby's individuation and brings her great joy.

"At about four and a half months, that's when I went for an ultrasound, that's when I saw the little legs and feet, and what it looks like when it crosses its legs, that this little thing can already cross its legs and that it's already alive. And that it moves its arms, legs, it swims, it enjoys, does acrobatics, that it has enough space. And again it all ended with 'so everything is as it should be, that's it'. That ultrasound was more interesting for me because you really see a lot there, the feet and the little toes were already more or less there. And everything was starting to take shape more or less. When he starts telling me that the baby already has a bladder, kidneys, and that baby is this big (show with her fingers). She's just 15 cm and that's really fascinating." (Teodora)

The baby on the screen sometimes even shows activities that are typical of a much older child (crossed legs, somersaults). Such insights often fascinate women, and they are surprised at how early the foetus' organs develop and it takes on a human form, even though it is only the beginning of the pregnancy and the foetus is still very small.

"And then, when I managed to recognise the baby on the ultrasound on my own, it was beautiful. It has already taken on human form. And I see that she is a girl, I see her moving. This is very interesting. The first time I saw a real baby, she was still so small that she could turn around and swim in the womb, it was the fifth month. And while we were watching her, she literally did a roll forward and then a roll back. It was incredible, she was really swimming in a circle like that. That was incredible, and the gynaecologist laughed, 'Oh, this baby is so restless!' and we realised that she's very active, that she is restless. It was something really cute. Truly wonderful. And she was waving her hands and legs like that..." (Saška)

It is very interesting that all three interviewees (Mirjana, Teodora, Saška) rely heavily on their embodied experience of pregnancy and the baby, and this does not seem to contradict their extremely positive attitude towards technologically mediated experiences. This insight is significant insofar as it problematises the fairly common view, particularly in the earlier feminist-oriented literature, of the exclusive relationship between these two modalities of experiencing pregnancy and the baby, which I will return to in detail at the end of this chapter. Even if the idea of their antagonism seems unlikely, can we assume that these two different modalities of experience play somewhat different roles for women?

One possibility, supported by the accounts of some women, is that the ultrasound experience of the foetus contributes to the individuation of the baby, but only to a certain extent. From the ultrasound image, the woman begins to understand that "this living thing inside her" has the form of a baby. However, it is a generic form, based on which her baby looks like all other babies. The woman cannot rely on the ultrasound image to tell her that it is not just *a baby* she is carrying in her womb, but *her baby*, a being with specific characteristics. Therefore, even the most positive reports leave an impression of fascination, similar to what we might experience, even those of us who are not pregnant, when we encounter the "magic of life" or the fact that "something of 15 centimetres already has a bladder and kidneys" or that "it can cross its legs".

> *"Well, maybe I'm not even fully aware of what's going on in there. I mean, I know it's a baby and that's all great and we're going to have a baby, but it's fascinating that from these two cells... It completely blew my mind. When I was in Belgrade and they did that 4D ultrasound, and when I saw his picture, you know, a real baby. He was like tossing around, putting his hands like that, it was just awesome." (Mirjana)*

A woman who is pregnant certainly experiences this image much more emotionally than someone who is not pregnant, because this "incredible" process is taking place in her body. But it is only when the embodied experience of the baby enters the stage that it becomes clear what women rely on first and foremost when it comes to appropriating pregnancy and bonding with the baby. Mirjana, for example, who was openly enthusiastic about the insights from the ultrasound, recognises only the embodied experience of the baby's movements as crucial to experiencing the foetus in the womb as her future child. This same participant talked a lot about being able to recognise patterns in the baby's activity and even interact with her baby based on embodied experience, which will be the focus of the next section.

"When it starts kicking you in the stomach, then you start to experience it as your child. Then you realise that it's... Because you see, on the ultrasound, it's all there, but it's still just an image. And this, when it starts shaking..." (Mirjana)

In a direct comparison of the two modalities of experiencing the baby, it becomes clear that they do not have the same status for the woman. The technologically mediated experience becomes the one that ultimately provides "just an image". And the image is perceived as less realistic, or at least less relevant information about the presence of an independent being compared to the embodied experience of "kicking in the stomach". After all, the image is "out there", displaced on a monitor that can reflect something unclear and deceptive, while the kick or "when it starts shaking" is something a woman cannot ignore, much like the signals from her own body.[27]

Interacting with "The Autonomous Being Inside Me"

Based on the changing patterns and quality of embodied sensations of the baby's movements, women typically construct an increasingly differentiated and complex picture of the presence, activity and characteristics of their future child. Pregnant women often try to recognise at what times of day and how often their babies "announce" themselves, and they estimate from this when the babies are asleep and when they are awake and active. These *sporadic* experiences of movement form the basis for the construction of the activity cycle and the notion of the baby's *constant* presence in the woman's body, even if she only senses it occasionally over several months. On this basis, women anticipate (and later recognise) the continuity between the baby in the womb and the baby after birth.

"He doesn't sleep when I want to sleep, that's normal. So, you get into a certain rhythm. (...) I think it's around six in the morning when I have to get up to pee, and then when I get back into bed he starts moving, fidgeting, and then he

[27] Leder (1990, p. 91–92) calls this a "telic demand"—in some states (e.g. illness, but also pregnancy) the body simply cannot be ignored, nor does it allow us to do nothing about what is happening to it.

calms down again. Then the same when I lie down, whenever that is, then he plays his little session. (...) Now, for example, he has just been fidgeting, and then he'll be quiet for two or three hours... Well yeah, now he has the baby's rhythm, and it will probably stay that way when he's born. To fidget a bit, and then sleep." (Ivana)

"She has her own rhythm, I know it now, she is more restless at night... There are exactly these intervals when she is more awake, and I guess she will continue like that after birth." (Sonja)

Recognising the rhythm of activity leads to further individuation of the baby for the mother, as the baby becomes a being with differentiated habits, moods and even character traits, receptive to the environment.

"He also has this trick, probably to annoy me, as if he's stretching with his arms and legs at the same time, so he's kind of splayed out on all sides. And you just can't sit down, you just have to stand up, move, you have to react somehow. (...) I think it's a kind of ***his need to do something*** *... because* ***he's either trying out his strength or he's just being saucy****, it's one of these two. (...) When I go to bed,* ***I think he senses that I want to sleep, so he won't let me****. Or he adjusts his position, I don't know,* ***but we really feel each other****. (...) And he reacts, he reacts. He doesn't like some positions at all... I mean, during the ultrasound, he argues with (the doctor)... he just feels the pressure and then he kicks, he tries to do something. (...) And I figured out that he reacts to other kids making noise, he kicks then, like he would like to play, which will probably be the case when he comes out..." (Ivana)*

In Ivana's experience and imagination, the baby is a completely autonomous being. She speaks of it as if it had already been born and attributes to it certain psychological states, motives and even character traits. The fact that the baby is separated from external surroundings by the skin of the belly and that it is actually inside her body seems to be a completely contingent (and irrelevant) circumstance. She also recognises that the baby sometimes reacts to her movements and positions, and she herself feels the need to adapt to the baby. Therefore, she imagines the baby as a psychologically complex being, receptive to stimuli from the environment, with feelings, motives, reactions, preferences, etc. That is, based on her embodied experience, she perceives it as an independent and, to a certain extent, developed subject.

Recognising the pattern of activity allows women to form certain expectations and develop some daily practices that seem to represent the beginning of a true relationship with the baby. Realising the baby's rhythm and adapting to it gives them a sense of community or togetherness ("then we go to sleep"), and discerning some expressions of the baby's activity as its attempt to communicate ("to say hello") provides a sense of real interaction with it.

"Then I feel her in the morning or when I wake up, it's as if she wakes up then too, that's the impression I got, and then she starts tapping on my belly. And I found that interesting. Every morning I would wake up exactly like that. I wake up and now I wait for her to kick me three or four times and that's it." (Teodora)

"And in the morning, after I wake up, after about twenty minutes, then he starts to wake up. ... Because after that, at some point I get hungry, maybe he get's too, I don't know, but that's when I feel him. (...) Somehow, even when I go to sleep, ***there he is, just to say hello, kicks gently two or three times, and then we go to sleep****." (Mirjana)*

As the process of individuation of the baby progresses, so does its separation from the mother, which also enables the highest degree of closeness (not symbiosis!) with her—as a woman has the baby almost constantly on her mind (and in her experience), she is receptive to its (imaginary?) needs and adapts her functioning accordingly. The gradual emergence of a baby as a relatively autonomous subject is a prerequisite for interaction and communication. What develops in this phenomenological space made possible by the embodied experience of the baby's presence and activity is what we might cautiously call the birth of intersubjectivity—although the other subject is still only indirectly and imaginatively present.

"And when I scratch the other side of my belly, she moves and comes there and kicks, 'I'm here!' And that's ***my first experience of communicating with my child****. Oh, I was totally thrilled.* ***She actually listened to me, she reacted!*** *And I'm just like 'This is full communication! We're seriously talking now!' I was*

over the moon. And on the other hand, ***I listen to her too****. I notice when my posture bothers her (…) She just starts kicking down here again and again. And then, well, 'I'm sorry', so I move and she calms down. And then I adjust to suit her and ask her to move a little bit to suit me, so we kind of adjust to each other." (Sonja)*[28]

Another participant, Mirjana, also describes something that represents a complex interaction with the baby. She interprets its movements as carrying certain messages and connects them with her own behaviour. She recognises that the baby reacts to some positions of her body, to her moods, and even believes that they dance together to music.

"And then you connect somehow, you understand each other. It's like a kind of inarticulate language *(nemušti jezik)…* ***And we react to each other****. That's clear. When I bend down, like when I'm putting on my shoes or vacuuming or something, and then when I stand up, he kicks me a bit up here, like 'what are you doing to me?' And when I, I rarely get annoyed, really, but when I do get pissed off, I can feel him 'tap, tap, tap'. These reactions are like 'hey, don't do that now!', you know. Maybe I'm imagining it now, but… Yeah, or when we listen to music, it's incredible. Man, I listen to music and now I'm looking for something and when I find some really good song, I turn it up a bit and we dance, I really love to dance. And then I dance with him, like 'wou, wou!' and when I stop, he keeps going 'fuf, pup, fuf'." (Mirjana)*

This woman describes her relationship with her baby as "extremely instinctive" and finds it difficult to explain, but from her descriptions it seems that she relies entirely on embodied experience.

---

[28] It is interesting to note that one experience from the ultrasound examination was a confirmation for Sonja that it is possible to elicit a reaction from the baby through the surface of her body. By observing the baby's reaction on the screen, she immediately realised that this type of interaction was possible: *"And now she (the baby) has turned away from the doctor and it is not convenient to him, and the doctor did this tapping thing, he was poking her pretty hard with his ultrasound wand, but on the screen it looked like he was shaking her. 'Hey, what's up?' 'Move your hand!' And she moved her hand. I was like, 'Did you just nudge her and she moved or what?' 'Yes.' That was my first insight that this was possible, and then the two of us, well, we had tried that scratching thing before, when she also reacted. But this version, like I'll nudge her a bit when she's quiet and then she goes 'bump, bump, bump', and she moves."* (Sonja)

"Well, you know what, you can feel the baby, but it's some kind of indescribable connection, it's really extremely instinctive. You can't say, oh, because of this and that, I know that it's this and that. Instead, you just know. You know. I know it and he knows it. 'Aha, okay, now you'll go a little bit to the side, no problem, come on now, move a little bit down...'" (Mirjana)

All these depictions point to a situation in which a woman shares her body with her baby, who occupies a significant place in her phenomenological space during daily functioning. This specific situation of embodiment, in which a woman is not alone in her body, can be experienced and interpreted in different ways, and the prevailing cultural representations serve as a normative framework for women's expectations, although their embodied reality may deviate from and resist them.

Sharing the Body: Invasion or Duality

"I watched some BBC show called 'Taking over the body'. It fascinated me terribly. The whole story goes about what happens during pregnancy, until childbirth. And they follow some woman who is pregnant and the whole story of what's happening to her. The whole story is about the baby being some kind of alien... Well, it's called 'Taking over'. The emphasis is on what happens to the mother's body. How it changes, the uterus expands, this is pushed here, that is pushed there, the diaphragm rises so she can't breathe. So everything is cramped now, you can't eat much. I really thought when I watched this some two or three years ago, 'Bro, this kid is so demanding, it won't even let you breathe'. Pregnant women breathe three times more often in a minute... ***And I was expecting the baby to attack me from all sides*** *because I'm always so pessimistic and always worrying about everything and seeing bad outcomes. You know, it just occurred to me recently how I haven't experienced anything like that at all. I really thought it's going to be worse than ever. (...) I feel it, yes, but it's like everything is happening so slowly...* ***It's definitely not an invasion of the body, but it's all duality, like we're in the same story together. I bother her and she bothers me, I suit her and she suits me, that's how I see it. ... I really, like, feel that we're hanging out, the two of us.*** *That's exactly how I experience it." (Sonja)*

The documentary programme Sonja mentions is called "Body Story: The Takeover" (Klein, 1998). It reconstructs the process of pregnancy, focusing on the active role of the foetus as it aggressively transforms the woman's body to ensure survival. Drawing on scientific discourse, this representation dramatises the entire process of pregnancy, anthropomorphising the future human being almost from the moment it is composed of a few hundred cells and is invisible to the naked eye, and portraying the relationship between mother and baby exclusively in terms of conflict, conquest and subordination. Furthermore, although the film follows the pregnant woman and the changes she goes through, at no point do we hear her voice or her first-person experience. She is entirely reduced to a natural scientific object. On the one hand, her body is made transparent by computer simulations of the internal processes allowing us to follow the changes inside her body—such as circulation and glandular secretion as well as the development of the zygote. On the other hand, we see her behaviours and reactions—vomiting, tossing and turning in bed because she can't sleep, eating large amounts of food, grimacing in pain when the contractions start and she goes into labour—but we never hear how she experiences them. Instead, we hear a male narrator commenting on the events in a disinterested and impassive tone, similar to a well-known nature documentary series "Survival". The BBC documentary is not an isolated case when it comes to this kind of portrayal of pregnancy and the roles of the baby and the pregnant woman. Sonja herself referred to other sources—she read in a newspaper article that it is quite natural for the mother's body to reject the foetus, as it consists of both the mother's and the father's cells and is therefore treated as a foreign body. The placenta is said to play an essential role in camouflaging the foreign cells so that the mother's body does not attack them, and Sonja commented: "Wow, what a fight is going on between the mother and the baby for nine months".

The medical representation of the numerous and significant changes that occur in a woman's body as a result of pregnancy is widespread and usually familiar to women. This representation accurately describes the processes in a pregnant woman's body—but only from a third-person perspective. This distanced perspective reconstructs the situation of pregnancy as a threatening and alienating experience for the woman. From the previous analysis of *lived* bodily changes, it becomes clear that most women do not experience pregnancy as alienating or threatening, despite the negative symptoms that correspond to the medical account. The fact that they manage to associate the negative symptoms with the process of pregnancy actually enables women to accept and interpret them differently, and even directly experience them as less unpleasant.

Sonja, for example, described her experiences, which in many ways correspond to what was shown in the documentary she talked about: the baby presses on her diaphragm and she cannot get enough air—she even gets short of breath when she talks during the interview; the baby presses on her bladder and stomach, so she cannot eat as much as she'd like and feels a frequent need to urinate; she feels an increased need for sugar and believes the baby is "pulling it all to itself" as Sonja's blood results show her sugar levels are at the lower limit; her hips are expanding and preparing for birth, and at one point in the interview she even explicitly said: "I give her more and more of my internal organs".[29] Although this "takeover" of the pregnant body by the baby can be portrayed negatively, e.g. as an invasion, it is generally not experienced as such. In a woman's body, it is not a stranger, the Other, but her baby, and she interprets and describes this taking of space primarily as an indicator of the baby's growth and the fact that "it is running out of space and wants out", announcing the impending birth. Thus, the woman depicts the situation of sharing the body primarily as "duality" and "togetherness", as it allows her to relate and interact with the baby even before birth, which is significant for the continuation of the processes of individuation of the baby and bonding with her.

[29] This is a very typical situation and most women reported it as I often interviewed them towards the end of their pregnancy. For this reason, they all chose to do the interviews at their home, as they knew that their mobility was limited, that it was uncomfortable for them to sit for long periods of time, that they had an increased urge to urinate and so on. They also often became short of breath during the interview and spontaneously reflected on it.

Outcomes of the Baby's Individuation Process

It seems that women anticipate the birth of their baby quite differently depending on how the process of its individuation has unfolded during pregnancy. To illustrate this thesis, I will present two, in many ways contrasting cases.

Compared to most of the other women I interviewed, a very small part of Maja's narrative about pregnancy was devoted to the experience of the baby's movements. She mentioned that her baby was very still, and although she felt movements from the end of the fourth month, she did not distinctly experience these movements as an embodied experience of the baby's activity. It is only when the almost fully developed baby starts to move in the ninth month that she can feel something "alive" in her body, which significantly differs from the experiences of other women I have analysed previously.

> *"The bodily sensation until the ninth month...well, you can't really have that feeling like you have a baby inside you. And then when the baby grows, like now when it's almost your due date, you feel when it starts to stretch, then you feel on both left and right sides that it's something big. When it stretches, I simply feel that there's something alive inside you, that... that something exists. So it's only in the ninth month when she becomes this big that you can feel something. When she's small, no, you can have absolutely no physical sensation that something is growing inside you. Nothing." (Maja)*

Maja also emphasised the importance of the ultrasound, which made the baby more real for her and allowed her to get at least some idea about it. Based on the embodied experience, she had a rather vague impression of something she could not even imagine. It is important to remember that Maja could feel the baby's movements weeks before the ultrasound exam she described:

> *"That image from the ultrasound is just... you can really see the baby, the picture of the baby, it's just... And it's a very strange feeling.* ***You're aware all the time that you're pregnant and okay, you have something inside you. But you can't imagine that something.*** *And then when you see it for the first*

time... I was a bit startled. You know, you get scared, like 'Oh, that's a baby!' ***Only then you become aware when you see it on the ultrasound.*** *(...) When I saw the fully formed baby in 4D, only then did I realise, like, 'Aha, that's a baby'." (Maja)*

In Maja's case, the role that ultrasound can play in the individuation process is obvious—"something" she is carrying inside her becomes a baby for her. When I asked why she thinks the ultrasound left such a strong impression on her, she replies:

"Ah, that's what I'm saying, yes, it's only then, when you see it, that you realise that what you have inside you is a baby. Yes, yes, yes. Until then it's something, you think, 'aha, that's something', something, but you don't imagine it as a human at all. That it has a human form. It's strange really, ***but you don't have a sense of what that something is...***"

Based on Maja's narrative, it seems that this participant did not go through a similar process of individuation of the baby as the other participants. Although the ultrasound image occupies a very important place in her pregnancy experience, it can only provide her with the idea of a generic and unspecified object/subject. Maja did not refer to any characteristic or specific aspects of her baby, nor did she describe any forms of (proto-)interaction that occurred in the accounts of other women. This indicates that the baby did not appear to her as an independent being during pregnancy, so she maintained a symbiotic relationship typical of the early months. As a result, this woman describes something that can be recognised as an expression of separation anxiety, triggered by the fact that the baby will become a separate being after birth.

"One thing that's funny to me when I think about it, I mean how silly I think about it. ***I kind of have the baby just for myself now. And she's inside me and that's it. So she's just a part of me.*** *And then I think when I give birth, I will then share her with everyone.* ***It sounds a bit crazy, yes, but like how am I supposed to share her with everyone, she's just mine now, and after birth she'll belong to everyone.*** *So that's how I understand it a bit. That's what came to my mind, she's in me now and she's only mine." (Maja)*

I will now consider a completely opposite example. Sonja has developed a highly differentiated image of her baby and perceives it as an independent being. In the following quote, we see her reaction when someone refers to the baby by the nickname she was given at the beginning of the pregnancy. This reaction makes it clear how much Sonja's perception has shifted and how far removed her idea of the baby at the end of the pregnancy is from the vague, undifferentiated being that was constituted at the beginning of the pregnancy on the basis of the ultrasound image.

> *"For example, my friend came over yesterday. In the meantime, at the beginning, we called the baby Smoki. And she, we hadn't seen each other for a while, and she calls me and says, 'what's Smoki doing?' I say, 'Man, that's not Smoki!' First of all, Smoki is a male, totally out of the entity. I can't relate at all. Now Milica (the name she chose for the baby) is a* ***totally different being. She's alive now, she moves, she has a temperament. She has a name. And she's simply just a little being on her own.*** *But Smoki was more of a fantastic invention. Of the male gender, slightly sexless, imperceptible. When she told me 'Smoki', it felt like two hundred years ago. You know, this is Milica now, this is a being now. You'll see. Only I know that. No one else knows yet. They'll see it when she's born." (Sonja)*

For Sonja, the baby is present as a totally independent and complete subject—someone with its own behaviour, personality and name. She also believes that "only she knows that", because the fact that she is carrying the baby in her womb gives her privileged access. Sonja even imagines that this relationship is not one-sided, that she also has a privileged position for the baby. She is convinced that the baby reacts differently to her than to other people, e.g. that it recognises when she touches the belly. This only encourages bonding and interaction with the baby even more.

> *"When I touch her, she doesn't stop moving immediately, she really wriggles. Sometimes she scares me, I really think she's about to jump out, she has these swings, swerves left, swerves right. But when others touch her, she stops immediately. I think she recognises... Or she senses the movement of my hand. (...) And usually when she moves, I don't move at all, apart from shaking her a little, giving her a stroke. I shake her harder if she really overdoes it.*

B: Does she stop moving when you shake her?
S: No. She seems to be stubborn and I get more and more lenient. And I give her more and more of my internal organs." (Sonja)

When the baby is unproblematically individuated during pregnancy, women usually imagine continuity between the baby in the womb and the baby after birth. The fact that the baby is currently in the mother's body, thus, appears as a completely contingent circumstance. The expectant mother often gets to know this new subject even before the birth, primarily based on her embodied experience, so when the baby is born, it is only a completion of a long process.

"I can imagine her whole body, her arms and legs and her facial expression, but I can't imagine her at all. The features of her face are completely blurred to me. She, Milica, already has an identity, and I can't imagine her as a copy of me or her dad. ... I can't wait for her to come out so we can meet. I mean, we already know each other, but to meet officially." (Sonja)

I consider this early beginning of intersubjectivity to be a necessary context that prepares the mother to treat her baby as an independent being—as a subject—once they are physically separated.[30] In the attachment literature, maternal sensitivity, originally defined as "the mother's ability to perceive and to interpret accurately the signals and communications implicit in her infant's behaviour, and given this understanding, to respond to them appropriately and promptly" (Ainsworth et al., 1974, p. 127), is considered one of the most important factors for establishing an attachment relationship with the baby. As we have seen, for most women, this process begins long before the baby leaves the mother's body.

* * *

[30] This process of individuation of the baby *for the mother* during pregnancy also serves as a precondition for the process of the baby's becoming a subject (or its self-individuation) after birth. The understanding of the genesis of subjectivity as an inherently social process that is fundamentally linked to the intersubjective relationship with primary caregivers, in psychology originates from Vygotsky's theory (1997, p. 105): "through others we become ourselves" or "the individual becomes for himself what he is in himself through what he manifests for others". This, of course, echoes Hegel's thesis on the genesis of self-consciousness (2018, p. 76): "Self-consciousness is in and for itself, when, and by the fact that, it is in and for itself for another self-consciousness; that is, it is only as something recognized".

The analysis in this chapter has attempted to show that the embodied process of becoming a mother is phenomenologically complex and temporally unique. It involves both embodied and technologically mediated modes of experience, as well as the changing process of their interaction and relative contribution. Medical technology can therefore play different roles in the woman's subjectivity, her bodily experience and her identification with pregnancy and bonding with the baby. As we have already seen, these roles change according to the stage of pregnancy, but also depend largely on the specific circumstances in which the medical examination takes place—the roles of the doctors, the patterns of communication, the material organisation of the institutional context, i.e. the situatedness of the technology, to which we turn next.

3.4 Ambivalent Role of Medical Technology in the Embodied Experience of Pregnancy

In the analysis that introduced this chapter, but also throughout the rest of the chapter, it is repeatedly pointed out that medical technology can play a dual role—the information it provides can both reduce and increase the uncertainty that women often feel in the early months and later during pregnancy. We have considered various cases where insufficiently present or unclear bodily signs make women feel insecure and lead them to seek a professional and technological resolution—which often reassures them and provides an appropriate interpretation or validation of their experience, even if it occasionally raises further uncertainties.

This does not only apply to those women who are used to mistrusting their own bodies due to their bodily socialisation and often need external (preferably medical) confirmation. In such a subjective constellation, it is to be expected that medical technology plays an essential role in eliminating the uncertainty caused by unclear and ambivalent embodied experiences. However, medical technology sometimes plays this role even in the case of women who are inclined to rely heavily on their embodied experience, as the phenomenological peculiarities of the reproductive body described in the introduction to this chapter present these women with a challenging epistemological task. For example, towards the end of her pregnancy, Sonja began to notice numerous unfamiliar bodily changes that she lacked the adequate resources to interpret. As a result, she felt somewhat insecure and found it useful to seek medical information to validate or appropriately interpret her condition.

> *"And what's scary inside is that I know something is happening, now that there are no more ultrasounds. Aside from the baby moving, I don't know anything else, that something in my body is preparing, finally. It's not that nothing is happening, a lot is happening, and it's happening all the time. And always something new." (Sonja)*

Sonja is fascinated by nature ("*everything is a miracle because of nature*") and how everything in pregnancy is spontaneously and adequately arranged ("*nature arranges everything beautifully*") so that the body adjusts on its own. This belief is the basis for her decision to give birth without an epidural and allows her to resist certain medical technologies. However, trusting in nature does not automatically mean that she understands everything that is happening to her and that she can fully surrender to what is happening. In situations where she is not sure how to explain what she feels, she seems to need medical reassurance. She is then inclined to rely on medical knowledge and technology to validate and explain her embodied experience.

> *"But I'm proud that some of my impressions are quite... two of them turned out to be true—that the baby really does have its legs down and is kicking me, and that my hips hurt for a reason. And that I'm not making this up, that it's not psychosomatic, I have some proof, it's written there, something's written down." (Sonja)*

The fact that Sonja is proud because of the medical confirmation of her condition can be interpreted in two ways. On the one hand, it could indicate a general attitude of distrust towards women's embodied experiences in the medical context, which should be understood here in a broader sense beyond the framework of medical institutions. Sonja reacts with pride because she is "right" and "has proof"—the only acceptable kind of proof in the medicalised world. On the other hand, Sonja could be proud because she has received external confirmation that she "reads her body well", which can only strengthen her confidence in her own embodied experience. In this case, technological knowledge only appears as a confirmation of embodied knowledge and contributes positively to the overall experience of pregnancy, although this role would probably not be possible without the privileged status it holds in the modern world.

So far, we have mainly focused on cases where the woman's feelings and her concerns or needs were the starting point when interacting with the medical interpretation. However, there are also cases where a woman feels well, has no worries or concerns and therefore does not need any additional insight or confirmation from the doctor. Then medical examination and technologically mediated information may seem completely external to her. In pregnancies progressing normally, scheduled examinations and tests can sometimes induce anxiety about possible abnormalities that could be detected. In these situations, a visit to the doctor can trigger or increase anxiety because women fear hearing "bad news" and they begin to question their embodied experience wondering if it is a reliable indicator of their baby's health. The use of technology, therefore, makes it possible to reduce anxiety induced by the examination situation in the first place.

> *"I never liked going to ultrasound examinations. Because before the ultrasound I would always get so so nervous, in that sense... I don't know... I always just thought about going there and hoping everything would be okay. That doctor would tell me everything's ok. And normally, when I don't go for an ultrasound, I just don't think about it, I just feel ok. And then when I have to go for an ultrasound, and then that just throws me into some thoughts about... Will everything be okay? But what if they see something on the ultrasound and it's not okay? I get some feeling of uncertainty in the sense that I might hear bad news now. That's why I didn't like to go. But then when I go and when she (the doctor) says that everything is ok, then of course it's easier." (Nevena)*

The capacity of technology to provide a resolution to the uncertainty it itself induced, by offering the possibility of making a baby's condition constantly available through technological means, has led to some entirely new and potentially problematic occurrences. Initially there were ultrasound Doppler devices for home use, which women could purchase to listen to their baby's heartbeat at any time, and more recently mobile applications. It seems that due to the dominance of the discourse of risk, the mere fact that their baby's current condition is potentially always accessible through medical technology, while their embodied experience only provides occasional and perhaps insufficient insights, creates and reinforces anxieties regarding the baby's condition when they have no "direct" insight into it. And if there is already a built habit to rely on technology and the information obtained through it as the only way to alleviate their anxiety, the intervals between check-ups may become too long. The problem with using home Doppler devices (or their mobile alternatives) is that, similar to bodily knowledge, the technological information is ambiguous and requires interpretation that can be more or less precise and adequate—e.g. it is difficult to distinguish the baby's heartbeat from one's own and other sounds from the body. As a result, expectant mothers may seek medical help too often because they fail to hear the baby's heartbeat, or they do not seek it when needed because they mistakenly believe they have heard it (FDA, 2014; Gornall, 2009). Interestingly, in this situation, the experts advise that women should try to rely on their embodied experience, i.e. the sensation of the baby's movements, and use this as an indicator of whether they should see a doctor and be examined using technology. This does not imply that one modality of experience is replaced by another, but that they are coordinated. So here we have a case where a technology developed with the aim of reducing uncertainty, and advertised as such, actually perpetuates and deepens it.

Finally, it is important to leave room to think about medical technology outside of the either/or dichotomy—as something that either introduces/amplifies uncertainty or offers reassurance and resolution, because the experiences of at least some women call for different understandings. In contrast to the case discussed above, in which the woman's lack of a spontaneous need for medical input means that the examination itself triggers concern and anxiety, Una goes to the check-ups (for which she has no spontaneous need) "routinely" and without worrying about negative outcomes. Nevertheless, she experiences the medical confirmation that "everything is okay" with the pregnancy and the baby as a great success and personal achievement ("like you've climbed a mountain"), even though she is, of course, aware that she "hasn't done anything".

> *"Every time I come back from a check-up, everything is good. Although I don't expect anything bad—I've been going to these appointments terribly routinely because they last two minutes and that's it. Every time they tell you everything is okay... and they don't say anything more than that, I mean they don't say 'wonderful' because it's not wonderful, it's just okay. And the whole day you feel like you've climbed a mountain, like 'yes!' You have no idea why, and you haven't done anything. But you just feel great." (Una)*

It should be noted that this is a woman who highly values her embodied experience, for whom the body is, in her own words, her "safe zone her whole life" and who feels admiration and fascination for the manifold bodily changes during pregnancy. So she is not someone who privileges the medical point of view and technologically mediated knowledge. After all, she is also the only research participant who defied the medical model and attempted a home birth. This is precisely why her reaction is interesting and relevant. When I asked her why she feels such happiness and excitement when the check-ups confirm that everything is fine, Una responded that it is because she "identifies a lot with the pregnancy" and "has become attached to the idea of being pregnant".

Her identification with pregnancy is therefore the reason why new pregnancy-related insights or experiences are extremely important to her and why she experiences them emotionally, regardless of where these experiences come from. This response suggests the possibility that there is a reciprocal relationship between the insights offered by medical technology and women's identification with pregnancy—that is, the more a woman identifies with pregnancy and the more central it is to her, the more intensely she will react to the check-ups and the new technologically mediated information, which in turn will strengthen her attachment and give reality to the pregnancy and the foetus developing in her womb. And surely, the same applies to the embodied experience of pregnancy.

Throughout the previous discussion of technologically mediated and embodied knowledge or modes of experience, it has been implicitly assumed that these two modalities are similar or analogous, differing only in their source or origin. In other words, the very fact that both ultrasound and feeling the baby's movements tell us something about its presence and activity at the same time suggests that they offer the same kind of insight. But is this really the case?

3.4.1 What Kind of Technologically Mediated Input Is Meaningful for Women? Doctors as Mediators Between Women and Technology

The analysis of the women's accounts indicates that, throughout the course of pregnancy, ultrasound is primarily important to them as a source of medical information about the baby. Women think primarily about the baby's health, especially possible problems or abnormalities, when they have an ultrasound examination—satisfying their curiosity, obtaining non-medical information or simply being able to see the baby are quite secondary. Thus they usually emphasise as particularly relevant (or even as the only important thing) the confirmation that "everything is fine".

> *"I always focus during these check-ups... neither my husband nor I are really concerned about whether it's a boy or a girl. No, that didn't interest me at all. That's the last thing I asked about at these check-ups. So I kind of always concentrate, I go for that check-up, and just wait for them to tell me everything's okay." (Teodora)*

The ultrasound scan is therefore not perceived as an opportunity to see the baby and obtain some non-medical information about it. The dominance of this attitude is best illustrated by parts of women's narratives related to 4D ultrasound technology. This technology offers the possibility of obtaining a 3D image of the foetus in real time,[31] which is why it is

[31] Hence the name of the technology, because time is regarded as the fourth dimension. What is actually obtained is a short film with a 3D image of the foetus.

often perceived by both pregnant women and doctors as something that primarily allows future parents to see the baby.[32] Although information can regularly be found on the websites of private clinics stating that this is the most detailed and therefore most reliable ultrasound with great diagnostic possibilities, the reference textbook for obstetrics William's Obstetrics concludes, based on numerous empirical studies, that there is insufficient evidence that 3D/4D ultrasound has significant diagnostic advantages over "ordinary" 2D ultrasound, which is also the official position of the American College of Obstetricians and Gynecologists (Cunningham et al., 2010, p. 361). In Serbia, doctors generally recommend 4D ultrasound to women as an optional examination, which is performed exclusively in private clinics. Some women decide not to undergo this examination if there is no medical indication for it. They are aware that this ultrasound can provide the clearest image on the screen—at this point the foetus "really looks like a baby", but looking at the baby is not recognised as sufficient reason, because this technology is treated primarily as a diagnostic tool.

> *"That 4D or whatever it is, how many Ds, when the yellow image looks like, I mean really looks like a baby. But thank God everything was fine with the pregnancy so I didn't have the need for those things. And they don't have that at the health centre (public practice), you have to pay for it and make an appointment and... forget it. Well if there was something problematic... then okay." (Ivana)*

Even in cases where women have opted for a 4D ultrasound scan in a private clinic after the doctor has recommended it, they often question whether it is justified and look for medical reasons. Not only do they insist on the importance of the information relating solely to the baby's

[32] On the website of a private clinic in Belgrade, the 4D ultrasound scan is advertised with the following words: "When you watch your baby scratching, smiling, crying, yawning or getting angry, you and the future father are already establishing close contact with her during pregnancy. Such images and videos are more than an obvious confirmation of the doctor's words that your baby is doing well. No wonder one little girl, a future sister, exclaimed at the end of the examination: 'Why don't we take the little brother home with us?'" (http://www.analife.rs/menu/1791/ekspertski-4d-ultrazvuk-od-20-24-nedelje-trudnoce/; accessed 11/09/2023).

health, but the fact that they are getting the most realistic picture of the baby's appearance is explicitly recognised as "least important".

> *"Then I asked him, 'Okay, why should I do this?' There's only one, and it's done exactly at the twentieth week, or around the twenty-first or second, because by then the baby is fully developed, a human in miniature. And to see that everything is as it should be. Because 4D is not about you seeing what your baby looks like, it's about them seeing if it has all the fingers, all that and the smallest details. (...) And to see if the skin as an organ is healthy, not for you to see what your baby looks like. Because that's the least important." (Sonja)*

What should the medical input look like so that a woman finds it informative and yet sufficiently reassuring? So-called expert ultrasound examinations (at least in private clinics), for example, involve a very comprehensive and detailed assessment of the development, anatomy and health of the foetus. This very detailed information follows a pattern we have already identified—it can induce anxiety and fear of discovering something problematic that the doctors may have missed ("Literally, as if they are looking for some anomaly, God forbid."), but at the same time, the absence of negative findings in such a thorough examination can alleviate the woman's fears and reassure her.

> *"And the doctor really looked at literally everything during that expert ultrasound. And then I realised that it's not just an ordinary ultrasound, but from counting the little toes on the feet, the hands, to the smallest capillaries in the head and heart. And like how long the thighbone is, let's see the spine, let's see the last vertebra down there and let's check the lip to see if it has a cleft.* ***They examine it down to the tiniest details. Literally, as if they are looking for some anomaly, God forbid.*** *(...) Such an extensive analysis is done.* ***And then you come out of there and you know that your child is complete, as they say. That means a lot, a lot.*** *(...) And then I really came out of there... phew (a sigh of relief)! Like that's it, now I'm at peace." (Teodora)*

However, we should not conclude from Teodora's account that the more detailed and comprehensive the medical information is, the more reassured and convinced a pregnant woman is that everything is fine with her baby. In most cases (including this participant), if the pregnancy is progressing normally and without complications, extensive and detailed medical knowledge can lead to uncertainty rather than reduce it. Therefore, most women just want a simple confirmation from a medical authority that "everything is fine". One possible reason for this is that they do not have established interpretative schemes into which they can assimilate information and assess its meaning and relative importance. Detailed medical knowledge that is not fully transparent to them can therefore create or increase uncertainty rather than resolve it.

> *"So these measurements from the ultrasound, they're such mini numbers, 1.6 of something. I don't know what they measure. But these things don't interest me in the slightest. Because I'll find something and then I'll start freaking out. I just need to hear if it's good. I mean, if I'm a straight A student in everything else, in this area I'm really... Just give me the simple categories of bad and good, the simplest... 'It's good - it's not good' does the job for me." (Sonja)*
>
> *"Well, basically, it wouldn't mean anything to me if the doctor had said the circumference of the head is this big, that wouldn't mean anything to me. But if he's like 'everything is okay'. That's the impression I had at the end, because I came out of his office feeling calm. So that's it. Heartbeats are good, everything is fine, and that was enough for me. Now, if he had gone into details, who knows what I'd have constructed in my head..." (Teodora)*

This has been discussed before—when a woman is not going through a period of uncertainty that technology needs to resolve, but that uncertainty may be induced by the examination itself, detailed medical information or sophisticated diagnostic techniques do more harm than good. However, if the initial situation is different—for example, when there is suspicion of a problem or negative symptoms have appeared - detailed information is welcome and only it can relieve women of uncertainty.

The problem arises when women cannot obtain this information from their doctors, who, as already mentioned, should act as intermediaries between them and medical technology. It is a misconception to believe that ultrasound provides something that is immediately understandable or relevant to women. For an ultrasound scan to mean anything to them at all, a process of accumulating experience, building competencies and adopting normative standards is required, on the basis of which vague outlines on the screen and incomprehensible marks and numbers in the medical report can represent relevant information about a baby.

> *"The doctor explained it quite well to me in the sense that he turned the monitor towards me and said, 'You see, this is the uterus, and this spot here is the pregnancy.' (...) Even though it's really nothing, I mean it's just a little spot. It doesn't have the shape of a homunculus. It's just a spot. And the monitor is bad. I mean, it's grainy and looks like snow on the TV. If he hadn't shown me what's what, I wouldn't have understood anything, what's going on." (Una)*
>
> *"That's all fine with me, but really, they're little aliens, you can't see anything there." (Jasna)*
>
> *"Oh dear, it looked strange, everything was, I don't know, he (the doctor) shows you... And the first, the second, the third, and the fourth time... I don't see anything there, because I'm trying too hard to see and then I get lost... And it was very strange to me. And we were looking at that picture like... how is that even there? Everything is somehow... I mean it's strange, I don't know, I have no idea." (Sofija)*

What women see on the screen often appears "strange" to them and doesn't meet their expectations, or they aren't sure what they are supposed to be looking at or how to interpret the unclear outlines. Many of them recognise how important the doctor's role is during an ultrasound examination and that the doctor essentially acts as an intermediary between them and the technology.

> *"When I go for an ultrasound, I see nothing. You see a spot, that's what you see—a spot. So, you don't see anything. Oh! That's a baby! Alright. It could be a foreign body, I mean, it's the same to me. I'm not a doctor, so I'm like - okay. You trust them. How they approach, or how they tell the story, makes you believe or not believe. (...) What they see there, I don't understand at all. And how they can see if something is wrong or right. But they can. I mean, that's something you learn." (Ivana)*

So "seeing the baby" is not something that happens by itself. First of all, a woman must have a certain amount of experience and knowledge about what to look for and how to recognise it. In addition, the doctor must be prepared to explain to the woman what she is seeing and guide her through the process. Finally, there are certain technical requirements—a sufficiently good ultrasound monitor on which even a person who is not a doctor and does not have the necessary skills can recognise something.

"Based on the ultrasound and this kind of visualisation, that's how you imagine the baby now, that's how little Johnny imagines it. Because with the ultrasound, I mean... They swipe that camera around and they, like, see something clearly there. I don't see anything there. Because you need certain experience and probably a better ultrasound that when you listen to the doctor you can say, 'That's it,' and to recognise what you're seeing yourself." (Ivana)

Therefore, even when a doctor, almost exclusively in private practice, has the willingness and patience to explain and show a woman what is on the screen and how to interpret that, repeated experience and practice are required for it to become clear to the woman herself.

"The screen is always facing me, and he (doctor) points out everything he looks at, even the more specialised aspects, with his finger. He is very considerate. And really, every little thing, 'oh, what's that?' he explains, 'this is this, that's that, everything is fine.' With a regular ultrasound, it's hard to see and understand when he shows you, 'look, there's the head,' and I can't see anything. But I managed, somewhere around the fifth month, I think, that's when he saw the gender and explained 'this is this, look.' And it took me two or three times to see, but on the fourth attempt I managed and saw the outlines, saw the head, saw the sex, it's a girl." (Saška)

It should be noted that most women who have repeatedly had the opportunity to see the image on the monitor and receive an expert explanation eventually begin to recognise some outline of the baby, but they all agree that the most important thing is "what the doctor sees" so that he can "tell them that everything is fine".

"He (doctor) always shows me. And I am free to ask him, but ***it is simply most important to me that he is satisfied with what he sees, so he can tell me that everything is fine****. (...) He has always explained, right from the start, what is what, even though nothing could be seen at the beginning. He looks*

first. I keep quiet; I don't like to ask him many questions. He looks, measures, does whatever he does. But when he's finished, he always says: 'Here's the heart, there's the hand', depending on how the spine is turned. (...) When the baby is smaller, it's easier to see; now that the baby is bigger, I can't quite distinguish before he tells me which part of the body it is. (...) It's not very clear; I mean, it's important for me that he tells me everything is okay." (Tamara)

Therefore, unmediated contact with the ultrasound image is not informative enough for women. They lack the framework to interpret the data provided by the technology, and therefore the doctor should act as a hermeneut and mediator, providing different types and extents of information depending on the circumstances. But what happens when a doctor fails to fulfil this mediating role?

3.4.2 Situated Technology: When a Mediating Role of Healthcare Practitioners Is Missing

As previously mentioned, at least part of the findings regarding the role of ultrasound in the experience of pregnancy can be explained by the specific circumstances in which women encounter ultrasound technology in local practice. All participants who had undergone an ultrasound examination in state medical institutions (health centres, maternity wards within a hospital or maternity clinic) consistently reported quite negative experiences, primarily related to the attitude of the medical staff towards them and the constellation of the examination itself. The examination scene typically involves the woman lying on a bed with her abdomen exposed while the doctor moves the ultrasound wand over it, observes the projection on the screen and dictates the findings to the nurse. The doctor generally does not address the woman, does not explain anything to her and is not concerned that she might hear what he is saying. The woman is therefore not included as a subject in the examination in any meaningful way—she is merely physically present, and the situation would not change a bit if she was lying unconscious on the table.[33]

[33] This configuration of the ultrasound examination is so normalised that, when it takes place under significantly altered circumstances in a private practice, some women perceive it as deviating too

The woman often does not understand much of what the doctor says when dictating the findings and does not know how to interpret what she hears, which leads to uncertainty as to whether everything is in order. As a rule, she does not have the opportunity to inquire in detail about anything that sounds unusual or worrying to her. She usually waits until the doctor has finished the examination before asking questions because she does not want to interrupt, but even then she either gets no answer or only a very brief explanation.

> *"They absolutely don't talk to you about anything. ... I don't know what it would be like if you went to their private practice and planned to get a connection,[34] then maybe they would devote more time. But there it's like an assembly line. They examine you, they don't even wait for you to wipe the gel off after the ultrasound, I've tissues lying next to me. And that's about it. Everything happens very quickly. And even if I ask something it is always in a second, it's getting dressed, getting undressed, the next one comes in, and that's it. ... I get up, wipe myself off, give it to her, she's already writing it down, they give you the report, you take it and leave. You don't have time to say, 'Doctor, can I ask you...' Yes, while she's working, I'm also trying not to ask her, she's looking at the ultrasound, I want to let her see what she needs to see, in those three minutes while I'm lying there." (Anđela)*

Furthermore, the monitor is usually not turned towards the woman, so she cannot even see what the doctor is observing on the screen or what part of her insides he is referring to. Often other people are in a position to see more than the woman herself, whose body part is projected onto

much from a normative medical encounter. If the setting is adapted to the woman and her needs—with friendly and informative staff and a screen set up so that she can also follow the examination—the impression is created that this is not an "expert examination" but rather a "show programme": *"And now they are incredibly friendly because it's a private clinic. And then the doctor really went out of his way and everything was set up to accommodate and please you. I don't have the impression of an expert examination as much as I have the impression of a show programme. I mean, he has his own monitor that he looks at and I have a fixed TV on the ceiling that I look at. I think they even have a pillow or something similar to make me comfortable"* (Sonja). Thus, for this participant, the fact that the examination is adapted to her implies that it is being performed *for her*, rather than *for the baby*, giving it a connotation of something unnecessary and non-medical.

[34] This strategy for ensuring the quality and continuity of care has already been discussed in the previous chapter.

the screen and who sometimes appears only incidentally and contingently as an observer.

"The doctor showed it to his nurse this last time, so he turned it (the monitor) a bit, so I managed to see it too." (Teodora)

"It seemed quite brutal to me in a way... I mean, I understand that I'm the millionth pregnant woman they've examined, but I don't know... that there's no humanity, no warmth at all, I don't know how to explain it to you. ... And it was horrible that the doctor doesn't talk to you at all. He doesn't say anything. Nothing. He only says some things to the nurse. ... During that ultrasound I couldn't see the monitor. But my friend went with me. And the door... there is the hallway where we're all waiting, and the door to that hallway is open. And she stood behind it to peek and watch the baby because she wasn't allowed to come in with me. And when I came out, she said 'I saw everything!' But I couldn' see anything." (Sofija)

The examination setting that Sofija experienced reveals a paradoxical relationship between privacy and exposure. On the one hand, no one except the woman and the medical staff is allowed to be present during the examination,[35] suggesting a situation of privacy. On the other hand, the door of the doctor's office is open so that everyone in the waiting room can see the inside of the woman's belly, which is simultaneously inaccessible to the woman herself.

The possibility to hear information without the opportunity to clarify it sometimes means that medical technology, because of its specific embeddedness in institutional practice, increases and deepens uncertainty and concern about the state of the pregnancy and the health of the foetus, rather than reducing it.

"At the first ultrasound in the health centre, the doctor told me... I mean, he didn't tell it to me, he said it to the nurse he was dictating to, and he was dictating all kinds of codes like ACGMLF. And then he said, 'Corpus luteum cyst on right ovary'. And I was shocked. But he said it so casually, like he was saying it's

[35] This applies to many state medical facilities, although there are some that allow access to escorts, but only the female ones. This effectively means that the organisation of practice and prevailing norms in public medical institutions prevent expectant fathers from ever sharing the experience of the examination with their partner or receiving medical information about their baby directly.

5 degrees outside. So I googled it and realised I shouldn't have done that. It's actually something quite normal, it's where the baby started, got separated, and got nourished until whatever. I've no idea, something like that. It's nothing serious." (Sofija)

Sofija's concern about the incomprehensible information she received (or rather overheard) during the examination and her subsequent reaction are typical of most women I have spoken to. In such situations, women either look for additional sources of medical knowledge—mainly on the internet, but also in books and by consulting a healthcare professional in their social circle; or for additional technology—for example, an examination with a better ultrasound machine; or for additional interpretation of the results—by seeking a second opinion, usually from a doctor in private practice.

"I mean, recently we had a problem with this. The doctor said to the nurse, 'Why are these plexias here?' And now you hear this sentence, and you don't know what plexias are, or why they're there, but you see she's looking at the head. And you think: what's wrong with the baby's brain now? I'm going to kill myself, or her, I don't even know. Her explanation wasn't, 'Let me tell you what it's' or 'Wait, I'll show you'... That's the craziest thing with doctors, to make you feel stupid. Whatever they say, you don't know. And then they shock you with some statement that something is wrong. I managed to ask a question or two, but then I was speechless. She said, 'I can't tell you anything, we'll see in three weeks.' 'Alright doctor, what does that mean?' 'Well, if it goes away, it's good, if it doesn't, it's not good.' And I get home and... maybe something's wrong with the baby. So I go on the internet, but how to know if I remembered the right word. And when you search for brain, brain development, you find problems, diseases, but nowhere does it mention plexias. Oh man, did I remember correctly what she saw? I spent two or three days browsing and then thought, 'Are you crazy?!' Then we went to see another doctor in private practice and everything was normal. He said, 'I don't know what she saw or didn't see. It's normal for one to be developing, it happens that they don't grow at the same rate, but by the end they should even out... It's all normal.' And then I had an anatomy lesson, 'this is this and this is that.' When you look, you can see that everything is normal. First, I could see the ultrasound better. It was a private clinic and they set up the screen so you could see while lying down. And it was a big flat

screen, somehow the image was clearer. You know, you can see everything." (Ivana)

So, instead of medical technology resolving some uncertain situation, it actually introduces additional uncertainty because the mediating role of the doctor is missing. Ivana even believes that they deliberately put women in this position "to make you feel stupid" and that "you don't know", as a way to exercise their power, i.e. to maintain and reproduce the unequal and hierarchical relationship between women and doctors that has already been discussed. The woman is expected to remain passive and simply wait for the next check-up, which implies that she has to spend a relatively long time in uncertainty about the health of her future baby. One of the ways for the woman to take an active role in this situation is to take control of the medical monitoring of her pregnancy. This is exactly what Ivana did. The inevitable consequence of this kind of exercise of agency is that the woman overcomes the negative effects of the medicalisation of her pregnancy by subjecting herself to additional medicalisation.

However, there are situations where a woman fails to take an active role in monitoring her pregnancy, and in such cases the absence of the doctor's mediating role can have quite dramatic consequences. At the end of her third month, Una received a wrong diagnosis from the doctors during an ultrasound scan that she was pregnant with conjoined twins. Not only did they present her with this very serious and extremely rare diagnosis[36] without any sensitivity or further explanation, but they also discussed the options for resolving the situation, namely the removal of the foetuses, in front of her. The doctors neither considered the impact this information would have on her, nor did they address her obvious fear and distress when she received the news. In keeping with their complete disregard for Una during the examination, apart from the image of her uterus they observed on the screen, the doctors left her to cope with the new situation entirely on her own, without offering her any resources.

---

[36] On average once in one hundred to two hundred thousand pregnancies (Cunningham et al., 2010, p. 863).

"The doctor did an ultrasound and he was like ok, but told me to come back in five days, which was very soon. But I went back... And then they told me, he was looking... The reason he asked me to come back was because there were twins. Yes, there were twins. He called his colleague to check if everything was okay. Then this woman, she is an ultrasound expert, his colleague, the two of them were sitting there. I lay on that table for fifteen minutes. She literally, without exaggeration, repeated five to ten times that they were Siamese... she didn't say it like that, but that they were twins joined at the sacral part. ***It was absolutely horrible, I started crying. I really started crying. It was awful. At that moment I realised... It was terrible for me. I was like a zombie.*** *And the way she said it... Do you know what it sounded like? I'm lying there and the two of them are there looking at the screen and saying 'yes, yes, yes, I'm 200% sure. Yes, yes, yes, you see, they are joined... wouououo. Should we use the hook?*[37] *Oh yes, oh yes, I'm sure they're joined.' And I'm trying to say something, but I'm completely stunned by the information that they are twins and that they are joined. It was horrifying, absolutely horrifying. And this woman just leaves the probe there and walks out without even saying goodbye. I was thinking what kind of person are you, what's going on in your head? And then I asked the doctor, the only thing I managed to mutter - 'Well, will they separate over time?' Which is a completely ridiculous question, but fuck, what can you do. And then he said, 'No, no, no, let's take it easy.' Actually no, he didn't even comfort me, he just said, 'Sit here and wait', and then he picked up the phone and tried to find some other doctors in the hospital. In another department where they have a slightly better ultrasound machine to gather around and check. But he didn't tell me that. He made the calls in front of me. And then he said, 'Come in on Tuesday morning at half past six'. And I walk away completely stunned, I say nothing, could not articulate a single question." (Una)*

Una felt so distraught that she could not even formulate a coherent question. It is important to understand that her helplessness in this situation was a result of the objective circumstances of the examination—the conduct of the doctors, the implicit and explicit norms prevailing in the institution, and such positioning of the woman that, despite being central in this situation, she has no insight or voice in it, and none of her

[37] The sentence "Should we use the hook?" refers to one of the embryotomies, obstetric operations in which the foetus is dismembered and reduced in size to enable its extraction through the birth canal (Mladenović et al., 2008).

personal or social characteristics matter.[38] The most serious consequence is that it is not easy for a woman to recover from such an experience of marginalisation and jeopardy of her subjectivity. It seems that the fact that she was basically prevented from being an agent during the examination made it difficult for her to be an agent afterwards and to actively engage with her condition in any way. She still describes herself as a zombie—a metaphor that vividly points to the consequences of desubjectification.

> *"I mean, that weekend was... I really was a zombie. (...) And basically all we needed to do was go to a private doctor and pay 50 euros for an ultrasound. But that didn't occur to me... it occurred to me five months later. Only then did it occur to me what I should have done to solve my dilemma. ... No, no, the worst thing is the three or four days you spend in this state. And your brain obviously doesn't work well enough to ... to simply realise what you need to check so that you know." (Una)*

Such a constellation of medical examination that disregards the woman's agency and subjectivity, combined with a potentially risky medical scenario, can leave her feeling genuinely vulnerable, with no discernible way to regain control. It's not just about lacking tangible resources; it's about being unable to adopt a position from which any action would be possible. The woman feels paralysed, or, as described in the quote above, "like a zombie".

Another factor that should not be overlooked, and which has been discussed extensively in this chapter, contributes to this situation—Una's case (like those previously examined) still concerns the early stages of her pregnancy, in which she still lacks concrete embodied insight into her condition. Embodied insight sometimes cannot reveal anything about

---

[38] Una is aware of this and emphasises that she is in a much better and more privileged position than many other women who visit medical institutions: she knew the doctor beforehand, and her education and background are potential resources for a sense of power and integrity (she is a middle-class woman from Belgrade, has a PhD and a research position at an academic institution). However, none of this was of any help: *"And besides, I keep thinking all the time, I mean, I got in there because of a personal connection... and I'm not some little defenceless creature. I told you that, I have this sense of inner strength, I really feel like I could do a lot to them if I wanted to. I mean, I understand it's not the same, but I mean, I'm not someone with no education, I'm not someone who came from the country and had to pay who knows how much money to get here just to get kicked around." (Una)*

specific health issues, but in the cases where it can, women are often inclined to relativise or disqualify medical knowledge much more readily when their embodied feeling tells them otherwise. Una, for example, reacted very differently to a doctor's misdiagnosis in her ninth month and defied her authority. At this point, she clearly felt the baby's movements and had a direct insight into its activity, so the medical technology and the doctor's interpretation were not the only sources of information. When the doctor told her, based on the CTG[39] results, that the baby was not active, i.e. had no heartbeat, she dismissed the medical technology as unreliable and rejected the doctor's interpretation without questioning the validity of her own embodied insight.

> *"CTG is the stupidest thing in the world. They buried my child once. I mean, they do it all the time in the healthcare system, nonstop. She did the CTG check-up and then, they love that motion, 'Oh my God!' [she mimics the doctor and spreads her arms out in shock and disbelief]. I'm like, 'What is it?' But I know everything is fine because luckily, the baby is incredibly lively. So my baby is moving, they're doing the CTG and she's like, 'Oh my God, oh, oh!' I'm like, 'What's wrong?' And I know everything's fine, but okay, let's hear this theory. 'The baby's not active.' I said, 'The baby is active, and while you were doing the CTG, you can hear everything, you can hear the heart all the time, and the baby is moving, I'm not crazy.'[40] 'It's not moving,' she says... That's because the CTG is an unreliable device and it seemed that way to her at that moment. Then they said, 'Now we'll call the doctor to check.' Then they called someone to do an ultrasound. And they said everything was fine. I mean, I knew everything was fine." (Una)*

The extent to which a woman is able to resist expert opinion and the technologically mediated representation of her condition does not depend solely on her decision or intention. Both the medical technology and the woman herself are always situated—embedded in an entire network of

[39] CTG or cardiotocography is a medical technology that enables the simultaneous monitoring of uterine contractions and the frequency and quality of foetal heartbeats (Mladenović et al., 2008, p. 232).

[40] Normally, the medical staff place the CTG device on the woman's body and then leave the room so that she can hear the heartbeat, while the doctors or nurses only read the printout at the end of the examination.

institutionally bound relations, norms and practices in a concrete material environment. Therefore, the analysis of the following case also serves as an introduction to the next chapter, which will focus entirely on the institutional network that produces particular birthing bodies and subjects. In fact, the CTG, which objectifies the presence of the baby and the contracting uterus, represents a typical example of technological mediation in an institutional setting between the woman as embodied subject and the physician. Unlike the ultrasound, which is only occasionally present during pregnancy and thus allows the embodied experience to have a more consistent and relevant role for the woman, the CTG is (almost) constantly present during childbirth and positioned in such a way that it completely eliminates the need to rely on the woman's embodied experience.

> *"CTG is a really good little device. It shows you whether to admit the woman to the hospital, what to do to her, whether to induce labour, and whether to perform a C-section. It shows you everything. But for an ordinary person, a layperson, it means nothing. Just some little waves on the paper. But when a doctor looks at it, he knows that a little square up or down means a lot and tells you what to do." (from an interview with a doctor)*

This device objectifies uterine activity, and the contraction curve appears as an intersubjective indicator, and often also as evidence, of the woman's experience. While the experience of pain or discomfort is a subjective category, the contraction of the smooth muscles of the uterus is an objectively measurable parameter and is the only one considered diagnostically relevant. As can be seen from the above quotation, the doctor's knowledge and competencies are essential for reading the printout of the device, which becomes the bearer of authoritative knowledge in the situation.

But what happens in situations where there is a discrepancy between embodied and technologically mediated information? It is not uncommon for the CTG to indicate one thing while the woman feels something completely different. I realised this during my fieldwork, especially when I talked to women in the waiting room of the maternity hospital. All of these women were close to their due date (or even past it) and came in for a CTG. It was relatively common for the CTG to show contractions even though the woman did not feel them, and she was then sent to the maternity ward. Conversely, it could happen that a woman came to an examination because she felt contractions but the CTG did not register them and she was then sent home. This shows the status of the woman's interpretation of her own condition compared to medical interpretations given by experts or mediated by technology—it is generally considered irrelevant.[41]

> *"And I kept expecting someone to come and do something. Because I had contractions all night and no one came. In the morning I could hardly wait for the ward round or whatever happens, for someone to come. (...) And I was finally happy to announce that the mother was in labour, the contractions started. 'Mother,[42] does it hurt?' I say, 'It hurts!' And she, some doctor, 'Let it hurt, we'll wait a little longer'. I said, 'What do you mean a little longer? You don't understand doctor, I've been in pain since three in the morning, every minute and a half, what should we do?' And then she said, 'Bring the CTG.' And they brought it five or six times that morning. And I told the nurse, 'I already have really strong contractions, they have been lasting for hours, and they are very frequent, could you tell someone that something is happening?' She was like, 'Don't worry about anything'. And after the third time, I said, okay, they come every half hour with the CTG, look and say nothing, 'Can the doctor come? Can she check the cervix? Can you tell me what it (CTG) says?' Give me something, some feedback. And then she said, 'Okay mother, well, ok. Now you're being impatient, it has to go as nature dictates, it has to, yes, yes.' And she kept talking as she walked out. And at one point, she did it (CTG) for the umpteenth time, I don't know, it was probably the fifth, but it seemed like too too many, and just at that moment I had a really strong contraction and I said, 'Now it really hurts!' And on that little piece of paper, it showed just a tiny bit (shows about*

[41] It should not be overlooked that medical knowledge itself is often incoherent and inconclusive—different devices can give different results (as in Una's case above, where the CTG and ultrasound gave different findings). Even the printouts provided by medical technology can sometimes be interpreted differently by different doctors. However, what is exclusively sought within the medical setting is to match different medical data (e.g. through a hierarchy in which some sources are considered more reliable and accurate), rather than to ensure that medical and experiential data match.

[42] This way in which the doctor addresses a woman in labour is very common in local maternity wards. The medical staff typically address the women in the maternity ward as "mothers" instead of using their personal name or another type of address. This form of address has largely become normalised, even if a certain number of women react negatively to it. In the quote above, Sonja uses this form of address somewhat ironically by repeating it often and even referring to herself in this way. "*And I was finally happy to announce that the mother was in labour, the contractions started*".

2 cm with her fingers), it was nothing, I expected this (shows about 15 cm with her fingers). And I said, as she handed out the paper output, 'Look, can you see that I have a contraction, can you see that I'm not faking it, I don't understand why no one believes me?!' And she was like, 'Well, it's not that strong.' Man, you know from the outside how strong it really is for me. And it really hurts. I'm not expecting them to sympathise with me, I'm prepared for it to hurt, and that's fine, I'm ready for that. But hear me out, at least look at the paper a bit longer if I say it hurts. That much, really. Put on an act, 'Oh mother, you are right, I see the peak.' And leave. Just comfort me that much." (Sonja)

Sonja is confronted in the maternity ward with the fact that the medical staff ignore her embodied experience. When they do decide to take it into account, they bring a device to validate this experience. Sonja herself has no insight into what the CTG is showing (as the doctor said in the previous quote, *"for an ordinary person, a layperson, it means nothing"*), and this makes it even more difficult for her to connect what she is feeling to a medical indicator or interpretation.[43] Finally, she manages to compare her subjective experience of pain with the graphic representation of the contraction recorded on the paper and is disappointed by the discrepancy. But, what seems to bother her most in the entire situation is the complete lack of acknowledgement of her condition by the medical staff. They are only interested in the objective representation of that condition and on that basis disqualify Sonja's subjective experience. As a result, her pain remains unrecognised and, therefore, unshared. At no point is her pain something she can relate to together with another person, something that can be shared in an intersubjective situation. That would bring her the comfort she desires. In analysing birthing experiences in the

[43] Very often the CTG is positioned outside the woman's visual field, i.e. it is inaccessible to her, although it could be used as a resource to gain insight into the baby's condition during childbirth. This is also indicative of whether it is assumed in the hospital that the medical technology is intended for the woman herself, or only for the medical staff: *"Well, you can't see it because it's on the side. You can not lift yourself up. You can't see it, you can't observe it. You can only hear it"* (Saška). Even when they have the opportunity to view the CTG printout, women often lack the competence or criteria to interpret the results—unless they have informed themselves online in advance or perhaps asked a midwife during childbirth preparation classes: *"That CTG, it's a device for them, not for me. (...) I don't know how to use that machine, I mean. (...) You hear something. But no one has explained this something to you. I mean, if I was from the country, I would not have a clue, I mean, I read a bit somewhere, so I kind of knew, so okay"* (Ivana). Therefore, the CTG remains informative only for the doctor, not for the woman herself.

following chapter, we will see that ignoring women's perspective during childbirth is the norm in our local institutional settings and leads to much more dramatic consequences.

To illustrate that it is the embeddedness of medical technology that is crucial and not some of its inherent properties, let us consider an example of a completely different constellation of the relationship between embodied and technologically mediated experience that allows for a mutual validation of both. This not only avoids alienating consequences, but actually allows the contractions to appear as something intersubjectively shareable between this woman and her partner.

> *"What is interesting, for example, the previous day, when I was feeling those contractions. When we went for that CTG and now I am lying down and my husband was next to me, they allowed him to be there that time. And now we are watching, and I tell him I feel this subjective hardening of the belly.*[44] *And he looks at that paper from the CTG. And he counts there, I don't know, let's say that value was at twelve, and I say to him 'how is that number behaving now?' And now as I feel it rise for me, I feel it rising, he says I don't know 'here it's fifteen, seventeen', it went up to twenty-five, and I feel how it is slowly decreasing now, how it is slowly easing, and he says 'here, it's decreasing now'. So literally just as it was recorded there, it was happening like that to me. And then I said to him, 'Now you've got it, that's a contraction!'" (Teodora)*

It may seem that Teodora is simply participating in the objectification of her condition and that she is pointing to the external indicator, marked on the CTG, as her contraction. But that would be an overly simplistic and inaccurate interpretation. In the situation described, what is relevant is that the CTG enables the objectification of the woman's physical condition in a way that is consistent with her subjective experience of that condition. As a result, her embodied condition is immediately shareable with another person—the one who is primarily interested in her experience, not just her physical condition. By having both perspectives—the external and the internal—this woman does not experience the objectification of her uterine activity as alienating, but rather the objectification becomes a resource and enables mediation.

---

[44] This is how labour contractions are typically described by the midwife in antenatal classes.

We have already discussed that a woman often has no direct and privileged insight into her condition, and particularly in these moments, technological objectification can be very relevant to her. But in this example, we see that technology can act not only as a mediator between a woman and her body, but also between her and other people. The reason why medical technology rarely plays such a role for women lies, as already suggested, in the specific circumstances of its institutional situatedness. Women are often denied insight into what medical technology offers, and when they do have insight, doctors do not act as interpreters to help them appropriate this knowledge and connect it to their embodied experience.

In the conclusion of the book, I will attempt to map different models of the relationships between technologically mediated and embodied knowledge and experience during the early transition to motherhood, based on the empirical analysis presented. It is clear that these relationships depend on the embeddedness of medical technology and the status of pregnant and birthing bodies in specific institutional choreographies that can lead to different possible experiences and practices. In the next chapter, we will look at this topic in detail and analyse the importance of appropriate networking of all actors present for the woman's subjectivity as well as the dangers of broken connections. While women establish expectations and patterns of behaviour towards medical authority and hierarchical relationships within the institution before and certainly during pregnancy, contact with the hospital setting remains only occasional and sporadic. As we shall see shortly, with the onset of childbirth, the socio-material network of actors comes to the fore in an often dramatic way, which is both productive and often destructive for the woman as subject.

References

Ainsworth, M. D. S., Bell, S. M., & Stayton, D. (1974). Infant-mother attachment and social development. In M. P. Richards (Ed.), *The introduction of the child into a social world* (pp. 99–135). Cambridge University Press.

Barber, C. C. (2012). Prelude to parenthood: The impact of anxiety and depression during pregnancy. In M. G. R. Castillo (Ed.), *Perinatal depression* (pp. 19–38). InTech. https://doi.org/10.5772/32076

Benn, P. A., Ying, J., Beazoglou, T., & Egan, J. F. (2001). Estimates for the sensitivity and false-positive rates for second trimester serum screening for Down syndrome and trisomy 18 with adjustment for cross-identification and double-positive results. *Prenatal Diagnosis, 21*(1), 46–51.

Butler, J. (2004). *Undoing gender*. Routledge.

Clark, A., Skouteris, H., Wertheim, E. H., Paxton, S. J., & Milgrom, J. (2009). My baby body: A qualitative insight into women's body-related experiences and mood during pregnancy and the postpartum. *Journal of Reproductive and Infant Psychology, 27*(4), 330–345. https://doi.org/10.1080/02646830903190904

Clement, S., Wilson, J., & Sikorski, J. (1998). Woman's experiences of antenatal ultrasound scans. In S. Clement (Ed.), *Psychological perspectives on pregnancy and childbirth* (pp. 7–24). Elsevier Science.

Csordas, T. J. (1994). *Embodiment and experience*. Cambridge University Press.

Cunningham, G. F., Leveno, K. J., Bloom, S. L., Hauth, J. C., Rouse, D. J., & Spong, C. Y. (2010). *Williams obstetrics* (23rd ed.). McGraw-Hill Medical.

DiPietro, J. A. (2010). Psychological and psychophysiological considerations regarding the maternal-fetal relationship. *Infant and Child Development, 19*(1), 27–38. https://doi.org/10.1002/icd.651

Duden, B. (1991). *The woman beneath the skin: A doctor's patients in eighteenth-century Germany*. Harvard University Press.

Everett, C. (1997). Incidence and outcome of bleeding before the 20th week of pregnancy: Prospective study from general practice. *British Medical Journal, 315*(7099), 32–34. https://doi.org/10.1136/bmj.315.7099.32

Gallagher, S. (2005). *How the body shapes the mind*. Clarendon Press.

Gallagher, S., & Zahavi, D. (2008). *The phenomenological mind: An introduction to philosophy of mind and cognitive science*. Routledge.

Gornall, J. (2009). The dangers of listening to the fetal heart at home. *BMJ*. Retrieved from https://www.bmj.com/bmj/sectionpdf/186393?path=/bmj/339/7730/Feature.full.pdf

Gracia, C. R., Sammel, M. D., Chittams, J., Hummel, A. C., Shaunik, A., & Barnhart, K. T. (2005). Risk factors for spontaneous abortion in early symptomatic first-trimester pregnancies. *Obstetrics & Gynecology, 106*(5/1), 993–999. https://doi.org/10.1097/01.AOG.0000183604.09922.e0

Healthcare for women during pregnancy: National guidelines for doctors. (2005). Serbian Medical Society.

Hegel, G. W. F. (2018). *The phenomenology of spirit: Translation with introduction and commentary*. Oxford University Press.

Heron, J., O'Connor, T. G., Evans, J., Golding, J., & Glover, V. (2004). Course of anxiety and depression through pregnancy and the puerperium in a community sample. *Journal of Affective Disorders, 80*(1–2), 65–73.

Kastratović-Kotlica, B. (2005). Dijagnoza trudnoće, nadzor trudnice i metode praćenja stanja ploda. In D. Plećaš, B. Stanimirović, A. Stanković, & M. Vasiljević (Eds.), *Ginekologija i akušerstvo: Udžbenik za studente medicine*. Medicinski fakultet Univerziteta u Beogradu.

Klein, L. (Director). (1998). *Body story: The takeover* [Documentary series, S1 E5]. Discovery Channel.

Kristeva, J. (1990). Motherhood according to Giovanni Bellini. In J. M. Thompson (Ed.), *Twentieth century theories of art* (pp. 441–467). Carleton University Press.

Kukla, R. (2005). *Mass hysteria: Medicine, culture and mothers' bodies*. Rowman & Littlefield Publishers.

Kuriyama, S. (1999). *The expressiveness of the body and the divergence of Greek and Chinese medicine*. Zone Books.

Leder, D. (1990). *The absent body*. University of Chicago Press.

Leifer, M. (1980). Pregnancy. *Signs, 5*(4), 754–765.

Lemieux, K. L. (2006). 13 short pieces, but not the whole [t]ruth. *Hypatia, 21*(1), 74–79. https://doi.org/10.1353/hyp.2005.0144

Merleau-Ponty, M. (2005). *Phenomenology of perception* (C. Smith, Trans.). Routledge. (Original work published 1945).

Mladenović, D., Mladenović-Bogdanović, Z., & Mladenović-Mihailović, A. (2008). *Ginekologija i akušerstvo*. Zavod za udžbenike.

Mujezinovic, F., & Alfirevic, Z. (2007). Procedure-related complications of amniocentesis and chorionic villous sampling: A systematic review. *Obstetrics & Gynecology, 110*(3), 687–694.

O'Dowd, M. J., & Philipp, E. E. (1994). *The history of obstetrics & gynaecology*. The Parthenon Publishing Group.

Pantović, L. (2022). Providing a service or seeking a favor? The role of private prenatal care on the continuity of care in Serbian public maternity hospitals. *Birth, 49*(3), 506–513.

Rich, A. (1986b). *Of woman born: Motherhood as experience and institution*. W. W. Norton & Company.

Sandelowski, M., & Black, B. P. (1994). The epistemology of expectant parenthood. *Western Journal of Nursing Research, 16*(6), 601–614. https://doi.org/10.1177/019394599401600602

Sartre, J. P. (2003). *Being and nothingness: An essay on phenomenological ontology* (H. E. Barnes, Trans.). Routledge. (Original work published 1943).

Slade, P., & Cree, M. (2010). A psychological plan for perinatal care. *The Psychologist, 23*(3), 194–197.

Smith, J. A. (1999). Identity development during the transition to motherhood: An interpretative phenomenological analysis. *Journal of Reproductive and Infant Psychology, 17*(3), 281–299. https://doi.org/10.1080/02646839908404595

Taylor, J. S. (2008). *The public life of the fetal sonogram: Technology, consumption, and the politics of reproduction*. Rutgers University Press.

Tone, A. (2012). Medicalizing reproduction: The pill and home pregnancy tests. *Journal of Sex Research, 49*(4), 319–327. https://doi.org/10.1080/00224499.2012.688226

U.S. Food and Drug Administration (FDA). (2014). Avoid fetal "keepsake" images, heartbeat monitors. *FDA Consumer Health Information*. Retrieved from https://shorturl.at/msCQZ

Ussher, J. (2008). Reclaiming embodiment within critical psychology: A material-discursive analysis of the menopausal body. *Social and Personality Psychology Compass, 2*(5), 1781–1798. https://doi.org/10.1111/j.1751-9004.2008.00151.x

van der Ploeg, I. (2004). 'Only angels can do without skin': On reproductive technology's hybrids and the politics of body boundaries. *Body & Society, 10*(2–3), 153–181. https://doi.org/10.1177/1357034X04042941

Vygotsky, L. S. (1997). The history of the development of higher mental functions. In *The collected works of L. S. Vygotsky* (Vol. 4). Springer.

Young, I. M. (2005b). Pregnant embodiment: Subjectivity and alienation. In *On female body experience: 'Throwing like a girl' and other essays* (pp. 46–61). Oxford University Press.

Zlotogorski, Z., Tadmor, O., Rabinovitz, R., & Diamant, Y. (1997). Parental attitudes toward obstetric ultrasound examination. *The Journal of Obstetrics and Gynaecology Research, 23*(1), 25–28. https://doi.org/10.1111/j.1447-0756.1997.tb00800.x

4

Distributed Subjects: Losing and Reclaiming Maternal Agency Under the Alienating Conditions of Local Institutional Practice

Throughout the early transition to motherhood, even independently of entering medical institutions, women undergo a series of potentially destabilising changes. These changes have already been analysed in the previous chapter, but they become especially prominent during childbirth, when bodily processes can appear intense and uncontrollable, and thus threatening to women's embodied subjectivity. It is important to understand the quality of these changes in order to fully grasp why and under what circumstances institutional procedures and medical practices sometimes have dramatic consequences for women. The analysis in this chapter will focus specifically on women's embodied subjectivity during *childbirth*, which is a complex process shaped by the interaction between constantly changing bodily events on the one hand, and the medical practices and techniques to which they are subjected in specific institutional circumstances on the other. This process is characterised by intense experiences of pain and loss of control, imposed both by the autonomous physiological process of labour and by the problematic model of its institutional regulation.

While the previous chapter has shown that the availability of expert knowledge and medical technology can provide women the opportunity

B. Stanković, *Giving Birth To A Subject*, Sociocultural Psychology of the Lifecourse,
https://doi.org/10.1007/978-3-031-77236-8_4

to experience themselves and their bodies in technologically and conceptually extended ways that would not be accessible otherwise, it has also indicated that medical encounters, at least in the Serbian context, very often lead to alienating and objectifying consequences for women as embodied subjects. Problematic aspects of institutional practices and organisation of care are thus present and visible throughout pregnancy, but their influence is much more pronounced during childbirth and their consequences are much harder to ignore or evade. To explain this, I will try to map the complex socio-material network of institutionally bound relationships, implicit and explicit norms, procedures and practices involving various actors and situated medical technologies. Due to the nature of the empirical reality in Serbian medical institutions, most of the chapter will be devoted to broken relationships, absent mediators and threatening procedures, which ultimately prove to be disruptive rather than productive for women's subjectivity. At the end of the chapter, however, I will focus on the constellations in which the various actors are related and coordinated in a way that supports women to maintain their integrity and a sense of agency.

4.1 The Emergence of the Body-in-Labour: Institutional Resolution of Embodied Uncertainty

The beginning of the last chapter (*Uncertain beginnings*) offers a detailed phenomenological reconstruction of the emergence of the pregnant body. As the woman approaches her due date, she undergoes an analogous process when it comes to the emergence of the *birthing* body, but with some relevant differences that are concerned with the specifically institutional resolution of her embodied uncertainty. Recognising the onset of labour appears to be an epistemological challenge of enormous importance due to its practical consequences. The woman is then faced with the challenging task of interpreting the vague and multifaceted visceral body—only now, unlike when recognising the onset of pregnancy, this task must be solved much more quickly. Although there is a false and unfounded belief among those around them, including medical staff, that "they will know when it starts", women do not have an *immediate* and *privileged* understanding of the bodily processes they are experiencing. As during pregnancy, to navigate this challenge they rely on medical knowledge widely available in popular books for expectant mothers, websites and prenatal classes,[1] simple techniques (such as counting) and everyday objects (such as a clock)[2] associated with the medical model, as well as the experience of close others. The physician's role in assessing the onset of labour is also of great importance and it relies on medical technology (CTG) as well as maternity hospital protocols (which dilation is an indication for hospitalisation) and certain contingent factors (how much time the woman needs to reach the hospital given her place of residence). All these various aspects contribute to the complex process of emergence of the body-in-labour:

> *"In the middle of the night I was awakened by contractions. I wake up and then wait. I take a watch and wait to see if the next one will appear. But the next one doesn't come for more than fifteen minutes, so there's no need. And then I fall asleep again. But in the morning, around nine o'clock, I wake up and see that the contractions are repeating, and they weren't strong. And then I started timing them. Now they were eight minutes apart, but exactly eight minutes apart, they were coming regularly. And I count now, one, two, three, and I get to fifteen, sixteen, seventeen, eighteen, and they stop. But they stop completely. As if nothing had happened up to that point. They just stop. And nothing, and nothing, and nothing.* ***And now I don't know what that means. According to the antenatal classes it was all very clear. Why did it stop now?!*** *And*

[1] Women generally learn three signs that signal the beginning of labour—the onset of contractions, the breaking of the amniotic sac and the expulsion of the mucus plug. The problem is that none of these signs are unproblematic—neither as a definitive indicator of labour nor as something a woman can easily interpret. The women who have attended psychophysical preparation classes have a much more sophisticated knowledge and rely on a more complex set of practices to determine whether their body has entered labour (e.g., they know how to distinguish true from false or preparatory contractions, and a complete from a partial rupture of the amniotic sac).

[2] Almost all of the women I interviewed relied on timing to judge the frequency of contractions and thus the onset of labour. Only when contractions occur at regular intervals does the birthing body maintain a stable presence in their experience. If they recognise that the contractions occur irregularly, and if they are not yet painful and uncomfortable and therefore do not require the women's immediate attention, they are ignored and the women continue with their usual activities. The body then recedes into the background once more.

for an hour, nothing, for two hours, and my husband sees that I'm getting restless. 'Let's go get you checked, honey, let's go get you checked and we'll see.' And we go, we get in the car, and go to the hospital. (...) The doctor puts me on the CTG, everything is okay. 'Lie down, let me examine you.' And she says, 'You're one and a half centimetres dilated, and the cervix is 0.75.' And now she already, 'aha, it's shortening, it's already started and you have some contractions there'. It's nothing serious, nothing is happening. She asked, 'Where do you live?', I said, 'I can be here in five minutes.' 'Okay, then nothing, you go home, and we'll probably see each other tonight.' (...) And they continued in the afternoon. Simply, the intensity of those contractions became such that around nine o'clock, I had one contraction that, I was like, I still wasn't even breathing because there was no need. But this contraction was so strong that, I think it was strong, I overcame it, it wasn't anything serious, but it was, I probably turned red or something because my sister said, 'Are you okay?' I mean, everyone knows, we're all sitting and talking, I turned on the stopwatch, I told them I was counting contractions, everyone is aware of what's happening. 'Are you okay?' 'I am.' 'Did you just have a contraction?' 'I just had a contraction.' 'Are you okay?' I said, 'Yes, yes.' 'Your face looked at that moment, and your colour looked like you were about to throw up.' So she noticed it just by looking at me from the side. And then I told her, 'Yes, yes, it was a stronger contraction.' And that was my signal to head to the maternity hospital." (Teodora)

We can see that the emergence of the birthing body is a process in the course of which one of its specific parts—the contractile uterus—appears and disappears from the woman's phenomenological field. At the same time, determining the onset of labour is also a process of assessing whether the manifestations of the birthing body are indicative and relevant. The woman closely monitors the quality and frequency of these manifestations as she recognises them as indicators of the onset of labour based on her previously acquired medical knowledge. However, the specific manifestations of the body are ambiguous and unpredictable, as they often do not fit well into the normative framework provided by medical textbooks or websites (Chadwick, 2018, p. 52). The final assessment often does not depend on a perfect match between embodied experience and expert knowledge, but is the result of an agreement between very different indicators present in the specific situation—some of which are observed by other people, not necessarily by the woman herself.

What makes the emergence of the birthing body extremely uncertain and different from the emergence of the pregnant body is that there is a problem in determining the onset of labour in an *objective* and not just a *subjective* sense. The reference textbook on obstetrics (Cunningham et al., 2010, p. 382) states that "the greatest impediment to understanding normal labor is recognising its start" since "this diagnosis is confirmed only retrospectively" (p. 384). In contrast to determining the onset of pregnancy, which is unequivocally registered by measuring hormone levels in the blood (despite all the uncertainties of outcomes that may follow), determining the onset of labour—defined as "uterine contractions that bring about demonstrable effacement and dilatation of the cervix" (Cunningham et al., 2010, p. 382)—is a complex process with an uncertain outcome even for medicine, i.e. doctors.

The physician's assessment of whether labour has begun takes into account a number of indicators, each of which is evaluated based on a specific medical practice or technique: cervical dilation and the condition of the amniotic sac are assessed by the doctor's fingers during a vaginal examination; the presence of contractions is assessed by reading the CTG printout; the size of the baby is assessed by ultrasound parameters; an overdue delivery date is assessed based on Naegele's formula. None of these criteria is unproblematic, and their application depends on the competence and knowledge of the doctor (and probably his or her previous experience), the precision of the medical technology, the good adjustment of the device to the woman's body, various diagnostic standards, etc. Finally, the decision to leave the woman in the maternity hospital also depends on contingent circumstances, such as the duty shift of her chosen doctor or her place of residence, i.e. the distance from the maternity hospital.

Considering that recognising the onset of labour is always, to a greater or lesser extent, arbitrary and tentative, in most countries it is formally linked to the time of hospital admission (Cunningham et al., 2010), in line with the approach advocated by the pioneers of active labour management (O'Driscoll et al., 1973). This criterion, which makes it possible to determine the onset of labour in each woman very precisely (to the minute),[3] naturally only conceals, and does not in the least resolve, all the diagnostic uncertainties. Sometimes the women themselves articulate this dilemma, i.e. the arbitrariness of the medical assessment, as they recognise how the beginning of their labour is only formally determined and even retrospectively they cannot estimate its duration:

> *"Well, I don't know anymore about my labour, when I replay the events and what I learned in the prenatal classes, I don't know if I could classify my labour as rapid or average. Because I started, it began the previous day. Now, I don't know, if we were to start measuring, from which moment they could tell me, you started labour then, and you were in labour for two, five, or six hours. In the maternity hospital from the moment of admission, which means they admitted me at 11:20, and I gave birth at 2:20. Exactly three hours later. That's rapid labour. Now, I had contractions from four in the afternoon the previous day, so that's average. So, I can't determine now." (Teodora)*

It could be said that today the body-in-labour is something that is typically constituted only within the medical institution, when doctors and techniques come into play, and does not refer to an embodied state of the pregnant woman that would exist prior to and independently of that. Despite all the uncertainty and arbitrariness of estimating the onset of labour, this act is also enormously significant because of its practical consequences: the woman is sent to the maternity ward and a series of practices begin—measuring the pelvis, shaving, enema, infusion of glucose and/or hormones to augment labour, etc. Once the process has started, it cannot be interrupted, i.e. there is no way to reconsider it. When it is declared that childbirth has begun, irregular contractions or their cessation are interpreted as an interruption of labour progression rather than a misjudged onset, and interventions are used to accelerate labour as doctors rely on the incorrect assessment of slow progression. For example, a woman may arrive at the hospital relatively late and be

[3] The importance of precisely determining the time of onset of labour is imposed by the way it is treated in modern times, primarily due to its institutionalisation. It is easy to imagine that for women in the past this problem did not arise in any relevant way and that they generally went about their usual activities as long as they could endure the pain associated with labour. It is also to be expected that the problem of precisely determining the onset of labour arises in a less dramatic manner in home births.

listed in the medical records as a patient who had a rapid labour as she will give birth within a few hours. And if a woman arrives too early and is admitted due to a misjudgement, she is considered to have had a prolonged labour and medical efforts are likely to be made to accelerate and shorten the dilation phase. Therefore, such operationalisation and formalisation of the onset of labour, which inevitably leads to a series of institutional procedures and medical interventions, may not only be arbitrary, but also completely disconnected from the woman's lived experience of going into labour:

> *"The due date was exactly the 22nd. I went to her (the doctor) for a routine checkup and again the CTG showed nothing. She examined me manually and said I was three centimetres dilated, the baby had dropped a little, and told me, 'Come on, we'll send you to...'. I thought, 'Three centimetres dilated... but I am not having any contractions, none at all.' I was expecting her to say, 'Just go home, nothing's happening', but instead she said, 'Come on, you'd better go to the maternity ward' I was like, 'What? To the maternity ward?!' And she was like, 'Yes, yes, yes.' She sent me away: 'Admission there, admission there!' So I went there, prepared everything I needed, had an enema, they took me upstairs to the maternity ward and laid me on the table.* ***I was completely clueless, I am giving birth, without a single symptom, absolutely nothing. Nothing. My waters hadn't broken, nothing at all.*** *I was totally bewildered, thinking, 'Why did you send me up here, woman?' Only then did the doctors come. They asked me: 'Who is your doctor? Why are you here?' I said: 'My doctor sent me, I don't know' Then they examined me. They gave me glucose or an induction, I don't know, some kind of infusion to see if anything would happen. (...) Then their boss, Dr. R., came and asked, 'Why did you come?' I said: 'I don't know why I came.'" (Anđela)*

The onset of labour is completely *externally* determined, and the woman feels confused and inadequate because there is such a discrepancy between her embodied experience ("I have no symptoms, absolutely nothing") and the situation she finds herself in ("I am giving birth"). This initial situation is highly indicative of the subsequent course of childbirth within the institution—the woman's perspective and her embodied experience are routinely ignored and considered irrelevant. Inside the maternity hospital, the woman is subjected, on the one hand, to a series of institutional procedures that have desubjectifying and alienating effects (which we will analyse next) and, on the other hand, to a series of medical interventions that only deepen and emphasise these effects (which we will discuss later).

4.2 Transforming Embodied Subjects into Objects of Care

From the moment women enter the maternity hospital, they are submitted to an array of disciplinary and regulatory practices resulting in the transformation of embodied subjects into desubjectified bodies that are the sole objects of medical practice. The desubjectification of women is prepared by institutional practices of deindividualisation and standardisation—their social identity and individual specificities become suspended and they get transformed into generic patients susceptible to a treatment consisting of a set of equally generic procedures. A woman's body (or specifically her uterus) is meant to be not only the central, but often the exclusive focus of monitoring and regulation during childbirth. Her experience and subjective involvement are thus actively rendered obsolete. She becomes objectified and partialised, reduced to a set of organs and processes that are not connected to her embodied self or her life projects. This leads to a number of problematic psychological, practical and ethical consequences for her subjectivity, that will be discussed in detail.

In the previous chapters we have seen that medical knowledge, practices and techniques are present throughout the entire process of pregnancy for women. However, entering the hospital introduces certain specificities that, although occasionally visible in situations such as the antenatal check-ups, were not so obvious or did not lead to such dramatic consequences. The aim of this section is to reconstruct the institutional positioning of women during childbirth and the impact this has on their lived experience and agency. By outlining the characteristics of the institutional environment, we can better understand the effects of specific medical practices performed on women during childbirth. It also allows us to view medical technology as situated, which facilitates a contextualised interpretation of its effects.

One obstetrician said in an interview during my fieldwork in response to a question about the role of women in childbirth: "Everything happens beyond the scope of women's volition or consciousness. Women give birth even when they are unconscious, they give birth while in a coma". Doctors in maternity wards often behave as if every woman were in this altered state, characterised by a complete absence of consciousness and agency. From an obstetric point of view, it even seems desirable for the woman's subjectivity to be completely excluded from the situation of birth.

There are a number of *institutional* practices and patterns of behaviour that testify to this, transforming women from embodied subjects into desubjectified bodies suitable as objects of medical practice. These come into effect as soon as the woman enters the maternity ward and accompany her throughout the entire birthing process and subsequent stay in the hospital. This process of desubjectification and deindividualisation occurs both through the exclusive focus of medical monitoring and intervention on the woman's bodily processes and through specific institutional practices that facilitate this process of objectification of the birthing body.

Maternity wards in Serbia are closed departments in hospitals and clinical centres, meaning they are physically inaccessible—only birthing women and medical staff are allowed to enter them.[4] This means that women are literally separated from their previous environment and close others (their partner and family members), which usually leads to feelings of isolation, abandonment and being "cut off from the rest of the world". Upon admission to the maternity hospital, women leave their clothes and

[4] Maternity wards are generally notably closed facilities with rigid borders—e.g. visits from the partner, family or friends are not allowed at all during the women's stay in hospital, or only for a very limited period of the day and always in a room outside the maternity ward (Arsenijevic et al., 2014; Pantović et al., 2024). Women I spoke to during the fieldwork in the maternity ward occasionally mentioned other closed institutions—prisons and psychiatric hospital wards—and pointed out that "even there, visits are allowed".

personal belongings[5] and change into hospital gowns.[6] Feelings of uncertainty and fear are very common in women giving birth for the first time, as the birth process is fraught with uncertainty and potentially negative outcomes. The institutional circumstances in maternity wards only exacerbate this situation. The fact that they are left alone and have their clothes taken away leaves them with the impression that they have no other choice but to stay where they are and submit to procedures that they cannot foresee or alter. All this intensifies the feeling of fear and makes them experience a kind of existential insecurity—as if they were "going to the front" and might never return home. These feelings are further aggravated by the fact that the women cannot express and share them because their voices are not heard.

> *"And then they took me upstairs and I got a bit scared. Because they take you somewhere, through some sterile elevators, I didn't see any stairs. It's a really closed ward.* ***You say goodbye to your husband as if you are going to the front. And then, with your things in a plastic bag,***[7] ***like an orphan, you go away.****" (Sonja)*
>
> *"When they admitted me, I couldn't sleep all night.* ***I had this feeling that I would never return home again.*** *I know it is that irrational fear, I heard a lot of women have it, but it is really awful. When my husband left me, and you know I am not one of those spoiled girls who always need someone around….* ***I was simply convinced that I would never get out again.*** *You know it is that... oh, I got goosebumps. He took me, left me, took my things, because you*

---

[5] When you are transferred to the delivery room, the rest of your personal belongings that you are usually allowed to bring with you (money, mobile phone, jewellery) are taken away, which is reminiscent of being admitted to prison: "*And then the nurse comes back and takes your phone and your money and you have to sign that they took it from you*" (Saška).

[6] In the cases where women are expected to bring their own gowns, it is not a departure from this institutional practice, but rather a practical necessity—the hospital does not have enough gowns or they are in too poor a condition. The same applies to the bedding that women in some maternity wards have to bring from home. This was especially prevalent during the Covid-19 pandemic (Pantović et al., 2024).

[7] A woman is allowed to bring to the maternity ward what she needs during her stay in hospital and what is not already provided there. This is a relatively standardised list of items (mainly hygiene products and diapers for the baby). In many large maternity hospitals in Belgrade, these items can only be brought in a plastic bag (not in a suitcase), which is justified by practical considerations—the lack of space in the maternity rooms. However, this rule further contributes to uniformity and the absence of individual specificities in the maternity ward.

change there and all your things are taken away. ***I was really like 'I am not coming back'****, because everything seemed so dreadful to me." (Sofija)*

"And then the nurse told me 'go behind the curtain and put on the gown'. And she gave me that hospital gown. I can't explain to you how frightened I was. ***I felt like the loneliest person in the world, like I had no one*** *and like I was going to fall on my knees and beg someone to send me home just so they would not keep me there. But I had to do it, I had to finish it. (…) 'Go, take off your clothes', you know, nobody listens to you. (...) I mean, I can't explain it to you, you feel... I would kneel down like a child: 'Mommy, take me home!' You know, I wasn't ready at all, but you have to be cool. Okay, I go, I take the bag, I take my things. I go out. Now I should say goodbye to my boyfriend, but like no, I don't want to. I'm not ready yet." (Saška)*

The sense of isolation and abandonment is so pervasive that it even appears in the narratives of those participants who, in their own words, were well prepared for what awaited them, who had secured support during birth (through personal connections I mentioned earlier) which ensured a more positive birth experience, and who showed no resistance to the medical model of birth or the institutional environment.

"I was well prepared for the birth and everything, but afterwards… I couldn't cope with that at all. I could not believe it when I came out that I was out. ***That they had let me out. That I was in the outside world.****" (Tamara)*

"I stayed in hospital for three days. And it seemed like an eternity. It's really hard, you know... that time in hospital. You have no... ***You are totally isolated from the whole world****, it was just us postpartum women. Each with our own thoughts and worries and so on. And it's not that we don't help each other and talk, but somehow we're just waiting for something. Maybe the hormones do the rest. Then, when it gets to seven in the evening, when the day calms down and each of us is lying in her own bed, and each one is crying." (Nevena)*

"And afterwards, in the hospital, ***I felt like I am on some desert island, and like there is no one there****." (Ivana)*

In addition to the physical removal of the woman from her social environment and the interruption or obstruction of relationships with close ones that institutionalisation entails, her social identity and individual characteristics are also suspended. Individual characteristics are only relevant to the extent that they allow the woman to be placed in a diagnostic category or risk group. The woman thus undergoes a process of bureaucratisation (Thompson, 2005, p. 199) and is transformed into a generic patient, a classifiable body that is monitored and subject to intervention. Upon admission to the maternity ward, she is required to provide adequately selected and concise information about her pregnancy history (and previous births), mainly in order to assess the risk level of the current delivery and, on the basis of this assessment, to classify her in the appropriate category.

The bureaucratisation of childbirth enables its standardisation, as the woman is subjected to specific treatment depending on which category she is placed in—as a first-time mother, obese, with high blood pressure or with a previous caesarean section. In the medical institution, childbirth is operationalised through well-defined phases, aspects and corresponding procedures, so that it is monitored and regulated according to established patterns adapted to the non-specific categories into which women are placed. In this way, childbirth ceases to be a process that involves the whole person with her particularities, preferences and lived experiences. The lack of an individualised approach to treatment and care[8] can lead to extremely negative consequences, not only for the woman's well-being and sense of agency—as the deindividualised and objectified childbirth is actually alienated—but also for her safety and the safety of her baby.

Finally, the desubjectification of women is significantly influenced by the fact that various aspects of the institutional environment and the organisation of childbirth—from the design of the beds[9] to the position of the woman's body and the rules governing her behaviour and clothing—are adapted to suit the doctors, who are positioned and recognised as the main actors in the entire process:

[8] The best example of this is the routine administration of hormones to augment contractions and the performance of episiotomies on all first-time mothers.

[9] Very high beds make it easier to examine women after childbirth during the ward rounds but make it considerably more difficult for women with stitched episiotomy or caesarean section wounds to get on and off the bed.

"And like it's really not fair. The beds are this high (shows a height of about one metre with her hands), prehistoric. It's really hard for a woman to get up after giving birth... instead they put up ones that are even lower than usual so you don't have to climb. If I lift my leg up like that now, I'm stitched up... I mean, it hurts, the stitches are pulling." (Sonja)

"Because we have wounds and because they, because the ward round is at seven in the morning, for example, and they enter your room and say, 'Come on, women, check-up!' And first they shout at you that you have to be bathed for that check-up, I mean… At seven in the morning and the bathroom is at the end of the hallway, and you can't walk. The beds are of course set up so that the doctor doesn't have to bend over, so he doesn't have to bend his back, and you can barely get down. And then they make you lie on that bed, spread your legs and pull your nightgown all the way up, and you lie like that and wait for the doctor to come. And there are seven of us in the room, all spread out like that... I mean, they put you in terribly humiliating physical positions. And then some nurse comes in and yells at you about why you're not ready... and it takes me three seconds to do that. I don't want to do it." (Una)

Everything in the hospital is adapted to the most efficient performance of medical practice, without regard to how the women feel—whether they feel pain, fatigue or shame. Women are transformed into disciplined bodies, stripped and positioned (on their backs, legs spread) to suit the doctor's gaze and unhindered medical manipulation. Like the bodies in the military, the birthing body is one "that is manipulated, shaped, trained, which obeys, becomes docile…" (Foucault, 1995, p. 136).

The process of desubjectification not only affects how medical staff treat the woman's body, but also how the woman herself perceives and relates to her body. Women often speak of a changed relationship with their bodies during hospitalisation—what is experienced as intrusive and uncomfortable under usual circumstances is no longer perceived as such in hospital and becomes normalised. The woman is exposed to the gaze of various unknown people while lying naked and with her legs spread—these are not only nurses and doctors, but often also medical students and pupils doing their internship on the maternity ward. These people change frequently and usually do not introduce themselves or ask for the woman's consent to examine her or attend the examination.

"So there were also these trainee nurses, third-year high-school students. And there were also a few medical students. And the doctors and those midwives. And they were all running around. And they brought me the bedpan to pee. And they all examined me." (Anđela)

"I mean, I'm not particularly shy, but it bothers you, this constant poking. And when you're there in the maternity ward and someone's sticking their hands in every hour, you're like, 'Come on, is there anyone else, come on!' I mean, you just get to a point where you feel like you're on display and whoever wants to look, let them look." (Ivana)

It is as if the body is not perceived as something *personal* anymore, so that certain treatment of the body is not simultaneously experienced as treatment of the person. The body is turned into an object of observation and intervention, which becomes a "normal" situation even for the woman herself. In addition, the arrangement of the hospital rooms, the organisation of work and the (implicit) norms often violate women's privacy.

"When you enter the toilet, the door is open and can't be closed. It's so embarrassing. Everything is open, literally. And that place where she (the nurse) shaves you, there are two more tables and people are passing by. Fortunately, no one was around at the moment, but when it's crowded, I can imagine how uncomfortable it must be. Everyone is passing by. I imagined they would shave me in some bed where no one could see... but no, they shave you in the hallway. Literally, it's like a kind of a hallway. Horrible." (Saška)

Medical practices and representations, as well as the specific circumstances in the maternity ward—the number of women in a room, the arrangement of beds, the protocol prohibiting the wearing of underwear, etc.—lead to the constitution of a desexualised and deprivatised body for women.

"There are no doors on the shower stalls, but the amount of nudity and the indifference to nudity, I've never seen anything like it in my life... I took off another girl's underwear to see if she was bleeding. She apologised to me for looking at her pussy, and I was totally not uncomfortable with that. Pussies were flashing everywhere. ***It was just part of the body, at that moment it really didn't matter.*** *This one is sticking his hands, that one is sticking his, it*

didn't matter anymore. Tits were also everywhere. I saw more tits than ever in my life. They were bringing the babies, they were nursing, this one woman was pumping milk behind me the whole time..." (Sonja)

Neither one's own nor someone else's body is perceived as something personal or sexual, and the absence of shame is an important indicator of this. As Sonja says, vaginas and breasts are just "body parts", biological organs, and all taboos associated with them in the cultural context (outside the hospital) temporarily cease to apply.[10]

"I had such freedom with the woman who was in the room with me that she eventually said, 'Let me see your wound, don't be shy.' Imagine... let me see your wound. What kind of freedom is that? 'Look, if you want, I don't mind'." (Sofija)

In a way, the women distance themselves from their bodies, which become object of surveillance and manipulation during their stay in hospital. As a result, their bodies become alienated and objectified for themselves. It seems that this is not only a consequence of the women's institutional repositioning, but also a coping response. This distancing protects them from feeling vulnerable and exposed, as their privacy in the maternity ward is systematically violated.

The process of desubjectification to which a woman is submitted in the maternity hospital seems to make her body more susceptible to partialisation and objectification, which is a prerequisite for medical monitoring and intervention. It is important to remember that the institutional practices mentioned are likely to be encountered in medical settings in circumstances other than childbirth. In the case of illness, the changes that the subject, his body and his social identity undergo serve to facilitate the person's smoother transition through the clinic and the resolution of their medical problem (Mol, 2002; Thompson, 2005). However, the situation during childbirth has its specificities. Pregnant women are not patients

[10] Desexualisation of one's own body often persists for some time even after leaving the hospital. The body is then something that is largely reduced to its reproductive function, i.e. to the nurturing function in the context of breastfeeding: *"The baby wanted to nurse on one breast, not on the other. So, I was constantly with bare breasts, like it was just us in the room. Sure, give the breast, take it out, eat, don't eat, you just don't have those barriers in your head anymore. And then when all that is over, they put the barriers up again. Like, 'don't walk around with bare breasts'."* (Ivana)

and, before entering the institution, are not typically identified with that role. This discrepancy between the self-positioning and the positioning they are subjected to in the maternity ward makes the negative aspects of the aforementioned processes of desubjectification even more pronounced. We will now turn to numerous other consequences of these problematic institutional practices—both for the relationship between medical practitioners and women (*Broken connections*) and for the way medical interventions are performed during childbirth (*Alienated birth*).

4.3 Broken Connections

Relational aspects of care—i.e. a close and caring relationship with caregivers who are supportive and understanding—are frequently emphasised in the literature as central to a positive childbirth experience (Baker et al., 2005; Elmir et al., 2010; Esposito, 1999; Larkin et al., 2012; Thomson & Downe, 2008; Waldenström et al., 2004), and can even serve as a protective factor when women are faced with pain or obstetric interventions (Andersen et al., 2012; Creedy et al., 2000; Hodnett, 2002; Nilsson et al., 2010; Olde et al., 2005; van der Gucht & Lewis, 2015), regardless of ethnicity, culture and socioeconomic status (Esposito, 1999; Lazarus, 1994; van der Gucht & Lewis, 2015). However, the situation in Serbian maternity wards is far from this desired situation.

The medical record of the woman giving birth, which is created upon her admission to the maternity ward on the basis of the medical documents she brings with her and the information collected at that time—and which accompanies her until her discharge, contains all relevant information about her condition and the interventions she has undergone.[11] Since selected information is collected from the woman in the

[11] Una's childbirth experience is a good illustration of how irreplaceable medical documentation is as a source of information about a woman. Even when a woman is present, knows the relevant data and is willing to share it with the medical staff, and even in reasonably urgent situations (as Una had begun to feel pushing contractions), she is not treated as a relevant and reliable source of information upon which the doctors would base their decisions and practices: *"And then, bad luck, in our panic we forgot my folder with the documents. So then I didn't have the documents. And I told them I was receiving prenatal care there, who my doctor was. They didn't care. They won't do it. They put me up in the delivery room, and they were terribly angry, terribly angry. The nurses and the doctors, the whole*

form of an "obstetric history", all that is relevant to her health status is either already noted in her medical record or is monitored indirectly (through doctor's checkups or medical technology such as foetal heart monitoring), so further interaction and communication with the woman serves no practical purpose and is often left out altogether.[12] And considering that for adequate monitoring and management of labour it is only relevant that the medical staff is informed about the woman's condition, but not the woman herself (since she cannot influence the process anyway), she is usually not given any information or explanation about the procedures and interventions she is undergoing.

> *"They generally have a policy during childbirth to stay silent, not tell the woman anything, and just have it their own way." (Ivana)*
>
> *"The doctor wanted to, she said let's go upstairs, break the waters, that was her plan, but the other doctor didn't agree. What was his reason, maybe he saw or was waiting for the contractions to do their thing in terms of dilation, I don't know, I have no idea. It's like that, you know, they don't tell you anything, and since you don't know and you are not informed, the only thing you can do is guess and try to reconstruct some kind of story based on a few things you do know." (Teodora)*

Since the information and explanation are withheld from women, they fail to create a framework for understanding and interpreting their birth experience, so they are unable to anticipate what will happen next or how long it will take. The process thus becomes completely opaque to them, and they may feel disoriented and disconnected from it. Without the possibility to rely on their embodied experience, they sometimes even

---

on-duty team, and I didn't have my papers and I arrived like that, shame on me, in the final stage of labour. (...) And they wouldn't examine me even though I was feeling the urge to push. They said no, not until the papers arrived, no. The doctor asked, 'What's your blood group?' I said 'A positive.' 'Are you sure?' I said 'Well, yes, I recently checked because of the birth.' 'Do you have the paper?' I said 'Well, I told you three times we forgot it at home.' 'Well, I can't start delivering you now, do you know how many women lie about their blood type?' And I thought, yes, sure they lie. What nonsense, that's the bureaucratic mentality. Why would they lie? Yes, they lie to deceive you and fuck up themselves and the baby. Sure, that's what they do. I mean, idiot. And they were very rude and didn't want to examine me until the papers arrived. So, I was lying there with pushing contractions." (Una)

[12] Communication and the provision of information during childbirth are left to the good will of medical practitioners and are treated as a "non-standard service", so they are usually omitted in practice.

wonder if "this is it", i.e. if the childbirth has actually started or if there are still some preparations to be made.

"She examined me and said, 'Excellent, take her down to the delivery room.' And she didn't say anything to me. And you know what's even worse? When she said, 'Take her down to the delivery room', I didn't realise I was about to lie down and give birth. I still thought something else was going to happen. I even asked the nurse if I could walk around a bit and not lie down and she just looked at me like, 'Yeah, yeah, you can (sarcastically), like there's something wrong with you, girl.' I didn't understand at all that I was about to give birth." (Sofija)

"It's all so uncomfortable and you don't know what to expect, where you're going next, whether you're going straight to the delivery table or... I did everything, the shower and all that. And then I waited. No one was there. I had done everything and was sitting in that gown on the bed, and no one appeared." (Saška)

Many women are not only unable to anticipate the doctors' actions, they also perceive them as arbitrary. They cannot relate them to their condition or to any reliable diagnostic information that might be available.

"They just leave you there and say nothing. I really don't know why they took me there at exactly half past eight. It's arbitrary, they didn't even examine me. They took me there arbitrarily at half past eight. The doctor examined me before the enema, which was before seven o'clock, and from then on they didn't examine me. Not even when they put me on the table did they examine me. They just started the induction." (Maja)

Similar to the ultrasound examination discussed at the end of the previous chapter, women usually manage to learn some things about their situation during labour by overhearing conversations between the medical practitioners. Although the doctors rarely address them directly, they exchange information with their colleagues or give instructions to the nurses, so the women can obtain pieces of information in an indirect manner (regarding what is happening to them and what interventions they will be subjected to). They are aware that the doctors do not pay attention to the fact that they are present and can hear them, so they might feel excluded and put in the position of an external observer of their childbirth.

> *"He did not tell me that he would break my water, but I kind of knew it from their conversation about what he was planning to do. And I felt the water running from my body, he didn't say anything like 'now I am going to do this' or 'your water broke.' And then he gave instructions to the nurses to turn on the induction drip. They started the induction, attached everything, and left." (Anđela)*
>
> *"He doesn't address me, no, he doesn't tell me anything. I just overheard when he said 'oh god, we overdid it with the induction, reduce it. The baby's heart rate isn't good.' So they reduced it. So they don't inform you about anything. They don't say, 'The baby is like this, so we'll do that.' No, they do everything on their own, among themselves." (Saška)*

The practice of not informing women is very common—not only do they often not know what is happening to them or what will follow during their childbirth, but they do not find out afterwards either.[13] The lack of relevant information about the childbirth process makes it difficult for the woman to integrate birth into the flow of her life experience and build a coherent narrative about it. Childbirth represents in itself a dramatic event that brings with it a kind of interruption to the normal flow of experience, and if a woman is not granted the opportunity to be properly involved in it, this can only deepen the dissociative effect. Furthermore, not knowing all the relevant facts about what happened during childbirth

[13] Some of the women recognise that withholding information from women giving birth is difficult to explain, as they are usually well informed and very interested (and unwilling to confront the doctors): "*And I really can't understand why they are not telling us anything? I don't understand why it's so hard for them just to say it out loud, when they know how much you care, how interested you are, they know everything, and yet they don't give you the opportunity. I don't know, if we were really saucy and started talking back to them, but most women are not like that, they are so scared. But in my experience - and it sounds silly to say this—almost all the women who were in the room with me were well educated, they had read everything and knew exactly what we were talking about.*" (Anđela) In other words, women cannot understand the reason for such distance and disproportion in position between them and the doctors, given the characteristics of (at least contemporary) healthcare service users who have largely adopted medical discourse (as discussed in the Chap. 2). While a change in the doctor-patient relationship and a shift in the distribution of power has taken place in large parts of the Western world in recent decades, the traditional model in which all power and knowledge lie exclusively in the hands of doctors still dominates in local medical institutions.

makes it difficult for women to construct an interpretive framework and normative standards for evaluating their postpartum experiences.

> *"And then this one nurse shouted 'placenta!'. And then the doctor came to look at the placenta. I was lying there. And the next thing I remember is waking up. I woke up, and there was some woman standing over me, completely unfamiliar. And the doctor was stitching the last stitch, and it hurt a lot. And I know that I literally jumped up from the table and he was like, 'there, there, I'm finishing the stitching, I'm finishing the stitching'. And I said to this woman, 'oh, I fell asleep'. She said, 'it's okay, it's okay, it's supposed to be like that'. So I said, 'Doctor, how did I fall asleep while you were stitching me?' And he said, 'because you have special treatment, so we gave you total anaesthesia while I was stitching you, but I stitch other women without total anaesthesia'. And I said, "aha, ok". And I believed that. How naive I was, thinking how cool the doctor is, he gave me total anaesthesia. In fact I wasn't informed at all about what was done to me under anaesthesia. And afterwards, in hospital, I had abnormal postpartum pain. I was in pain for three days. At times it hurt more than during the birth. And I cried for two nights. The woman next to me couldn't sleep. I wept at night. I begged someone to come. Nobody gave a fuck at all. A nurse came and I said it hurt a lot. And she said, 'Of course it hurts, everything hurts, you are so spoiled, of course it hurts'. And I was scared, why does it hurt so much. No, you can't imagine, I felt incredible. And I started to take an interest in my case, why it hurt so much. And I looked at the bed list. And it said placenta defecta revizio. I called my mother-in-law, who is a doctor, and asked 'what does that mean?' She said, 'it means the part of the placenta remained in your uterus, that they did a revision'. And that's why they gave me total anaesthesia, he did a revision, but he didn't tell me. He made me look like an idiot, saying I had special treatment, while stitching me up. In fact, that's why it hurt so much, I don't know. I have no idea. I was in shock. I found out by myself that a revision was done to me, no one informed me." (Saška)*

Saška was not only deprived of information, she was also misinformed and what the doctor did while she was unconscious was concealed from her. For this reason, she could not explain the severe postpartum pain nor could she assess whether it was a common symptom and whether she was only reacting to it because she was "spoiled". The information she didn't get from the doctor, she got from reading her medical records, in a completely indirect way. The fact that the information was written in Latin, the language of medicine, indicates that it is intended for doctors and that the woman needs an interpreter to understand it. Anđela had a very similar experience, but did not even manage to get indirect information about what was being done to her body while she was anaesthetised immediately after giving birth.

> *"I remember vaguely that this woman anaesthesiologist came to ask me something, and then they put me under. And then, I woke up. And there was some bottle of ice between my legs. And I looked up,* ***lifted the sheet, saw my belly was gone, completely flat. And you don't even know where you are****, and I am looking, I saw him, the doctor, still there, commenting 'take her blood, see, she's as white as a sheet'.*
>
> *B: And they didn't tell you - we did this and that?*
>
> *A: No, nothing. Absolutely nothing. They just took me to the room without any... And that's it. They left.*
>
> *B: Did you find out why they gave you anaesthesia after giving birth, what was done to you?*
>
> *A: No, I didn't find out and no one told me anything.*
>
> *B: Did you maybe see your medical record?*
>
> *A: The record is only there during the doctor's round and then they take it away. And then they gave it to us when we went for the gynaecological exam. I started flipping through it while we were waiting, and just as I started reading it when one nurse -* ***'That's our private document, don't look at it, close the record!'***
>
> *B: Who told you that?*
>
> *A: The nurse. She even shouted,* ***'That's ours, it's not yours, why are you looking at it? Close the folder!'*** *As if they had something to hide. And I didn't manage to see what happened at the end of the birth. It was only after a month, when I went for a gynaecological check-up here at the health centre, my doctor read it to me. I mean, it was written in Latin, I didn't understand it. But she said that my cervix had ruptured during the birth." (Anđela)*

The nurse's reaction, forbidding Anđela from looking at her medical record, reveals that withholding information from women is not just an accidental oversight or something that is omitted for the sake of efficiency, as informing women requires some time and commitment of the staff. The wording of this prohibition ("it's ours") raises the question—who owns the information about the woman and her body? In the maternity ward, there seems to be a paradoxical rule that something containing information about the state of a woman's body is considered a *private* document of the medical institution. This seems to be the ultimate expression of the specifically Cartesian division of labour and authority in hospital births—solely the doctors are responsible for the physical body and what happens to it, and therefore they also own the documentation on the treatment of that body. The woman as subject is generally excluded during (almost) the entire birth process, her body is objectified and left to the interventions of the medical staff. This *real* alienation is accompanied by a *symbolic* alienation. The information about the woman's body does not belong to her, but to the medical institution.

Furthermore, the fact that the information is not communicated has important consequences for the procedure of informed consent, which is one of the standards of contemporary professional care. The right to be fully and timely informed about the medical status and all planned medical interventions, as well as the right to consent to or refuse medical treatment, are among the guaranteed patient rights in the Serbian healthcare system (The Law on Patients' Rights, 2013).[14] Performing obstetric interventions without informing the woman in advance, explaining the options to her and asking for her consent is considered an indicator of a violation of rights or abuse in healthcare (Bowser & Hill, 2010; D'Oliveira et al., 2002), because: "The doctrine of informed consent is, in a very real sense, a protection of the subjectivity of the person involved—that is, it is an acknowledgment that the body can never be regarded merely as a site of quantifiable processes that can be assessed objectively, but must be treated as invested with personal meaning, history, and value that are ultimately determinable only by the subject who lives 'within' it" (Bordo, 1993, p. 73–74). Denying women the right to informed consent in local public maternity hospitals is another important indicator of disrespectful, instrumental and non-person-centred care that leaves women feeling

[14] The existing national guideline for good clinical practice during childbirth (Physiological Childbirth, 2009) also calls for informed consent and recommends that women should be properly informed about all planned interventions, medications and procedures and that their consent should be obtained, but without prescribing a specific procedure.

completely powerless, vulnerable and non-involved into the process of birth.

There is another important aspect that should be taken into account. The distanced relationship between women and caregivers is not only influenced by social factors such as prevailing norms and modes of interaction, but also by *material* aspects of the institutional context. The very structure and organisation of the delivery rooms embodies institutional norms that prescribe constant monitoring of the birthing bodies, coupled with a detached gaze and the avoidance of direct contact with the women giving birth. Many large maternity hospitals (especially within clinical centres in larger cities) have glass walls to facilitate the monitoring of women in labour without having to enter the ward or come into direct contact with them. This also allows multiple women to be monitored at the same time, which is just another manifestation of the approach to childbirth that is insensitive to individual needs or specificities.[15]

"We are in the ward, it is all in glass, and they are there in their room, but it's all in glass so they can see us. We lie and wait. I mean, we are giving birth. They oversee us and enter from time to time, lift the sheet, see how much we are open, put the sheet back..." (Nevena)

The largest maternity hospital in Serbia has perfected this principle of cost-effective monitoring[16] by organising the main delivery room in accordance with the principles of Bentham's panopticon (Foucault, 1995, p. 200).

"This delivery area in the hospital is very modern. It has recently been renovated. And it looks like a very long corridor. You have five delivery tables on one side and five on the other. It's all in glass and you see all the tables across you, on the other side. So you can see every woman giving birth and they see you. So it's all glass and you can see everything live. And in the middle, between these two rows of birthing tables, there are desks and doctors are sitting there. They have

[15] An additional consequence of this is the complete violation of privacy, since women giving birth can often see other women across them.

[16] Since it allows the number of medical staff to be reduced and involves less work for them, because they can oversee the progression of labour of multiple women at the same time.

set it up like that so they can sit, talk, drink coffee, because it lasts for hours you know, so they can just glimpse from the table to see what is happening." (Saška)

For the doctors, the monitoring process is extremely facilitated by this arrangement of the hospital setting, as they can keep an eye on a number of deliveries with little effort. Even if we, for a moment, leave aside the invasion of privacy in this situation, women in labour can see that medical staff are often preoccupied with private matters. This contributes to their feelings of loneliness, neglect and isolation (despite paradoxically being surrounded by people), but also to the impression that they are irrelevant and sidelined, as those who are supposed to take care of them are actually focused on something else.

"And my doctor was watching, she had a laptop and she was watching Suleiman [TV series] through the whole time. So I was giving birth, and I could see her watching Suleiman the whole time. And when something happens she just presses the pause button." (Anđela)

"And the doctors are there hanging on Facebook, and you see it. Some computers are between the birthing tables." (Una)

"The woman who was crying out was actually across from me. I could see that she was in severe pain, worse than what I had experienced so far, and I secretly hoped I wouldn't have to go through the same. I was watching her, and I was really like, 'Oh God, now this will happen to me too, this awaits me.' And then she started shouting, suddenly convulsing and yelling, 'It's going to come out! It's going to come out!' She must have been having pushing contractions. A young doctor was sitting at a desk, watching her over his shoulder, and he's like, 'It won't, it won't, what are you on about, it won't, chill out.' The woman was trembling all over, I swear, clearly having contractions, it was really... 'It's going to come out! It's going to come out!' And he was mocking her, 'Did you practise breathing exercises, did you learn?' And she couldn't even speak. And he was like, 'Well, breathe like this.' They were only five metres apart, and he was shouting instructions at her instead of getting up and going to her. It was awful." (Saška)

Since the doctors are "present" all the time and can prevent any risky or negative outcome, it seems as if they are fulfilling their role. Taking care of the woman, her emotional state and her needs does not fall within their remit. Combined with the routine handling of a large number of women giving birth on a daily basis, this probably leads to the insensitivity displayed by the doctor in Saška's account. The organisation of the delivery room further supports the detached relationship between the women and the doctors. The glass partitions separating the delivery tables from the doctors' room allow this relationship to be fully exposed—the caregivers are present primarily as a disinterested and distant medical eye, solely monitoring and controlling the medical status of the women (or more precisely, their bodies) and the babies yet to be born.[17]

A clear indication that the care is not focused on the woman, but exclusively on her body and indirectly on the baby to be born, is the fact that women are regularly left alone for long periods during the birth, since the presence of labour companions is predominantly not permitted and medical practitioners are only there to perform check-ups.[18] Doctors and nurses tend to manage bodily processes and conditions appropriately, with little interest in whether the woman needs anything, how she feels, or how much easier it would be if someone were there to help or support her. They monitor the women through the glass or appear at certain intervals to read the CTG and manually check cervical dilatation.

"And now, that last phase began, I was holding back, already getting annoyed. In fact, I called for them, but of course no one was there. They come at their own... As we were taught in antenatal classes, when this phase begins, you call the doctor, the midwife, and I started shouting there. 'Doctor! Midwife!', a bit

[17] The question can be raised whether this kind of relationship is necessary in the medical context or merely historically contingent. Foucault (2006, p. 2), for example, argues that: "The condition of the medical gaze (regard médicale), of its neutrality, and the possibility of it gaining access to the object, in short, the effective condition of possibility of the relationship of objectivity, which is constitutive of medical knowledge and the criterion of its validity".

[18] Previous studies have shown that the presence of a labour companion might serve as a protective factor against neglect by medical staff (Lundgren et al., 2009). However, the vast majority of maternity hospitals in Serbia do not allow the presence of fathers during childbirth and the presence of other possible birth attendants is prohibited in all institutions (Pantović et al., 2024; Stanković et al., 2017). Practical obstacles are usually cited as a reason (lack of private maternity wards and thus possible violation of other women's privacy), but ideological reasons should also not be neglected due to the patriarchal and conservative climate. A few hospitals that allow the presence of fathers have a special set of rules and restrictions. For example, fathers are obliged to bring the results of laboratory tests that are not older than 7 days, and in some hospitals they have to pay a fee for their attendance.

like I was losing strength, I couldn't even shout that much anymore. And I'm calling for the doctor, the midwife, but they weren't there, they weren't there. Now I can't even remember how long the corridor was. Could they hear me? And the doctor comes and asks, 'Why are you shouting?' I said, 'It's starting!' 'Why are you shouting so much, we're here.' 'I know you're here, but it's starting to push.' 'Well alright, just lie down, you'll have to wait. You're not dilated enough.' And they leave. ... This phase lasted exactly twenty minutes. And what an incredible thing that was. They seemed to have calculated, 'Aha, it's started, she started feeling the pushing contractions, so we'll come and check her in twenty minutes'. They know how long it takes, it can't be longer, it has to be like that. And they arrive at the moment when I'm experiencing the most intense contraction along with holding off, really intense." (Teodora)

Teodora is a "prepared" birthing woman. This means that during her pregnancy she took part in a birth preparation course, where she learned that she should call the medical staff as soon as she feels the urge to push, as this is a sign that the birth is nearing its end, and that she should hold off pushing until the doctor and midwife arrive. It is clear from her description that the staff visit the woman giving birth according to their schedule ("they come at their own") and not when the woman calls them. What matters to them is that they do not miss any significant physical changes. The doctor's remark, "We're here," means that they are there to ensure that nothing medically significant happens without their insight (and, if necessary, intervention), which is the only presence women should count on and which falls within the staff's "job description". Teodora's case shows that practical circumstances (e.g. too many women giving birth and lack of staff) are not the reason why they are not more present during childbirth, as she is alone in the entire delivery ward. Nor can this be explained by a lack of goodwill and interest—because Teodora has a good relationship with the midwife, and especially with the doctor who is her chosen physician.[19] For the medical staff, adequate care simply

[19] This doctor monitored her pregnancy in a private practice, which is a typical way for Serbian pregnant women to ensure continuity of care and a personal connection in the public maternity hospital (Pantović, 2016, 2022). She also paid several hundred euros for "her" doctor to attend her childbirth (since it was not his regular shift), which is a special service that this maternity hospital offered to women giving birth (this amount corresponded to the average salary in Serbia at that time).

equates to adequate care for only the woman's body and the baby to be born.

Finally, it is important to emphasise that women who give birth in local public healthcare institutions not only often lose *insight* into the process that is happening to them, but also any *authority* over it. The health professionals are the ones who take absolute control over the birth from the beginning, and the women play a passive role in it, as previously discussed in the Chap. 2. This is not only laid down as a normative standard in medical textbooks—"Modern childbirth management involves complete control in all its stages" (Momčilov, 2005, p. 345)—but is also consistently implemented in practice:

> *"You see, you have no control over anything that is happening, just forget about it. Literarily anything. Everything is just happening to you and the only thing you can do is wait for it to end." (Ivana)*
>
> *"All you have to do is lie down, shut up, and spread your legs." (woman interviewed in the maternity hospital)*

As a result, women's competence to make certain decisions is completely devalued (Beckett, 2005, p. 255). Their feeling that they might want to eat, drink or walk around at a certain moment is not treated as an indication of whether they should actually do so.[20] They are certainly not consulted regarding the procedures they will undergo, which is their right guaranteed by law, although from their narratives, it seems that the majority of women would not be prepared for any confrontation with the doctors or questioning of their decisions. However, women are losing control over even the most basic—their physiological needs.

> *"They brought me a bedpan to pee in. And I maybe peed by myself twice, but then I couldn't anymore. They would put it under me every half hour. I was like, 'Come on people, what are you doing...?' And every half hour they would put it, 'Pee, pee.' 'I don't need to pee.' 'No, your bladder is full, your bladder is full.' They kept insisting. I was like, come on... But they were like, 'Come on,*

[20] In Serbian maternity wards, women are not allowed to eat or drink anything during childbirth, and once they have entered the delivery room, they are not allowed to move or leave the bed.

pee, pee, did you pee?' 'No, I didn't.' Then they'd feel my stomach down there, it's full, and they were like 'Let's put in a catheter.'" (Anđela)

"I tell them I have to pee. And the midwife says, 'It's impossible that you have to pee, you just have this feeling'. I tell her 'I really need to pee'. And she says, 'Okay, now we're going to straighten you up to ninety degrees and bring you that bedpan, and you sit on that bedpan.' (...) I peed, even though she was telling me, 'No, no, you don't have to pee.' (...) And she's like surprised, 'Look, she really peed' 'Well, I told you, I'm not making it up.'" (Saška)

As can be seen from these two experiences, the woman's embodied experience is not taken as a reliable source, but her condition is checked indirectly, even when it comes to bodily processes where she normally relies on how she feels. So not only are the women not informed about anything, they are also not expected to report anything. It is therefore irrelevant whether the woman giving birth is even present as a conscious subject.

Finally, the widespread practise of medical treatment and disciplining of the female body, while neglecting that the woman is an embodied subject, favours a highly depersonalised attitude of medical personnel that sometimes occurs. Some women therefore experience that they are not only ignored and overlooked, but that they are also treated in an extremely harsh manner that undermines their dignity.

"That hospital is terrifying. It's a prison. It's a torture chamber. When we came for the ultrasound, there was this young doctor doing the examination. We were standing in a line like in a concentration camp, and they were saying 'Come on, come on, come on!' And because the women walk slowly and it takes a while for them to reach the place where that young doctor is doing the ultrasound, she shouts at them. And she says, 'Move faster, come on, faster!' And then I lie down like this and they tell you to bring a pad. And now I have a pad between my legs, because you're not allowed to wear underwear during these examinations, and you hold it between your legs and walk with it. And I have a pad between my legs and she says to me, 'Lie down I am lying down and I forget to remove that pad.' And she says, 'Move that! Do you expect me to move it?!' You know, like we're some kind of cattle and she's like some important doctor... I can not believe, whether she's ever given birth or ever will. In the last two days, I think I have been... like I have been in a psychiatric hospital. That's how I felt. You

know, they mess with your head so much, you can't believe it. Imagine a woman who is so sensitive after giving birth, physically, psychologically and mentally. You need them to be not just nice, but extra nice because you're so fragile. No, they are extra nasty. I can't explain to you what it's like. It's such arrogance, as if we're cows, they treat you like cows there, like cattle, giving birth on an assembly line. And there are so many births that it really goes like on an assembly line." (Saška)

The above description is very dramatic and will perhaps only resonate with some of the women who have given birth. However, it contains elements that can be considered typical based on the experiences of most of them: the feeling that everything in the maternity ward runs "like an assembly line", due to the large number of women and the highly routinised approach (which is particularly true of the largest maternity hospitals); the lack of sensitivity to the specific psychological and physical needs and limitations of women who have just given birth; the distant and disinterested attitude of most of the staff. These circumstances contribute to the fact that the openly hostile and disrespectful behaviour of certain healthcare workers becomes to a certain extent normalised and is not sanctioned within the healthcare institution.

Insights in this chapter are consistent with the abundance of studies on childbirth experience coming from different research traditions, which emphasise that the quality of the relationship with caregivers together with a sense of control[21] and active involvement during birth are essential for a positive birth experience and women's subsequent well-being (Baker et al., 2005; Czarnocka & Slade, 2000; Elmir et al., 2010; Esposito, 1999; Green & Baston, 2003; Hallam et al., 2016; Hauck et al., 2007; Hodnett, 2002; Larkin et al., 2012; Learly, 2006; Mathews & Callister, 2004; Nilsson et al., 2010; Swahnberg et al., 2007; Thomson & Downe, 2008; Waldenström et al., 2004). The most relevant relational aspects that are seen as crucial for positive birth experiences are support provided by the medical staff, provision of information, responsiveness to women's

[21] While this aspect is almost universally recognised as crucial, there is some evidence that the importance of control may be subject to class and regional differences (Lazarus, 1994). It is also suggested that for marginalised women, control is even more difficult to negotiate in the context of institutionalised care (Chadwick et al., 2014; Esposito, 1999).

needs and a caring and empathetic relationship. At the same time, it is noted that a distant, disconnected and fragmented relationship with caregivers and instrumental-focused care are associated with negative and even traumatic birth experiences (Andersen et al., 2012; Creedy et al., 2000; Czarnocka & Slade, 2000; Harris & Ayers, 2012; Olde et al., 2005; Thomson & Downe, 2008) and to the feelings of neglect or even abuse in healthcare (D'Oliveira et al., 2002; Schroll et al., 2013; Swahnberg et al., 2007). When women are ignored or neglected, their needs and preferences are not taken into account, and they are not allowed to gain sufficient insight and control over the process of their birth—they feel objectified (Swahnberg et al., 2007), alienated (Learly, 2006), powerless and vulnerable (Elmir et al., 2010), "nullified" (Swahnberg et al., 2007) and use the metaphors of the "lump of meat" and "slab on a table" (Thomson & Downe, 2008) to illustrate the objectifying and dehumanising practice of care.[22] The further analysis will strongly testify to this.

4.4 Alienated Birth: Disrupted Embodied Subjectivity as a Consequence of Medical Interventions

The exclusive focus on the body and the neglect of women as embodied subjects is not only expressed through the institutional norms, practices and relational patterns described in the previous sections, but also manifests itself through specifically medical procedures. This section will focus on a paradigmatic case of such medical treatment of the birthing body by analysing the widespread practice of hormone augmentation of contractions, which probably represents the most radical form of neglect and endangerment of women as embodied subjects and leads to a number of problematic consequences for their safety during childbirth and the well-being of their babies. This treatment not only affects how women feel and

[22] These problematic relational patterns are not only typical of the medical treatment of women during pregnancy and childbirth, but are generally present in local healthcare institutions and are perceived as particularly threatening in situations that are sensitive in themselves (e.g. women undergoing abortion, see Skočajić & Stanković, 2020) or when directed at members of vulnerable groups (see Vidić et al., 2022).

how they experience childbirth and the postpartum period, but also influences their sense of agency, which is particularly significant in the final stage of labour when their active involvement is required and expected. It is important to keep in mind that the embodied experience of childbirth, regardless of its treatment, can be unsettling and alienating due to the intense physical sensations, pain and loss of control. However, rather than facilitating the integration of this embodied experience and establishing (mediated/extended) agency, the way in which institutional maternity care is provided often deepens the woman's dissociation and alienation, rendering her utterly helpless.

4.4.1 Body in Pain: Inducing Dys-Embodiment

My everyday functioning is predominantly characterised by the absence of my body from my phenomenological field, as already described in the introduction to Chap. 2. However, I am often focused on my body or its parts during everyday practices such as dressing up, looking at myself in the mirror or mastering a new skill. But at certain times, my body is not only present to me (*body-as-object*), but it is excessively "in front of my eyes" because the body becomes the sole or dominant focus of my attention. This is paradigmatic of the overwhelming and intrusive presence of our own bodies in our experience. Just as we only become explicitly aware of the tools we use to achieve certain goals when they fail or let us down, we usually only become acutely aware of our own body or one of its parts when something goes wrong. Drew Leder (1990) refers to this specific type of bodily awareness by the term "dys-appearance",[23] to emphasise the fact that the body then comes to the forefront of our consciousness as problematic and dysfunctional. Actually, each time the body becomes explicitly perceived and thematised a certain distancing move in relation to the self is being introduced. Yet, unpleasant or painful experiences involve an alienating dimension that is not typical of neutral or pleasant

[23] Unlike the term "disappearance", which refers to the body receding from a person's focus during normal functioning, "dys-appearance" denotes a specific mode of the body's appearance in situations of bodily discomfort (the prefix "dys-" in Greek means bad, difficult, or diseased). Despite the apparent homonymy of the terms, these two concepts are in many respects antonyms.

experiences. In these situations, "the body itself can impose otherness and indignity" (Gadow, 1984, p. 64). Emergence of strong pain puts me into a situation where "my own body may feel away from me, something problematic and foreign", that "can come to appear 'Other' and opposed to self" (Leder, 1990, p. 70).

Body dys-appearance, therefore, implies its objectification, but the moment of dysfunctionality permeates this state with a character of *demand* (Leder, 1990, p. 91)—the body simply does not allow us to ignore it, nor does it allow us to do nothing about what is happening to it. This is important to bear in mind when criticising the medical approach. The objectification implied by medical treatment in many cases builds on the objectification that has already taken place independently of medical treatment and which already leads to alienating effects. The medical approach to the body can of course *deepen* the alienation that has already occurred, which very often happens, but it is to be expected that the relationship between the two kinds of objectification is more complex, at least in some cases. We will see that this analysis is particularly important for understanding the phenomenological experience of birth when dys-embodiment is prominent, and the potentially alienating effects of medical practice are widespread.

Although pain is a paradigmatic embodied experience and appears to be unmediated, the empirical analysis in this section will challenge this assumption. I will try to show that different actors are involved in the production of pain, especially in the medical context. Pain is therefore not simply an internal sensation, a manifestation of an isolated body to an isolated psychic subject. It has its place and origin in the whole situation of birth, and we will try to analyse it by looking at this phenomenon as complex and distributed.

The onset of contractions usually marks the appearance of the birthing body for the woman, and their occurrence is usually accompanied by pain. When women experience pain for the first time, they are usually still at home. The quality of this pain is specific and differs in many ways from the later experience of contractions that are chemically augmented after hospitalisation. Women often refer to this difference by introducing a distinction between "my" (and sometimes "natural") contractions and "artificial" contractions. They regularly describe "their contractions" as "bearable"—they are accompanied by pain that is not of great intensity and that increases gradually, has a familiar quality (similar to menstrual pain), is localised (usually in the lower abdomen), lasts for a relatively short time and has breaks during which women can rest.

"It starts with mild pain, then intensifies and lasts for a certain period, and then it stops. And then for a while, yes, for a while... And then again. I remember thinking at one point, well, the pain isn't that bad." (Tamara)

"These pains are like menstrual cramps, more intense, more frequent, but nothing unbearable." (Ivana)

"I felt it in the lower part of my abdomen where the ovaries are, it was just like when I get my period. It still wasn't painful, I just felt it and noticed it, and it was recurring. I was walking around normally and everything was okay..." (Nevena)

"And the pain at that moment was no stronger than menstrual pain. It was like that, but it can't be compared because during my period it lasts continuously for two hours. Here, the contraction lasts up to about thirty seconds at most, then it subsides and lets go. And I don't have that feeling like with menstrual pain, which is there all the time and torments you." (Teodora)

"Contractions were coming every four minutes, but I was able to stand and shower without any problems. I had contractions, but for the first four or five hours, nothing really hindered my functioning. (...) And they got stronger and stronger. Incomparably stronger than when they started. I mean, they were more painful and spread across my back and so on. But somehow my experience was... for me it was nothing terrible at all." (Una)

The experience of spontaneous contractions, especially in the first hours of labour, is not perceived as a disruption of embodied subjectivity, which also implies that women's ability to respond to them is not impaired. Women deal with the increasingly stronger and more frequent contractions in various ways, often relying on different knowledge, skills and tools—looking at the clock, counting, breathing techniques. The intensity of the pain is such that it can be endured and overcome, if not directly, then through the mediation of various means which, even if they do not reduce the pain, focus their attention elsewhere and make it easier to cope.

"These exercises from birth preparation classes helped me, the breathing, I think it's not so much about easing the contractions, it's about mentally preparing yourself, you know, 'now I'll do this, I'll breathe like this'. You just mentally shift your focus to breathing instead of thinking about the pain." (Ivana)

"Breathing helped me. (…) And then I got tired, and I slept, which was incredible… I was sleeping between contractions that were four minutes apart, then I would wake up and count to twenty because they lasted twenty seconds or twenty of my counts, I don't know which. And you know how they went, I knew exactly when I counted to ten, I knew I was halfway through, that around thirteen it was the strongest, and then the intensity would drop. And in the meantime, I slept. Incredible. I slept for two hours like that. I would wake up, count my way through it, and sleep." (Una)

Counting or looking at the clock as coping techniques help women because the contractions are then divided and put into a time frame. In this way, they are precisely objectified as an unpleasant experience with their regularity, frequency and duration and thus become less threatening. This is a good example of non-disruptive objectification—because here the deliberate objectification performed by the woman takes the place of the spontaneous and threatening dys-appearance of the body itself.[24]

The previous analysis indicates that a very important thing that helps women cope is the ability to anticipate the onset of contractions, their frequency and the gradually increasing intensity of pain, a possibility that is completely lost after the administration of induction. The quality and intensity of "natural" contractions therefore do not lead to dys-embodiment, i.e. they are not perceived as particularly threatening to the embodied subjectivity, even if they are experienced as painful and unpleasant. After a medical or pharmacological intervention, this situation changes radically.

In many local maternity wards, a synthetic version of oxytocin, a hormone that induces labour, is routinely administered to augment "natural" contractions and to speed up and shorten the second stage of labour (Birth incentive strategy, 2018; Pantović et al., 2024; Stanković et al.,

[24] See the chapter Clockwork birth (Chadwick, 2018) for a more critical appraisal of the medical normative and interpretative framework.

2017). This practice, known by both women and doctors as "giving induction",[25] is routinised because it is applied indiscriminately to a large number or even all women, i.e. without monitoring the progress of their childbirth and the speed of cervical dilation. Due to the routine application and high frequency of the practice, women usually expect to receive induction and the procedure is largely normalised.

> *"I know why they do it. Because they're overwhelmed, and everything is like on an assembly line, and they have to speed things up to deliver all the women. And I expect it... I mean, I expect it because they give it to everyone. I don't know anyone who went into labour and didn't get it... And I wouldn't like it. I would like to give birth slowly, naturally, but what can I do when I know they'll give me an induction anyway" (Teodora)*

Since the intervention is often performed without (clear) medical indication, women themselves associate it with the institutional organisation of maternal care—overcrowded maternity wards where a large number of births take place ("assembly line" metaphor), making the acceleration and shortening of labour a practical necessity. This view is confirmed by some doctors.[26] However, my fieldwork insights and the conversations with the birthing women question this organisational necessity as the sole explanation for the routinised practice—many of them gave birth when the ward was not overcrowded and there was more than enough spare capacity (e.g. Teodora received an induction even though she was alone in the delivery room that night). If we keep in mind the previous analysis of institutional practices that lead to desubjectifying effects, such medical

[25] In medical terms, induced labour refers to a labour that did not start spontaneously but was initiated with the help of uterotonics. For most interviewees in this research, labour did start spontaneously, and syntocinon was administered to accelerate and shorten it. The appropriate term for this would be "chemically augmented contractions" rather than "induced contractions". However, considering that the term "giving induction" is consistently used in the women's accounts, and given that chemically enhanced and induced contractions have the same effects on the subjective experience, i.e., they are phenomenologically equivalent, we will disregard this terminological difference which is only medically relevant.

[26] At a major obstetric conference in Belgrade in 2022, the head of one of the largest maternity hospitals in Serbia explained to me (in a private conversation, i.e. off the record) that the frequent and routine administration of induction was precisely for this reason—he stated that he had to clear the maternity ward and beds quickly because the next women in labour were already waiting.

treatment of women logically follows as a paradigmatic example of the exclusive focus on the body and the neglect of the subjective aspect, i.e. the woman's experience. When I ask doctors whether induction intensifies pain, the usual answer is: "*Induction intensifies contractions—the experience of pain is subjective*"—i.e. something that is not relevant to the obstetric situation. I will now try to analyse this "subjective" effect of the common medical intervention on women's experience and agency, i.e. their embodied subjectivity during birth.

When administering induction, a member of the medical staff practically hooks the women up to an IV drip or gives them an injection without asking for their consent and often without any explanation or information about what they are receiving. Shortly afterwards, the women experience extremely strong and painful contractions that occur almost without pause. They are usually completely unprepared for this, as their previous contractions had allowed them time to rest and had gradually intensified, so that they are now confronted with a completely different quality of pain. This pain is characterised above all by its *immense intensity*. A specific indicator of this is the difficulty the women have in describing and depicting it and finding an appropriate comparison, as they have never felt anything like it before. This pain is not only perceived as unpleasant and threatening, but also as overwhelming and unbearable.

> *"Actually, by far the worst thing is that induction, which unbelievably... I mean, when those induced contractions start, it hurts incredibly. And because it stretches you all of a sudden, because it shifts your bones... It's really horrible. I didn't even know it hurt so much, this induction. And I told you, I have incredibly painful periods, and so I thought my pain tolerance threshold was very high. But... It really is like being in mortal agony... The whole pain, it's like when you get your period, but it's thirty thousand times more painful, I can't even compare that pain. It's unbelievable. And it really can't be compared." (Sofija)*
>
> *"And the doctor then said, he told another doctor, not me, they were looking at the CTG, 'look how she has nice natural contractions'. At that point, I was feeling pain that was completely bearable. That means I could have had that pain for ten hours. I could bear that. When they give you the induction, I*

couldn't bear that anymore. ... I don't know, if they cut your finger, you would bear it, that's how strong that pain is." (Saška)

However, it is not only the intensity of the pain that leads to an overwhelming effect. A very important factor is the *suddenness*, i.e. the women's *inability to anticipate* what will happen to them and prepare for what is coming. The sudden onset of severe pain (because they were not told about the induction) and the abrupt change to a completely different quality of pain are often described by women as a transition from contractions they could handle to those they absolutely could not bear.

"They didn't even examine me. They examined me upon admission, and from that moment they didn't examine me anymore. And they just switched on the induction. But at that moment I didn't know what they gave me, or how much I had received, I really don't know. They just inserted the cannula and didn't tell me anything. All I know is that the pain started within a few minutes, maybe two or three minutes. Suddenly extremely strong. It's a shift from those contractions you can handle to those you absolutely can't overcome. I couldn't... I thought my stomach was literally going to rip apart. And the pain is so intense that I wouldn't know... I don't even know how to describe it." (Maja)

"But what struck me there was the sudden increase in pain, after that induction. Because I think that at least, it doesn't matter, let them naturally be like that in the end, but let them be at the end and let them be gradual. So, from those that are almost just annoying you and like cramps, you can tolerate it and you don't even have to complain that it hurts, to the point where you completely lose it..." (Sonja)

The extremely threatening effects are therefore not only concerned with the intensity of the pain, but with the complete removal of any possibility of predicting the pain, adopting an attitude towards it and possibly enduring or integrating it. The techniques that helped women cope with "natural" contractions—such as timing and counting—no longer have any effect after induction is administered, as there is no gradual increase in intensity of pain—either from one contraction to the next or during the duration of a single contraction.

"And suddenly there is no more peak, the peak lasts all the time. You have a little break when it stops completely. But when it hurts, it's always at its peak, there are no stages." (Saška)

"At one point it was most intense, it reached its maximum and then this maximum simply continued. When it reached its maximum, it stayed that way, maybe it was just more frequent, I can't say for sure about what happened afterwards... I just know that at one point it literally felt like there was no hope and 'just please just take me...' I thought to myself: 'please, just... just take me for a C-section, I can't take it anymore.' I looked at the clock, it had only been half an hour and I was like, no, no, this will never end. It seemed to me like it would never end..." (Anđela)

The subjective experience of time and its objective passage diverge radically. Although the clock shows that only thirty minutes have passed, for Anđela it feels like a painful eternity. She experiences it as if the suffering "would never end" because the childbirth could (objectively) last several more hours. This is a result of the fact that pain leads to a *spatio-temporal constriction*: "We are ceaselessly reminded of the here-and-now body" (Leder, 1990, p. 76). Pain has a "centripetal" effect on our field of consciousness—our experience of space is also heavily altered as "we are no longer dispersed out *there* in the world, but suddenly congeal right *here*" (p. 75).

Another feature of this pain that contributes to its overwhelming effect is the *inability to localise it*. Women regularly describe that their whole body hurts. There is no part or aspect of the bodily experience that is not absorbed by the pain.

"And this pain is menstrual, the basis of the pain is menstrual, but it is so strong that you lose the sense that it's menstrual. You feel like your whole body hurts. From head to toe, your whole body hurts. ***You feel like your whole body is falling apart. You feel like you are falling apart.*** *I literally went numb... I closed my eyes, leaned my head back, I was all sweaty and I wasn't looking at them anymore. I just lay there moaning 'Aaaaaah!!!'" (Saška)*

"That's when the agony started. At that moment it seemed as if there were no pauses, no nothing... I was absolutely unconscious for any communication, except to scream when I had contractions and that was it... And the pain overwhelms me. It started from down there, from the uterus, from the lower

abdomen, but it seemed ***like my whole body was cramping up and falling apart.*** *" (Anđela)*

"I felt like I was falling apart. *I had the impression that my back was splitting and that I was going to fall to the ground and die at that moment. It was terrible." (Sofija)*

"And then I just started screaming and felt like I was being electrocuted and projected onto the ceiling, to the extent... I think when it starts to hurt, it was like my heart was thumping, like it was going to jump out... There are pauses of about a minute, and that's the most agonising moment, when it subsides, absolutely nothing hurts. You could fall asleep at that moment. And that's the most blissful moment I've ever experienced. And then when it starts, you're in a kind of spasm the whole time because you know another one is coming, and as soon as it starts, ***I can feel it starting from my ovaries, and it lasts a millisecond where I can tell exactly where it starts from and then suddenly whoosh! Goodbye! To the tips of my toes, everything hurts, it burns, my skin burns as if I'm being electrocuted.*** *It's so unpleasant. You know, when you get an electric shock from a lighter and your whole hand hurts, that's how my whole body felt. And it doesn't let up... The break lasts maybe a minute. And then again. And then it seems even stronger. But you know, just like when it's cold below minus five, it's the same cold all the way for me. That's what it felt like, it hurt me to infinity until there was no further... I wanted to jump out of my skin." (Sonja)*

In contrast to the "natural" contractions, the quality of which is familiar to women and which they describe as menstrual pain, the quality of these chemically enhanced contractions is something unknown that they find difficult to describe. They cannot rely on the usual experience that most women share ("you know how it hurts when you get your period, it's that kind") and therefore resort to metaphors and comparisons that are often relatively unusual ("like being electrocuted", "projected onto the ceiling", "my back splitting"). Women often feel that the intensity of the pain has exceeded their upper threshold, which means that they can no longer differentiate possible changes in its intensity. But this extreme intensity is only emphasised by the contrast during those very short pauses when the contractions subside.

What options are left for women to *(re)act* when their lived experience is like this? Screaming and crying out are the most common indicators of their inability to cope with the situation and to endure the pain. Many women mentioned that they had expected to be able to hold back and not "let their voice out", but they lose self-control and the screaming becomes the ultimate expression of helplessness and overwhelm. The extent to which gender norms (to be nice, polite, cooperative) are internalised, even in relation to disruptive birth experiences (Martin, 2003), is evident from the frequent disclaimers in their accounts, as they feel the need to justify their behaviour and emphasise that it is not typical of them.

> *"And I screamed. I should have... it was that I couldn't keep it in... I thought there was no way, if I had contractions, there was no way I would scream. Like at the dentist, I never let my voice out, never made a sound. My mum told me that when I was little, I never cried, I kept everything inside. Even when I'm at the doctor's without anaesthesia, if I have a minor issue, I completely calm down and think about, I don't even know what, and I calm myself as much as possible, to be okay. I thought... but no way, there was no way, everybody heard me." (Anđela)*
>
> *"And they gave it to me. And then it starts to hurt intensely, and I think I endured three more contractions, hissing and doing my shhh shhh shhh, like I learned in childbirth classes. And my pain threshold had already been passed. From that moment on, I screamed at the top of my lungs and screamed to the end. The woman next to me was moaning very loudly, but she was just moaning, and I was screaming, I know I was screaming as much as my throat could take. I was screaming. Because I felt absolutely helpless, I had no other way of communicating with anyone. No one paid any attention to me. And... I don't know what else I could do except to show how much it hurts. Not even to communicate, but maybe to ignore the pain. It was a primal scream, I had never screamed like that in my life. When something hurts, I usually stay quiet." (Sonja)*

It seems that in such a situation, screaming is all that remains. It appears to play a double role—on the one hand it is an expression of physical suffering, and on the other, it is the only means of communication available. Intense pain poses extreme challenges to expressing in language and sharing with others. The disrupted subject often regresses to a pre-verbal level. As Elaine Scarry (1985, p. 4) describes: "Physical pain does not simply resist language but actively destroys it, bringing about an immediate reversion to a state anterior to language, to the sounds and cries a human being makes before language is learned". The subject is reduced to a body tormented and controlled by pain, causing nothing more than almost reflex reactions.

"And then they hooked me up to the induction. From that moment on, I thought I was going to fall apart. You think your guts are going to burst. I really can't describe this pain, it's ten times stronger than the contractions I was enduring. They were terrible, but I endured them. And I started to toss and turn... My husband asked me: 'Did you cry?'. How could I cry? Oh, I wish I could cry... My body was tossing and turning on that bed. And the pace was a disaster, I thought I was going to die... I was frantic, literally frantic... the contractions then were non-stop, there was no pause. It was literally only pain, pain, pain and just pain! Break of a few seconds, and then a new one would start and only pain and just stronger, stronger, stronger, stronger! And it was a disaster, I thought that's it, my belly was going to burst. The baby would come out through my belly button. That's how I felt..." (Maja)

Even though crying is an expression of powerlessness, it still implies maintaining a minimal distance from the stimulus that threatens us in some way. The ultimate indicator of being extremely endangered is that this woman cannot even cry. Crying is a reaction to a threat or disturbance, a way for the self to respond, no matter how weak that self may be. The quoted statement testifies to complete overwhelm, a self that does not have even the small margin to distance itself and react. The pain simply throws the woman's body around the bed. When the inner attack is so pervasive that it occupies the entire body and thus the entire phenomenological space, such a protective response no longer seems possible. This is what causes the experience of being overwhelmed and the radical dissociation that prevents the elementary integration of the embodied experience.

Why is the aversive feeling perceived as so threatening and overwhelming? This is clearly expressed in the transition from "your whole body is falling apart" to "you are falling apart" that was explicit in some of the quotes from the women above. Leder (1990, p. 77) speaks of dissociation in the phenomenological field that arises as a reaction to the sensation of pain: "Aversive, involuntary, and disruptive, the painful body emerges as a foreign thing". The painful part of the body positions itself as the *Other* in relation to and in opposition to the embodied subject, and Leder points out that such dissociation can have a protective function for the subject. The internal aversive factor is positioned as something external and thus becomes less threatening, and the attempt to escape from it—as one would flee from external unpleasant or threatening stimuli—represents a very common reaction. This evasive reaction is inevitably doomed to failure, as the enemy from which one is trying to escape is attacking from within.

> *"I know I was trying, walking down the corridor with that drip stand, and as it has these four legs, I tried to climb it when the contraction hit. It was like standing on something hot, it's burning. So I tried to climb it, and I'm climbing it... and I'm in slippers, and it is so uncomfortable, so I was climbing and thinking I might fall and hurt myself, but I kept trying. At some point I realised it was absurd that I wouldn't be able to climb it. But I had this idea that it would actually make me feel at least a bit better. Anything that might work, I'll try it. ... And you know how in schools they paint the walls with oil paint and then put a piece of wood moulding to prevent scratches. At some point I found myself there, going back to the delivery room and I tried, I gave up trying to climb up the stand, but when it hurt, I tried to hold on and pull myself up to where the wall and the moulding meet and tried to climb the wall. As if I could escape. Horrible." (Sonja)*

Even when there are no desperate reactions in the form of a futile physical escape from their own bodies—Sonja's experience convincingly shows how absurd this can seem, while vividly illustrating how she feels—women try in every possible way to avoid the pain and somehow alter their situation. This is why they often have escapist reactions—by seeking (or fantasising about) medical interventions that they were previously strongly against (such as epidurals or C-sections) but which they now see as potentially life-saving.

> *"And when they came to take me to the delivery room, I said I definitely didn't want an epidural. And they hooked me up to induction. From that moment, I thought I was going to fall apart. (…) And then at some point the anaesthesiologist came in and asked me from the door: 'Are you sure you don't want anaesthesia?' And I was like, 'Can I have it now?' I was desperate, literally*

desperate. (…) You can't imagine it, in that moment, if they offered you anything, literally anything, and tell you it would make you feel better, you would take it. Absolutely anything they say, I don't know, if they offered you anything, you would say 'yes, yes, just give it!' Just to make it stop. That's it, you can't think anymore, the pain literally destroys you, so your brain stops working. You just think about it to make it stop. That's all that's in your head, it's unbelievable." (Maja)

"'For fuck's sake, why didn't I ask for a C-section?!', you know, all sorts of thoughts running through your head, everything you were against all along. I was against the C-section and the epidural and everything. At that moment I thought what an idiot I am, what am I doing pretending to be brave, all these flashes..." (Sofija)

Thus intense pain, "even though it occurs within oneself, it is at once identified as 'not oneself,' 'not me,' as something so alien that it must right now be gotten rid of" (Scarry, 1985, p. 52). This must be taken into account when trying to explain raising epidural and caesarean section rates. These are regularly discussed primarily in terms of *choice* that is concerned with the aspects of *risk* and *control*, thus ignoring the role of childbirth *pain* in women's birthing decisions. We discussed in Chap. 2 (*The naturalness ideal within the medical model of birth: the case of epidural*) that Serbian women regularly choose not to undergo anaesthesia in order to preserve the ideal of "natural" childbirth, which is reinforced by the patriarchal model of self-sacrificing motherhood. And to understand the change in this "decision" when the actual birth takes place, it is crucial to account for "the material or embodied conditions where birthing women engage with discourses of risk while 'making' decisions" (Maher, 2007).[27]

When the subject feels extremely threatened, everything else becomes less important and the world recedes into the background. Even the most

[27] The widespread opinion among doctors completely ignores this aspect, as requesting an epidural during childbirth due to severe pain is interpreted as an expression of selfishness and self-centredness: "*Selfishness is the central factor. For them it is somehow most important to get that epidural. It's most important for them to get the epidural, and it's so stupid and so irrelevant... You know that when a woman gives birth, she calls on the phone, calls her husband, and the first thing she says is, 'It didn't hurt at all!' That drives me crazy, it gets on my nerves when I hear that. 'It didn't hurt at all!' They don't say 'I gave birth to a healthy child, this heavy, this long, boy or girl', as if the child didn't exist*" (from an interview with a female doctor).

important part of the world up to that moment—the baby. This is because intense pain leads to an *intentional disruption* (Leder, 1990, p. 73)—while I normally live from my body towards the world, when in pain, my body itself becomes the (sole) focus, something I am primarily attending to. Depending on the urgency of this "affective call" even projects that occupied the top of my existential priority list just before the pain arose can lose their significance and fade into the background. Pain can instantly shift our entire focus inwards, leaving the world of things we were previously focused on in complete haze since it "annihilates not only the objects of complex thought and emotion but also the objects of the most elemental acts of perception" (Scarry, 1985, p. 54).

> *"And I had statements like, 'Will you take her out finally?!' When the doctor came, she said, 'Shame on you! That's your child, and you're talking about her like that.' 'Aaaaa', I said, 'it's useless, mate.' I said 'I can't, I'll kill myself with the baby! I can't, come on already!' Like, 'how can you talk like that?!' But yes, I would have sold my own mother if they asked me, I would. I admit, I admit everything. If I were a terrorist, I'm a terrorist. I have no rank, anything goes, and this baby does not matter anymore, almost none at all. I'm hardly focused on the baby anymore. Just fleeting thoughts like 'I shouldn't say that'. But no way, in three seconds, goodbye, I'm in a different movie." (Sonja)*

Such a reaction, even if it sounds very unusual and unexpected, is not uncommon in women who have experienced an extremely painful birth due to induction. Women who have spent months concentrating on the development and well-being of the baby in their womb are put in such a threatening state during childbirth that they fail to focus on anything outside their immediate bodily situation.[28] Their reactions after induction, therefore, reflect their inability to maintain a minimal integrity of self and preserve any part of phenomenological space that is not filled with pain. It is not even a body in pain or a painful part of it. There is only pain. Overwhelming, omnipresent pain that does not cease and leaves no room for anything else. As Sylvia Plath (2006, p. 90) poetically described the phenomenological situation of the birthing women she

[28] From conversations with medical practitioners, it can be concluded that they see such behaviour in women giving birth as an indicator that they are "spoiled and selfish" and "only think of themselves and not of the child".

observed: "...that long, blind, doorless and windowless corridor of pain waiting to open up and shut her in...". When this happens, the only possible reactions available are bodily convulsions or moaning and screaming, inarticulate automatic responses of a broken and overwhelmed subject. The overwhelming pain of childbirth, which a woman experiences as extremely threatening, results from her inability to *maintain an adequate distance and dichotomy between the embodied self and the body*, i.e. to preserve a minimum integrity in the face of internal assault.

4.4.2 Deepening Dissociation

To better understand the state women are brought into during childbirth under existing institutional conditions, we will examine another medical practice that often follows the administration of hormones to augment contractions and further compromises the integrity of the woman's subjectivity—the administration of sedatives (typically benzodiazepines such as Valium).[29]

"And then the doctor said, 'Give her Valium' and they gave me Valium. It was chaotic, but I really can't explain how chaotic... What probably made things even worse for me was that every time the contractions eased off, I started to feel sleepy. Then the contractions would start again and I would jerk awake. I didn't know what was happening to me. It was really messed up..." (Sofija)

"He gave me something for the pain. He gave me something because I remember that halfway through childbirth, I fell asleep. But I was so scared that my fear even overcame the sedative. He gave me some sedative. But I'm not sure, everything went through the IV. I didn't even see it. They would just come and put something in, I had no idea. Nobody tells you anything, nobody explains anything. They just come and put something in, inject something. And I would fall asleep, but I was so scared. I was afraid of what might happen. You

[29] If they were informed about the medication at all, the women were told that they had been given something to help "ease the pain". From conversations with doctors, however, I have gained the impression that these drugs have effects that are completely independent of the women's subjective well-being and are related to the relaxation of smooth muscles and the facilitation of cervical dilation. Due to the pain they endure and the anxiety they feel during the pauses between contractions, women find it difficult to relax, which makes dilation difficult—some participants reported that medical staff frequently told them during childbirth: "Relax, why are you so tense".

lie there and have the feeling that you are all alone in the world, like you have no one. And you're just afraid of what's coming next, what's next, what's next?" (Saška)

As a result, the woman's experience then becomes divided into two clearly distinct phases—intense pain alternating with falling asleep, making the contrast even greater and the onset of pain even less predictable. It becomes even harder for women to anticipate and follow what is happening to them, and the sedative makes it difficult for them to maintain any sense of control or focus on the childbirth process.

"Then the doctor said to the midwife: 'Do it now.' And they gave it to me. The midwife said, 'This is something to relax your muscles, it will ease the pain a lot.' And it knocked me out so much that I was actually sleeping between contractions, and then this terrible pain would wake me up, it was so awful. It continued to hurt the same, but I was incredibly sleepy in between. I think it was Valium. Because that stuff really knocked me out. I was... well, I was actually asleep. You sleep and then you scream, and then you sleep and then you scream, and that's how it goes." (Sonja)

It seems that administering tranquillisers to women whose integrity is already compromised only increases dissociation. The intense pain comes as an even greater shock than before, because it is the only way in which both the world and their own body appear to them—in the moments when they are conscious, they only experience the overwhelming pain and have no way of anticipating or preparing for it. If we want to schematise the situation in which the women as subjects find themselves at this moment, it could be reduced to alternating exclusive positions—absent subject, then overwhelmed/threatened subject, then absent subject and so on. Probably the degree of dissociation is highest in women who do not even know that they have been given a tranquilliser and who suddenly find themselves in a situation where they do not understand what is happening and cannot prepare for the next painful attack.

"Up until that moment, I was aware of my surroundings and could follow what was happening. It would hurt, I would endure it, and it would pass. But then I became completely unaware of my surroundings, I didn't know who was

> *there or what was there. None of the breathing exercises... when those painful contractions started, they were so intense that between them I would like fall asleep, I was so exhausted that I would literally fall asleep.* ***I couldn't even think, 'I'll start breathing with the next one.' I couldn't prepare for the next one, I felt like I was actually sleeping.*** *Two minutes, but you like fall asleep. Then when the contractions started coming every two minutes, I couldn't believe it. Did I fall asleep, did I pass out, what happened? Then the pain would hit me with full force, and I'm awake, waiting for it to pass, my body spasming, and then it would start all over again." (Anđela)*

For women who have attended childbirth preparation classes and mastered breathing exercises, it is crucial to anticipate the onset of the next contraction and prepare for it. This is necessary for the techniques they have learned to be effective so they are not overwhelmed by the contractions. Therefore, even when sedatives do not lead to highly dissociative experiences that are difficult to integrate, they hinder the woman's active engagement and her reliance on the coping techniques she has used up to that point. This is particularly evident in the following case, in which the woman managed to establish a degree of active involvement and control over her childbirth despite severe pain, until she was given medication that significantly hindered these efforts.

> *"I had severe pains, I can't say they were minor. (...) But I think she [the baby] was less at risk because I was aware of what was happening to me. I was leading in a way, despite being confused at that moment, I was leading my birth. And that's very important for her. (...) And then, at one point, the doctor said, 'We'll give you an injection to calm you down. It's nothing serious, it'll just hurt a bit less. And during the pauses, feel free to sleep if you can.' But no way, there was no sleeping. And I carried on, but after he gave me that shot (...) I didn't like that he gave me that shot, I think I would control myself much better without it. Now, what his reasons were for giving that injection, I don't know, I really don't know why it had to be given. Anyway, he gave it to me, and it made my head spin. And I think that spinning in my head pretty much muddled my concentration because of that injection. I wasn't as focused, and I didn't hold on as I should have. Anyway, there was no sleeping, the contractions were strong, how could I sleep for a minute when... And I didn't even want to sleep, I just*

wanted to wait, so when it (contraction) started, I could immediately start breathing." (Teodora)

Therefore, even for women who manage to maintain a considerable degree of control and integrity during childbirth, sedatives are an impediment. Teodora relied on the technique she had learned during her birth preparation classes and managed to maintain an adequate distance from the pain. The drowsiness and dizziness caused by the medication only hindered her concentration on the upcoming contractions and her efforts to manage them. Unfortunately, hindering the use of coping strategies is not the only problematic consequence of tranquillisers. Overall, the way in which a woman is treated as a subject from the moment she enters the maternity ward, particularly given the pharmacological interventions she is subjected to, has a direct impact on her agency and thus on the outcome of the birth, as we will see below.

4.4.3 Push! Struggling for Agency in an Alienated Birth

The dominant medical model of childbirth, perpetuated both in discourse through medical knowledge in books, as well as in medical practice and beliefs of physicians (as discussed at the beginning of this chapter) and sometimes even by birthing women themselves, assigns a marginal role to the woman as an agent during childbirth. It might even be incorrect to call this role marginal because in medical practice it turns out to be extremely important, but it is associated with a very short final period of labour—the pushing phase—when the woman is expected to push and support the body's reflex physiological response so that the baby can be born as quickly as possible. The question arises as to why women often fail to push, i.e. to be agents in the only situation during childbirth where they are called upon to do so in the medical context and are actively encouraged to participate. The problem lies in the fact that in the local institutional circumstances, by the time this phase is reached, the woman's subjectivity has undergone such a transformation—or rather we can say it is so compromised—that the expectation of her active participation is completely unfounded.

As we have already seen, through various procedures, women are positioned as external observers of their own childbirth from the moment they enter the maternity ward. Birthing process is turned into something that occurs beyond their knowledge and control, managed by the medical staff through their influence on the physiological mechanism. This external perspective is evident in the narratives of some women, who rely solely on the behaviour of medical staff (or objects in the environment, such as a clock) to understand what is happening to them and how their childbirth is proceeding.

> *"Generally, at that point when it was like, is it going to happen, I was looking at him (the doctor), three hours, nothing happening… I have no idea, they come in… nothing. I mean, they were commenting, but it meant nothing to me, like eight centimetres. (...) They had adjusted the bed into that birthing position, and he was then commenting on nine centimetres, and I thought okay, now I'm going to give birth, and after that, they probably saw the baby hadn't descended, and they put the bed back. And then I thought 'there's no way, I'll never give birth'." (Anđela)*

Anđela fails to rely on her embodied experience to guide her during childbirth. She tries to interpret when she is "giving birth", i.e., when the pushing phase that leads to the birth of the baby will occur, based on the doctor's comments, the fact that they adjusted the bed to the appropriate position, and the passage of time on the clock in the room. Therefore, it seems to her that she will "never give birth" since the external circumstances immediately reverted to the previous state. The childbirth process is obviously alienated for her—she has neither insight into it nor does she participate in it. The process simply happens to her and she is forced to endure it. Not only does she not have a privileged position compared to others, considering she is this body-in-labour, but her position is extremely underprivileged. Everyone else has a better insight and more involvement in this process that is taking place inside her (not only to her). In an epistemic sense, Anđela would be in the same position if she were watching her childbirth from the side or even observing another woman's labour.

The final stage of childbirth should actually be announced to the woman by the feeling of pushing contractions.[30] These contractions are experienced very intensely, like strong spasms and a powerful urge to empty the bowels. Based on their embodied experience, women then inform the medical practitioners that the final phase has begun.[31] Part of the problem lies in the fact that it is not uncommon for women whose contractions have been induced or significantly chemically augmented to not feel this urge[32] and then be encouraged by medical staff to push anyway.

"And now this doctor asks, 'Are you getting them? Do you feel the urge, do you feel like you need to go? Do you feel like you need to poop?' For the last hour she's been asking if I need to go, and I know when she asks that it means the baby has descended and the pushing is starting. I want to tell her I feel the urge, but I feel nothing at all. 'Well no, I don't feel like I need to go.' But deep down I want to say, 'I do, I feel like I need to poop, just deliver me already!' I have no idea. I felt nothing, nothing at all. It was literally in vain." (Anđela)

"They say, 'push when you feel it coming, push!', but I don't feel it coming, you know. 'Push like you feel you need to go!' I didn't feel that at all." (Sofija)

[30] Pushing contractions are contractions of the woman's abdominal muscles and diaphragm caused by the pressure of the anterior part of the foetus on the cervical ganglia located in the cervix (Čutura, 2005; Mladenović et al., 2008).

[31] In childbirth preparation classes, the midwife instructs pregnant women to call the doctor and midwife immediately if they are not present in the room as soon as they feel the urge to push.

[32] In this study, it turned out that all the interviewees who reacted extremely strongly to induction (which could be a consequence of the exceptionally high dose of hormones, although this could not be determined) also had problems with pushing contractions in the final phase of labour. Without delving into the details of the physiological mechanism of labour here, I would like to hypothesise as to why women often do not feel the urge to push after induction, which I understand to be a result of the actual absence of the urge. I believe that this is due to the way childbirth is managed in local maternity wards. Childbirth is understood as a strictly mechanical process, and as such it becomes subject to compartmentalisation. This implies that it can be divided into smaller processes, which can then be treated independently of each other. As already mentioned, pushing contractions are a reflex reaction to the pressure of the baby's head on the bottom of the cervical wall. The rotations and movements of the foetus that allow it to enter and descend through the birth canal occur in parallel with the uterine contractions that dilate the cervix. In the medical practice of local maternity wards, the dilation phase, i.e. the opening of the cervix, is treated completely separately from the pushing phase. Since hormones are used to intensify and accelerate contractions and thus shorten the dilation phase (sometimes drastically), the foetus might literally not have enough time to reach the cervical wall and trigger the pushing contractions. This results in a disharmony in the mechanism (or better—the process) of birth.

"And they said, 'when you feel the urges, push!' Now I watch these American movies, you know, where they say, 'come on, three, four, now! Push!' And they push. But I don't feel anything. And I'm pushing like an idiot. Nowhere." (Sonja)

"And then they tell me, 'Saška, push!'. But I say, 'I don't feel the urges!' And I have to tell you, throughout my entire childbirth I didn't feel the urges. I didn't feel a single urge, I swear I was pushing on empty because they told me 'come on, push!'. I say, 'I don't feel the urge', they say, 'how can you not feel the urge?' I say 'I really don't, doctor'. Believe me, I ended up lying. And in the end, because they kept asking and forcing me, I finally said, 'I feel it, I feel it!', but honestly, I felt nothing."[33] *(Saška)*

Women who are encouraged to push but do not feel a spontaneous bodily need to do so and cannot rely on their embodied experience describe it as pushing "in vain" or "on empty". They have no sense of agency like women who push along with the body's natural tendency. When a woman feels the urge, her real challenge is actually to refrain from pushing, which medical staff sometimes ask her to do.

"The pain in my groin from the pressure, I have to push, I can't hold back, I have to push. And indeed... it was unbearable for me to hold back from pushing because I was... the natural posture of my body, everything was telling me 'Push!!'" (Nevena)

But when the key embodied aspect of the experience is missing at the end of labour and the medical staff encourages the woman to push even though she feels no spontaneous bodily urge, these instructions are perceived as external demands. This aligns with everything else done to her during labour—she has been subjected to a series of invasive practices throughout the process, performed without any regard for what she feels and her lived experience. Although she is encouraged and given the chance to finally do something, to participate in her birth, she does not feel like an agent. She actually feels frustrated and helpless because she cannot respond to the demand. And she cannot respond because the process of alienation and dissociation is already so far advanced that she

[33] This situation is highly paradoxical—instead of the woman informing the doctor that she feels the urge to push based on her bodily experience, the process is almost reversed here. The doctor informs her that she should feel the urge to push, and due to social pressure and a desire to conform to the norm, she decides to completely falsify her bodily experience and lie about it.

has the feeling of being "not conscious", of "not knowing where she is" and of being "completely numb". These are all indicators of the subject's vulnerability, disorientation and detachment from the birthing process.

> *"And then everything became blurry,* ***I honestly wasn't fully conscious anymore.*** *I know they were coming in and out, telling me 'turn this way, turn that way, spread this, do this, do that!'. They asked, 'Saška, are you feeling the urge to push, like you need to poop?' and I said, 'No, I don't feel anything.' And then he said, 'Well, push!' but how could I push when I didn't feel anything. And everything hurt, it was killing me, I didn't know where I was anymore. ... And then they shouted at me, 'Saška, push!' But I couldn't feel the urges. And I started, you know, pushing, pushing... Yes, this was the worst. Then you really... you're not fully conscious, maybe from fear, maybe from the pain, maybe from exhaustion, or maybe from all of it. And then I didn't know anymore what I was doing or how... I tried once, but I didn't have the strength. 'Try again!' but nothing, nothing. And so I kept trying, trying... At this point,* ***I was completely numb*** *and I remember they were shouting, 'Push, push!' and I said, 'I don't feel the urge.' 'It doesn't matter. Push!'" (Saška)*
>
> *"A: And then, they were coming and going, I absolutely didn't see any faces. I didn't see a single face, nothing.*
>
> *B: So did you have your eyes closed while this was happening?*
>
> *A: No, I was looking. You can't see anything around you. In those moments, I was... you could say I was asleep, I don't even know. They were gathering... I think there were seven or eight of them in that room. And they were shouting, 'Push, push!' but at the crucial moment of birth...* ***I was completely absent.*** *'" (Anđela)*

Anđela's experience of being "completely absent" at the end of her childbirth, despite being expected to play an active role then, illustrates very well the consequences of the desubjectification that women often undergo in the local institutional circumstances in which they are treated as mere birthing bodies. The following quotation shows an even higher degree of dissociation in this woman, a lack of orientation in the situation and, as expected, a complete inability to act in any way.

"A: And now the doctor comes to me and says, 'Anđela, now just listen to the midwife, she's on the right side, just listen to what she says and do that.' I was like, 'Okay, fine.' By the way, I still couldn't see her, I couldn't see anything.

B: What do you mean you couldn't see her?

A: Well, they weren't there. ***It's like I was unconscious.*** *And now I'm expecting those urges to come, but at the same time, I'm very scared, I'm so scared, in the sense of being scared of the pain. Scared of the pain in the sense that I'm afraid of how much it's going to hurt when the next contraction comes. Even though it had stopped at that moment, I kept expecting it to come and I was all tensed up. And at that moment they were like, 'Push, push!' And I know the midwife from the prenatal classes said you have to deliver a baby within two or three pushes at most. And I try the first time, nothing, the second time, nothing, and then they say, 'Come on! Now you have to!' And I start to push, try to push, and I try to take a breath to start pushing. And I take a breath and start, and then I fall asleep and start dreaming I am in my living room watching TV.* ***I fell asleep in the middle of pushing!*** *And they were like, 'Come on, come on, what happened Anđela, come on!' I wake up, look around,* ***I don't know where I am*** *and just through my head 'Oh god, you're giving birth'... literally. And then I jerk myself awake and try to push..." (Anđela)*

The doctors were urging Anđela to push, but she was completely out of sync with her body. She didn't even realise the contractions had stopped and was anxiously waiting for the next painful contraction. She felt no urge to push, and the contractions were the only thing keeping her awake despite the sedatives. Anđela was therefore literally unable to stay present and conscious during the birth, in the phase in which her active participation was necessary and required. The doctors' demand was directed at a person, an embodied subject with at least some preserved integrity and capacity to act, while in front of them often lay a woman who was overwhelmed and whose integrity was impaired to the maximum. And what happens when a woman fails to push the baby out? Then the birth is completed by those who were actually the agents all along.

"At one point, you no longer know what's happening to you. And anyway the doctor told me once more, 'push!' and then, that last time he was like, 'it's not gonna happen, forget it' and I thought again of a C-section... And then he literally started swearing and mumbling, 'Every shift there must always be the one

that needs forceps.' And now they're preparing the forceps. And I knew they were preparing the forceps. Because I kept thinking, oh oh now it's going to be a C-section, and when he said forceps, prepare the forceps, at that point ***I didn't have the strength to be scared, total numbness.*** *" (Anđela)*

The fact that doctors appear as the main agents at the end of labour instead of the women themselves is a natural consequence of the whole process of taking away the woman's agency and imposing the doctor's agency from the moment she steps into the maternity ward. Anđela's experience is a paradigmatic case of a birth in which the woman is extremely passive and the doctor appears as the sole actor. The interventions necessary to complete the birth are an expected outcome of such a distribution of activity and responsibility. Reliance on "instrumental completion" of labour (as referred to in medical textbooks), through the use of forceps or vacuum extractors to deliver the baby, is only one way in which the active role of the doctor manifests itself. Much more common is the reliance on the simpler practice of applying pressure to the abdomen to help push the baby out with physical force. This is an extremely painful and distressing experience for the woman and carries potential risks to her and the baby's health.[34]

[34] In professional texts, this practice is referred to as the Kristeller manoeuvre: "If the birthing woman does not cooperate well and does not push sufficiently, the assistant or midwife presses on the uterine fundus, during a contraction, with a hand or compress with both hands (Kristeller manoeuvre)" (Ristić, 2001, p. 134). The practice itself is controversial and, according to a report by World Health Organization, its effectiveness has not been confirmed by current research (WHO, 2018), so the application of manual fundal pressure to facilitate childbirth during the second stage of labour is not recommended. The way it is performed is also very important when it comes to assessing its impact: "If non-consented, or applied indiscriminately and with excessive force, applying fundal pressure could be considered an abuse of a woman's human rights" (WHO, 2018, p. 157). Even some of local authors warn that aggressive management of the second stage of labour can lead to uterine rupture, especially during the Kristeller manoeuvre (Mladenović et al., 2008). Moreover, this practice is very common in Serbia, and even two-thirds of participants in a large survey reported having experienced it (Stanković et al., 2017). Sometimes the practice is extremely violent and involves uncontrolled physical force, as illustrated by a quote from an interview conducted as part of a recent research project my colleagues and I conducted on women's childbirth experiences and (dis)respectful maternal care (Pantović et al., 2024, p. 64): "*And then I pushed, but the doctor was trying to push him down and wasn't succeeding, and at one point she said, 'Bring some man, any man!' so like a stronger person could help. And then some man came, I don't know what he was, he could have been a janitor, he could have been anything, he came and he was literally ruthless. (...) And he was pressing on my stomach without letting me breathe. I thought I was going to suffocate, I was telling him, 'I can't breathe, I can't breathe!', and he was saying to me, 'You have to push, you have*

"I didn't know how to push at all. She (the doctor) was pressing my belly because the baby was very high up, they were all pushing her (the baby), you know... This younger doctor, she was pushing and pressing. She literally leans on you like this, with her elbows. And she's pushing hard with her hands and elbows." (Sofija)

"And then I wasn't pushing properly at first and then the doctor came and pressed on my stomach. That's what I didn't want to happen, but, well, it did happen. And it's a disaster. You know it's so painful... Because he puts all his weight on you, no matter how big a man he is, he leans on you, they take like this, with their forearms, and they literally press down hard on this part and squeeze your baby. Man, when he leans on your ribs, on your belly, it hurts, I mean it really really hurts! That's when I screamed. That was the moment I screamed, even though I had controlled myself perfectly the whole time." (Teodora)

A series of practices that are often applied at the end of childbirth—pressing on the belly, shouting and threats, tying up the woman's legs—are not only perceived as inhumane and violent by the women themselves but also when witnessed from the side.

"And I watched the entire birth of the woman next to me before I gave birth. You could see everything clearly. And then the doctor and the midwives come, and now, of course, they're all around her. And then they came and then 'push, come on!' Yes, and then, it seemed awful to me, the doctor leaned on her stomach and pushed, and to me, it seemed... he was pushing on her stomach, and she was screaming, and I was like 'Aaaah!' (...) And it looked like the scariest thing to me, and then all this pushing and yelling. And then also, what surprised me was that they tied her legs because she was jerking so much from the pain. (...) Yes, yes, yes, she was like 'I can't, I can't!' and then they started shouting at her. Which also seemed inhumane to me. 'What do you mean you can't?! Do you want your baby to suffocate, is that what you want, for it to get stuck?! Come on, you have to do it!' And then, 'Don't give up now, what do you mean you can't, push, push!' And it seemed quite brutal to me... But it also seemed like the doctors were really worried that she would hurt the baby by stalling. I didn't get the impression that they overreacted in trying to pressure her, their

---

to push!', and he was violently pressing on my stomach. And then about ten young people came, probably some students, I don't know who they were, they all gathered around me, I didn't see anything but their heads and then all of them pressed on my stomach, about ten people were pressing at once."

reactions seemed genuine, like the baby was really in a pinch and they had to get it out." (Nevena)

Nevena's impression at the end of this quote seems to me to be quite accurate. In a way, the doctors themselves are, if not victims, at least unreflective actors in this whole situation. Based on their behaviour at the end of labour (as revealed in the interviews with the women) and from what the doctors themselves told me, they are very concerned about the baby's well-being and it is extremely important to them that the woman "cooperates" and pushes at the end of labour when the baby begins to move through the birth canal. They are often deeply frustrated and unhappy about having to take an active role in this phase, as there are numerous medical risks involved.

"Later on, when they need to use their strength, the strength of their will and their muscles to help push the baby out, they don't care. Then the birth comes to a standstill. They don't know how to push and they don't want to push and just lie there as if they were on the beach. At this point, the baby is already in distress, so it has to be delivered one way or another. And we are a little sorry and reluctant to use the vacuum or forceps, which we should use, because we're all so fed up with it already that we will do that more often. But we're more likely to end up lying on the woman's stomach and pressing and risking a prolapsed uterus, everything to just leak out. First, it's not nice to push like that, and then there's the possibility of uterine rupture and other complications, which, fortunately, has never happened to us. But in 90% of our deliveries, we end up pushing because the women won't progress, I mean they won't participate in their own labour at all." (from an interview with a female doctor)

Doctors do not realise that the situation women often find themselves in Serbian maternity hospitals significantly hinders or prevents them from being agents in the final stage of their labour—the only stage where they expect them to be active. Their demands are then directed at an imaginary, fictional agent, while on the table before them lies a woman who is overwhelmed and shattered and who lacks the integrity to respond to such demands. Thus, as has happened countless times throughout history, the woman who, as Adrienne Rich says, "has no final say over how her body will be used" (Rich, 1986b, p. 30), is expected to affirm the essence of her identity through suffering and sacrifice (Griffin, 2001), showing she is capable and ready to be a *mother*. Otherwise she is "selfish and spoiled". This infantilisation of women giving birth as not "trying hard enough" or not "willing to endure enough" is a common response, with no willingness to question the oppressive and alienating conditions of the birthing environment. The additional problem is that the women themselves often do not comprehend the situation they are being placed in.

> ***"I also felt some irrational gratitude towards the doctor because he managed to do everything right.*** *Since I didn't do anything myself. Nothing happened naturally. Neither the contractions, the doctor broke my waters and induced contractions, and he pulled the baby out. I didn't do anything naturally. And when people say that the doctor isn't important and the midwife does everything. Well, I mean, the doctor did everything for me, nothing happened spontaneously, not even the pushing." (Anđela)*

Women rightly see doctors as (sometimes exclusive) agents of their birth, but often fail to recognise their role in the genesis of the entire situation. The fact that the balance of power and authority is extremely disproportional from the beginning allows doctors to assume the position of the main (or only) actors in the birth, which, as a result, becomes alienated. The previous quote is interesting because it intertwines different, seemingly contradictory discursive frameworks. The woman simultaneously has the feeling that she "didn't do anything herself" and that "nothing happened naturally", which merges in the following sentence into "I did nothing naturally". So both the spontaneous tendencies of her body and her deliberate activity are missing—and these two are, as I have already argued, very closely connected. And the doctor, towards whom she feels an "irrational gratitude", has done everything and "done everything right" (well, hasn't he?). The choice of the adjective—irrational—is so fitting, and yet the logic of the birth situation is far from the woman's grasp. The reproduction of this model of childbirth with a completely unequal power and responsibility distribution, an externally imposed regulation, the exclusive focus on the woman's body, and with the radical exclusion and endangerment of her embodied subjectivity, is probably facilitated by the fact that both main actors in the situation—the women giving birth and the medical professionals—are generally unreflective about its unfolding and its consequences.

In the preceding pages I have attempted to show the effects of routinised medical interventions (through the combined use of uterotonics and sedatives) not only on the woman's birth experience, that is, on the subjective aspect of the process, but also on the medical outcomes of childbirth, that is, on its objective aspect. I believe that the distinction between the *subjective* and the *objective* aspect can only be drawn conditionally and that the problematic treatment of childbirth arises precisely because this distinction is *ontologised* in medical representation and practice.

The usual constellation of actors in the maternity ward—the woman, her body-in-labour, medical professionals, material aspects of the environment (walls, beds, etc.) and medical technology (IVs, CTGs, medication, instruments)—is organised and networked in such a way that it completely excludes the woman as subject. This not only interrupts (or prevents the establishment of) the connection between her and the medical actors—both human and non-human—but also between herself and her body. The result is a radical inability to integrate the experience and establish agency, i.e. the disruption of her embodied subjectivity. The end of this chapter, however, will be devoted to analysing rare but nevertheless existing constellations that clearly deviate from this pattern and lead to markedly different outcomes.

4.5 Women as Embodied Agents Across Socio-material Networks

This final section looks at the possibilities of different outcomes for women's subjectivity that exist, at least to some degree, in the current local institutional constellation, despite of all its shortcomings. Various actors—healthcare professionals, bodily processes, material aspects of the environment, technological means, as well as the experiences, competences and actions of the individual person—are sometimes interrelated and aligned in ways that lead to coordinated, shared activity and positive outcomes for the subject. In some cases, new actors are introduced (e.g. epidural) that intervene in the relationship between the embodied self and the body. In other, already present actors are organised and connected in ways that open up the possibility for new modes of experience and agency. This altered ontological choreography—in the sense of "the dynamic coordination" of various aspects "that are generally considered parts of different ontological orders (part of nature, part of the self, part of society)" (Thompson, 2005, p. 8) enables working socio-material networks to emerge and women's agency to appear as distributed. To illustrate this, I will discuss case studies exemplifying different constellations of networks—primarily a functioning network of a physiological hospital birth, but also alternative ones such as a caesarean section and a home birth.

> ***"And I was telling them, 'Here it comes!*** *Here it comes, let's go now!' So I would take a breath, and then push (...) And I was really pushing well.* ***It was exactly how it should be.*** *And every time I would be like, 'Is it coming? Can you see it?' And the midwife would shout, 'I can see it, I can see the hair!' (...) So I started pushing and by the fifth push, it began, 'Come on, come on, hold on, hold on!'* ***And with each push, what needed to happen was happening. I couldn't feel if I was bringing down the baby myself. I kept asking them, 'Has anything moved? Have I made any progress?'*** *so I could know if what I was doing was having any effect or not. If it wasn't effective, I just wanted to know. But no, no, it was 'Here it comes, here it comes!' (...) The midwife would literally say,* ***'Come on, push! Hold on, hold on, hold your breath!' and then she would say, 'Switch!***[35]***' That's all she would say.*** *During one push, you hold the muscle all the time, but the midwife tells you when to switch because she is watching what's happening all the time. She knows what she's looking at. She watches, watches, and then says, 'Come on, switch!' and I hold my legs and she said, 'Let go!' Then I let go, and we start again.* ***It was really interesting, honestly. Overall, the whole experience was really great."*** *(Teodora)*

Based on Teodora's narrative, it seems that she is positioned as the central actor in the situation, having the insight and control over the whole

[35] Meaning that the woman should exhale and inhale again.

event, making her feel like an agent. However, she wasn't doing things *on her own*—she did not solely rely on her spontaneous bodily urges and the skills she had previously acquired—she relied on the competence and participation of the midwife. Therefore, her agency was distributed, with some activities delegated to another person, and there was a coordinated activity to achieve the shared aim. This coordination was possible because the woman and the midwife were constantly communicating with each other and both the woman's experience of pushing contractions and the midwife's perspective played an important and complementary role in the situation. The midwife's perspective was completely different from that of the woman, and she monitored the baby's progress from the outside. This external view of the progress of labour did not have an alienating effect. Instead, it gave Teodora an insight that she would not otherwise have had and provided her with valuable feedback on her own activity.

This image is strikingly different from the one in Sheila Kitzinger's quote given in Chap. 2, which states that a woman in labour "has withdrawn in her own separate circle" and "knows exactly what to do, she does not need instructions, because she is totally tuned to her body and to the energy that waves through her with coming and going urge to push the child out" (Kitzinger, 1984; as cited in Akrich & Pasveer, 1998, p. 109). The woman is depicted not only as the central agent, but also as the only agent, promoting the idea that her agency is maximised (or perhaps only possible) when she is left to herself and her embodied experience, as well as the intuitive knowledge and competence that enable her to act spontaneously and in perfect harmony with her body. However, an analysis of women's experiences shows that things are in fact not that simple. To rely on spontaneous bodily tendencies to push the baby out, they need much more than confidence in their innate abilities. I will try to explore in detail, aspect by aspect, what is present in the situation of a collective and coordinated birth and what things look like *when one of the actors is missing or is not adequately connected and networked.*

One obviously significant aspect of the situation is the *coordination between the woman and the midwife*, which requires them to actively communicate with each other and their perspectives and activities must complement each other. When this is not the case, the woman will perceive the midwife's insights and instructions as completely external—they will not help her to regulate her activity and may even disrupt her functioning:

> *"She (the midwife) came, stuck her hand in me in the middle of the strongest contractions, through stimulation, and told me, 'Push now!'. But she didn't tell me what would happen next and I completely lost it because everything started happening at once and I lost control.... because everything started happening and I wasn't prepared for it and then I was completely lost. What now?! Where are my hands?! Where are my legs?! It took me a few minutes to pull myself together to see where everything was.... and she didn't tell me why she was doing that, when I pushed, the baby started coming out immediately, that very second, and I completely lost it..." (from a recent interview with a woman who gave birth in a central maternity hospital in Belgrade)*[36]

It is important to emphasise that very different constellations—e.g. both home birth and caesarean section—can serve as models for a functioning socio-material network and adequate coordination between the birthing woman and medical practitioners. Una was the only participant in my study who opted for a home birth in the presence of the midwife (although she ended up in the maternity hospital due to unforeseen complications at the end of the birth). The midwife, together with Una's partner, acted as a collaborator in her birth, supporting the spontaneous unfolding of the process rather than managing and controlling it. She was very non-directive[37] and openly encouraged Una to rely on her embodied experience and act accordingly.

> *"The midwife didn't give me any instructions on what to do. She was like, do whatever feels good to you. And in some moments it felt good for me to stand by the bookshelf and lean my back into that position. (...) And I was having*

[36] This citation was extracted from an interview conducted as part of the recent research project my colleagues and I carried out on women's childbirth experiences and (dis)respectful maternal care in Serbian maternity hospitals during the Covid-19 pandemic (Pantović et al., 2024, p. 63).

[37] However, it is important to bear in mind that Una is a specific participant who has a lot of confidence in her body and identifies with the idea that childbirth is a natural process that happens on its own and that one only needs to "surrender" to it. For women who do not share this belief, such a non-directive birth environment could be more threatening than helpful. Therefore, there is a possibility that many women would not have such a positive experience with a home birth, and some studies confirm this (Akrich & Pasveer, 2004).

contractions all the time, but it wasn't that bad. And my boyfriend prepared for the birth, he looked up acupressure points online for labour pain relief. And then he pressed those points for me. And then I would get into the pool... So then it started to hurt a bit and I would lie down either in the pool or on the bed, and then I would just raise my hand and one of them would rush to press this point for me. And it really helped me. I don't know if it was a placebo or what, I have no idea. But it helped me a lot. I had a bruise there because they pressed so hard, but it felt really good. Maybe it took my mind off other things, I don't know."

Una relied on alternative pain reduction techniques—acupressure and spending time in a birthing pool, where warm water helps with cervical dilation and reduces discomfort. It is also clear from her account that she was in the focus during the birth. She reported to her partner and the midwife about how she felt, relying on her embodied experience, and they responded to her cues and tried to help her. Thus, birth appears as a collective endeavour in which both the woman and others are actively involved. As a result, none of the indicators of suffering and distress that we observed in the section on alienated birth are present here, despite the intensification of pain.

"And it was such a beautiful day for me. I mean, very beautiful. Because we were somehow functioning really well together and ... I didn't do anything except just lounging around. Because I really didn't say a single 'aaah'. And it's not like it didn't hurt, I mean, I didn't find it terrible, I don't know how to describe it to you." (Una)

Let us also consider a radically different birth constellation—a caesarean section under general anaesthesia. Due to numerous health problems that she had been struggling with for years, Tanja succeeded in carrying a pregnancy to term for the first time at the age of 49 with the help of in vitro fertilisation. Because of all the possible health complications, she was scheduled to give birth by caesarean section, but she experienced the entire procedure in a highly collaborative way, primarily due to the excellent communication and cooperation with the doctor who supervised her pregnancy and performed the C-section. This doctor not only showed exceptional care and dedication, but also actively involved the woman in all decisions relating to the birth. Besides asking for Tanja's opinion and explaining her own views on the timing of the caesarean section, she encouraged her before the operation and was there to support her afterwards. Finally, she wanted to give the woman back some of the experience she had missed by photographing the baby immediately after birth.

> *"I trust this doctor. I am very fond of her because she has proven to be very dedicated. And she's really immersed herself in my case and truly takes care of me, whether I am there (at the hospital) or at home, and whatever happens, I can text her and she will respond immediately or call me. (...) And she's very conscientious, responsible and has done everything well. She managed my whole pregnancy well, monitored me on time and told me when to do what. So I really came to trust her. (...) And when I was admitted to the hospital, I waited for her so that we could make the arrangements.* ***She came and we discussed everything. And we agreed on things. She asked me: 'What do you think?'*** *'Well, whatever you say, however you assess the situation.' And she was like, 'I don't want it to happen over the weekend, if the childbirth starts, so that I have to come in and then you have to pay for that or someone else delivers you', which I didn't want. (...) So, we thought about whether to do it on Friday or Monday and eventually decided on Friday. Then they prepared me and took me to the operating room and delivered the baby. (...) When they undressed me and I was on the table, I started to tremble a bit. She said, 'What's the matter, are you nervous?' I said, 'A little.' 'Don't worry.' (...) And later when I woke up, I saw she was there with my husband and mother-in-law. She showed me pictures of the baby. She had taken photos when he was born so that I would have them as a memento." (Tanja)*

Therefore, no mode of childbirth—or a medical procedure or technique—is inherently alienating to a woman. What makes them alienating is the specific way they are institutionally situated, which is essentially connected to how the woman is treated by the medical staff. This woman experienced the caesarean section as a fundamentally collective and non-alienating endeavour that enabled her to realise her life projects (a safe childbirth and a healthy baby), even though this constellation of birth is the most striking expression of the medical model—the involvement of technology, the agency of doctors (it is practically an operation) and the general anaesthesia (a common procedure for C-sections in state maternity hospitals) literally excluded her consciousness and participation.

Let us now return to the case of Teodora, which we presented at the beginning of this section. In addition to the role of medical practitioners, another important aspect of the situation that may not be apparent at first glance, and that requires us to consider Teodora's birth experience in its entirety, is the fact that she was a *prepared birthing woman*—i.e. she attended childbirth preparation classes. This helps her to be an active participant in the collaborative constellation of birth. In the Chap. 2, we have already discussed the significant role that the medical knowledge about birth taught in prenatal classes—its course, its phases and its physical indicators—plays in organising the often chaotic experience of birth and thus in structuring the narrative about it. An additional resource she receives are breathing and relaxation techniques that she can use during the dilation phase of labour. These resources enabled Teodora to reach the final phase of childbirth with her integrity and strength preserved, as they helped her to cope with the painful contractions and exhaustion.

A very important resource from the birth preparation classes for the final stage of labour is the pushing technique. From the beginning of the ninth month, women do pushing exercises to strengthen the abdominal muscles needed for the expulsion phase and to learn the correct posture and pushing technique. As we will see, this can be extremely important in situations where the bodily urge to push is absent, either due to an excessive dose of epidural anaesthesia or due to a disturbed labour mechanics because of its acceleration.

In the antenatal classes, the woman is also *prepared to cooperate* with the doctor and midwife and to listen to and follow their instructions. The birth situation is presented in detail—the position of all actors involved, what they say, and what the woman's appropriate reactions are.[38] When

[38] It is important to emphasise that "training" for cooperation is only associated with the phase of childbirth when the woman's participation is required—when she has to communicate what she feels and make an active effort, i.e. during the pushing phase. In contrast, for example, it is mentioned in the class that the doctor will probably administer induction at some point. However, when a pregnant woman wanted to inquire about this in more detail, the midwife's response was: "You do not need to know that, the doctor knows". Thus, birth preparation classes reproduce the usual institutional division of labour and responsibility—the doctor knows the indications, timing,

women are prepared to cooperate with medical staff during childbirth, and have maintained sufficient strength and integrity until the final stages, birth can appear to be a truly collective endeavour involving mutual communication and coordinated activity.

> *"The midwife helped me a lot. I pushed well and didn't allow myself to let go in the middle of a push. I bent my head properly. I was afraid I wouldn't have enough air. That was a problem for me. Because I don't think I practiced pushing well enough in the preparation classes. But I remember the midwife standing at my right side and telling me whether I was pushing properly, how I should push. When to push and when to breathe. (...) At one point she says, 'Push, push, push!' and then suddenly she says, 'Breathe!' And this way she helps me so that I don't tear much." (Tamara)*

The knowledge and skills acquired in childbirth preparation classes therefore first help the woman to reach the pushing phase without being overwhelmed or too exhausted by the pain during the dilation phase and then also prepare her to coordinate her activities more easily with the medical staff at the end of the birth.

However, it should be noted that these effects also depend on the entire network present in the institution. It is not just about the individual skills and knowledge that exist in a vacuum and that the subject can rely on independently of other aspects of the situation. In fact, how effective the preparations can be in real-life circumstances, i.e. how much they can serve as a resource for women, depends largely on how well the institutional environment is attuned to the knowledge and skills of the woman giving birth. This attunement was already recognised and emphasised by the first proponents of the birth preparation in Serbia: "The staff who come into contact with a pregnant woman prepared for a pain-free birth, from the doorkeeper to the midwife, must also be trained" (Milošević & Prica, 1968, p. 35). But even today, this is often still far from reality.

In the birth preparation classes themselves, the importance of the role of medical staff in the successful application of skills is recognised and the specificities of the local situation, where there is a lack of communication

dosage and type of medication, while the woman's knowledge, activity and preferences in this regard are deemed unnecessary and she is not consulted.

with birthing women, are taken into account. The midwife in the class prepares the women for the fact that the doctor will remain silent during and after the examination and instructs them that they need to be proactive and ask how dilated they are so that they can act according to the stage of labour they are in.

> *"The doctor examines us and stays silent. We ask how far we are dilated so that we know how to behave." (midwife leading a birth preparation course)*
>
> *"Yeah, for example, they say in the preparation classes that up to five centimetres you breathe like this, and after five you breathe like that. I have no information at all about when it's five centimetres. So my measure of pain was completely off. In those classes, you learn how it's supposed to go. And to ask, she (the midwife) said we must ask how dilated we are. But after that first doctor who said nothing, no one came to check anything." (Sonja)*

The feedback provided by the doctor or midwife is a cue for the women's learned responses. However, sometimes there is not only a lack of cooperation from the medical staff, but they also have a negative attitude towards women who rely on some skills from the preparation courses and actively prohibit women from using them.

> *"And that's when I start breathing the second type because it really hurts a lot already. And it makes it easier, it distracts you, you know. And at some point I stopped and was breathing that second type, it is quite louder. And one midwife came up behind me, patted me on the back and said, 'You won't be doing that in the delivery room.' I said, 'Why, what?' Like, 'Whoever taught you that, forget it.' And that was my only defence at that moment, the only thing that protected me from the pain, and like, 'You're going to forget that.' And at that point, I completely broke down." (Sonja)*

In addition to maintaining the hierarchical relationship, it seems that at the heart of such a situation is also a conflict between two models of childbirth. On the one hand, there is the medical model, in which childbirth is a mechanical process and does not rely on the woman's activity, so accordingly the preparatory courses cannot have a significant role in it. On the other hand, although birth preparation courses are largely adapted to the medical framework and are based on medical knowledge about childbirth, even specifically tailored to the particularities of the local institutional environment, their basis is a natural model of childbirth where there is a place for the woman as a subject and her activity. This discrepancy between the two models leads to the fact that in reality the preparation classes and the birth itself often remain "disconnected", making it difficult for the woman to fulfil the role for which she has been prepared.

> *"I think it would be much better if they were also informed. And that they could tell me, for example, 'Look, the baby is high up, turn to the side as you learned in the preparation class, to lower the baby.' You know, just to give me a cue, it will be my conditioned response to do it, but if he knows that I can do it and reminds me at that moment, I will know what to do. I think that would help a lot. (...) And then those two things, preparation and birth, would be connected. Otherwise, I have to be the link between the two sides (midwives at the preparation classes and doctors in the hospital) because they are not connected." (Teodora)*

For a woman to be able to apply the techniques learned in the preparation classes during childbirth, besides the adequate adjustment of the institutional context, she needs to maintain sufficient integrity and a sense of agency. In the last section, on alienated birth, we examined Anđela's birth experience in detail. She was a prepared pregnant woman who had attended classes very diligently, and before giving birth she told me how well she had practised pushing: *"The midwife told me 'you hold the muscle well,' she asked if I had done any sports. It seems to her that I can push hard"*. However, a combination of induction and sedatives during labour put her in a dissociative state in which overwhelming pain alternated with falling asleep, so that she could not use the breathing technique or prepare for the next contraction. Anđela was in such a state at the end of her childbirth—exhausted from the pain, dazed from the effects of the sedatives and without the urge to push—that she could not push at all and the baby was delivered with forceps. Thus, there was no subject with sufficient integrity—i.e. with an adequately maintained body-embodied self-dynamic—who could practise any skills or rely on any techniques. We have seen that some women (like Teodora) manage to maintain this dynamic by relying on various techniques they have learned in the preparation course. For other women, this dynamic is maintained by introducing a new actor into the situation—the epidural—and I will analyse this constellation a little later.

In addition to an appropriately embodied self of a birthing woman, and medical practitioners who are ready and willing to communicate and coordinate activities with her, the functioning socio-material network of birth also requires *specifically material aspects*—body-in-labour with its autonomous reactions (pushing contractions) and the material support for the birthing woman's actions (adequate birthing table).

The importance of autonomous bodily reactions becomes clear when we consider the experiences of women who tried to push but did not feel the urge to push. As we saw, they reported that they pushed "in vain" and did not perceive themselves as agents. This shows that when one element of the network is missing, the outcome is completely different. However, it is not enough for the bodily experience to be present. The entire situation must be organised in such a way that the autonomous response of the body can form the basis for the active role and actions of the embodied subject. In the example with which this section began, Teodora feels the urge to push and relies heavily on this feeling in her activity. However, she does this together with the midwife, as they both adapt and coordinate their activities to the rhythm of the pushing contractions. This is in stark contrast to situations where medical staff encouraged women to push completely out of sync with the experience of pushing contractions.

> *"Then he (the partner) comes with the documents*[39] *and then they say, 'Let's go now! Push!' I say, 'Well, okay, of course, but I don't have contractions at the moment'. And they start delivering me completely out of rhythm. And that was completely terrible for me. They don't wait for my contractions, even though I tell them 'here it comes, in a minute,' they just start 'let's go, push!' But... I say to them, 'But why am I pushing now?' And I don't know how to push, I start pushing but it's not right. And they are shocked that I don't know how and I say,*

[39] This woman and her partner had forgotten the medical records when they came to the maternity hospital. Her case has been discussed earlier in this chapter, at the beginning of section on *Broken connections*, because medical practitioners refused to assist her give birth before her partner returned with the documents.

'But I don't know.' 'How did you get this far?' Well, damn, I got this far, it just happens, it's not something I will sit and do... (...) And then I push, and then they get angry at me for not pushing well. And then I push by taking a very deep breath and straightening up and filling my lungs with oxygen, and then they... No, they clench my teeth and squeeze my head like this, which is completely opposite of what I had been doing all day, clench your teeth and now push. And I can't do anything. And I just look at them like, what the hell is wrong with you people. It was really ridiculous." (Una)

Therefore, the social aspects of the situation must also be adapted to the unfolding physical events so that the woman's body-in-labour can emerge as a significant actor in the situation and empower her to act.

Finally, there are some seemingly banal and thus often less noticeable actors whose role in the working network of birth is nevertheless very important. Teodora's experience of pushing described at the beginning highlighted the role of one significant material aspect of the whole situation—the delivery table. The table can be adjusted in such a way that it allows the woman to maximise her strength by leaning on the almost upright position and supporting herself with her hands. The table therefore literally serves as a physical support and assistance during pushing.

"Actually, it's great there, those birthing tables. They immediately contracted me like this,in the proper position, like a dentist's chair, that can be put in all sorts of positions. So, this one too, you can literally bend it in any direction you want, and they put me in the position I needed to be in. And that was great for me. And you also have two handles on the sides to hold onto. Wow, that was great! Legs up, they tie your legs to that thing and now come on! And it's much easier than in the class exercises. And when you feel the urge to push, you know what to do." (Teodora)

Another woman's experience shows what happens when various elements are in place and adequately connected—the woman is prepared for the birth, knows how to push, feels the urge to push, and the medical staff encourages her to rely on it, but this time the final element is missing—she lacks the physical support for pushing because she is lying on her back on a table that is completely unsuitable for her current activity.

> *"I was like, 'But guys, I can't take this anymore.' It's pushing from all sides, it wants to come out and that's it. And they are like, 'Let's go!' And then it starts. But the problem is, I was getting these cramps from the position I was in. There's nothing to hold onto, it would be easier if I had something to hold onto. To have somewhere to place my legs. In the end, it's like you can barely give birth in that bed. Lower part of my body, everything down there, it is kind of numb, you don't really have control over it. And you want to, but you can't, there's just nothing you can do, even though you should. Then this one (nurse) says this, another one says that, the third one says that. And then this one lays on your belly, 'Blow like this! blow like that!' I mean... And then she presses, pushes, and the baby comes out." (Ivana)*

Ivana feels the contractions, but lacks adequate physical support during pushing. Her body is numb because she is forced to lie on her back. She also has nothing to hold onto with her hands or brace her legs against to support her body and make pushing easier. In such a situation, the medical staff takes the lead role in the delivery by exerting physical pressure on the woman's abdomen to push the baby out. With regard to the woman as an agent in this situation, both elements appear to be external—the pressure she feels from within as a result of pushing contractions and the pressure on her belly exerted by the midwife. Although this is all happening to her, she herself is somehow excluded from the situation and can do nothing. This is an example of a lack of cooperation and coordination, i.e. the absence of an adequate socio-material network of birth that is constitutive for the birthing woman's ability to act.

In contrast, Teodora's birth experience, with which we began this section, is an excellent example of a well-connected and functioning socio-material network that leads to the desired outcome. The favourable outcome is both objective and subjective. Teodora delivered the baby in a few pushes, it received a good Apgar score and was not deprived of oxygen in the birth canal for long, and Teodora is the only participant who was "not cut", i.e. did not have an episiotomy. Additionally, she evaluates her experience very positively and feels successful and proud because she has accomplished something very important to her. Both outcomes are, therefore, the result of the work of the entire network, which includes the activities and competencies of both the midwife and the woman giving birth, as well as the material, i.e. embodied, aspects of the situation—the appropriate delivery table that physically supported Teodora while pushing, and the reflex urges of her body that helped her deliver the baby. As already suggested, the prerequisite for this functioning network is an adequate body-embodied self-relationship, which can be mediated by knowledge/techniques (described above in Teodora's case) as well as by medication, the intervening role of which may be particularly appropriate in cases of its seriously disrupted dynamics.

4.5.1 Contested Self-Body Dynamics and the Role of Epidural

We have already discussed the detrimental effects that severe pain during institutionalised childbirth inflicts on a woman's embodied subjectivity. Both she herself and her world can become completely overwhelmed by the pain—it "begins by being 'not oneself' and ends by having eliminated all that is 'not itself'" (Scarry, 1985, p. 54). The woman is thus prevented from maintaining an active dichotomy and an adequate distance between her body and her embodied self, which have a protective function in this threatening situation. In such circumstances, the techniques of muscle relaxation and breathing mastered at the birth preparation classes may prove insufficient and the introduction of a new actor—the epidural anaesthesia—that intervenes into the dynamic between body and embodied self may become necessary.

Through the analysis of two contrasting cases of participants who gave birth under the influence of epidural anaesthesia, we will attempt to demonstrate how epidural can, but does not always, act as a mediator and allow for a more adequate form of embodiment for a woman giving birth. Both cases share some aspects of the experience—primarily in terms of the radical change in the sensation of (chemically intensified) contractions, i.e. the contrast between the intense and invasive pain they feel before anaesthesia and the "bliss of non-pain" (as one of them described) they feel afterwards.

"And then, the moment it started working, and it started working very quickly, maybe just two or three contractions more, and then you don't feel anything anymore. Nothing, nothing at all. I mean, I could have fallen asleep at that moment, that's how I felt after those pains where you think 'aha, now I have to scream', and then suddenly you feel nothing, you just lie there relaxed. (...) And I didn't feel anything until the end. (...) And everything was so painless, and I felt so rested." (Nevena)

"Literally within two to three minutes everything completely stopped. I mean, I can't explain it, it's like I'm not giving birth, like I'm at home in my bed. I just lay down, completely relax, completely, completely. And I literally slept for about two hours, literally slept. (...) But thank God this anesthesiologist came in, I don't know what else to say, really, that man literally saved me. I thought it was over, I was going to die... But when he came in, it was like the sun was shining on me... Salvation, literally salvation." (Maja)

The onset of anaesthesia, especially considering the contrast it brings to the previous bodily experience, is perceived as a significant break and transition to a completely different state of relaxation and calmness. The fact that they "feel nothing" was not perceived as threatening by these women, because this state is similar to the usual one, in which the body is completely absent from our experience—in contrast to the threatening presence just a few minutes earlier that leads to dys-embodiment. Both participants who gave birth under anaesthesia thus saved their strength for pushing, but the difference that emerged in this final phase indicates what needs to be fulfilled for the epidural to appear as a technology that has a mediating and therefore positive impact on both the birth outcome and the woman's sense of agency.

For Nevena, the epidural was well-dosed, meaning that although she did not feel pain during contractions, she did feel the urge to push and relied on her embodied experience when expelling the baby. Therefore, the relationship between the body and the embodied self was preserved. Being well-rested and composed at the end of the birth made it easier for her to cooperate with the midwife, to coordinate her activities according to the midwife's instructions, to use the spontaneous bodily urge to push and to expel the baby in a few pushes—something that women who had to endure pharmacologically intensified contractions without anaesthesia generally did not succeed in doing.

"And really, they didn't yell at me either, I mean, they tied my legs, probably as a precaution. ***I was so focused on those urges to push and that body language*** *that it all was so... And absolutely, I mean, every word they said and like, 'push!', you push, 'okay, stop!', 'come on, push!', 'push!'.* ***Somehow it worked, I mean they didn't have to repeat the instructions, and no one was pressing on my belly, and no one was shouting****. From the moment the doctor came in, I think I gave birth within five minutes." (Nevena)*

The situation in Maja's case was completely different. She probably received an overdose of epidural anaesthesia and felt no urge to push, which meant that she could not rely on her embodied experience. The connection between her body-in-labour and her embodied self was disrupted and hindered. Despite this, she managed to rely on alternative resources that enabled her to be an agent—the knowledge and techniques from birth preparation classes. The theoretical knowledge about how pushing contractions feel like enabled her to recognise very mild and undifferentiated bodily sensations that she would not otherwise have been able to "identify". And the pushing technique she had practised in the prenatal classes helped her to expel the baby, despite not feeling a spontaneous bodily urge.

"Absolutely nothing, I didn't feel anything. And then just at one point, but the exercises helped me with that, because ***if I hadn't taken the preparation classes, I wouldn't have noticed it or known how to recognise it****. At one point I thought I felt the urge to push. That was exactly what the midwife had described. You feel the urge like a pressure on the pelvis, starting to push downwards. It's a very light pressure that you can't really feel because of the anaesthesia. The first time I thought I felt it, I called the nurse and told her that my pushing urge had started because I knew the midwife had explained it in class. When she came and said everything was ready, the baby came out in three pushes. (...)* ***But because of the anaesthesia, you can't feel it, and you can't push effectively****; you don't have the feeling for pushing. I pushed with all my strength from my stomach, just like the midwife taught us, and I think the exercises helped a lot, really a lot.* ***I knew the technique and then pushed on the basis of this knowledge, from the head, not based on my feeling, I didn't feel it****. The first push, nothing, the second push, nothing, and the third push, in the middle of it, I remembered the midwife saying to stick the pelvis*

down onto the floor. When I did that, the baby came out. It's incredible! The exercises just helped me a lot. When I pressed my pelvis to the floor and pushed hard, the baby came out." (Maja)

It should be noted that Maja's ability to act and feel as an agent was made possible by a combination of two completely different techniques—the epidural and the knowledge/skills from the birth preparation classes.[40] Without the epidural, she would have been overwhelmed by pain in the earlier stages of labour and would likely have experienced the pushing phase in a similar state of inability to maintain minimal integrity as Anđela, whose experiences were described in an earlier section and who also learned techniques from birth preparation classes but could not rely on them. On the other hand, if she could not rely on the resources from the preparation classes, the inappropriate embodiment, i.e. the loss of connection to her body and its urges, would have prevented her from actively participating.

During my fieldwork on the maternity ward, I had the opportunity to talk to women who had given birth under epidural anaesthesia and experienced birth as alienating because their embodied experience was not sufficiently connected to the sensations from their body. Not only did they not feel the urge to push, but they also received no feedback from their body as to whether their efforts "from the head" had any effect. They often described feeling "numb" and "paralysed" even though they received feedback from the midwife about their progress. As a result, these women did not feel in control of the situation in which they should be actively involved, but experienced this phase of labour as chaotic and externally regulated:

[40] There is a common misconception that psychophysical preparation is unnecessary when a woman undergoes epidural anaesthesia, implying that these two types of techniques are mutually exclusive. In conversations with doctors, I have heard that "with an epidural, these exercises do not mean much" as they are primarily seen as an alternative technique to anaesthesia to help women cope with the pain and get through the dilation phase. However, Maja's case suggests the opposite. This coincides with the opinion of the midwife who carries out the birth preparation course: "*I believe that these women with an epidural need the preparation even more than those who give birth naturally. Above all, they need to learn how to push when their body does not naturally prompt them to do so*".

> *"I remember they didn't give me any handles to hold onto, everything went in a kind of chaos. The doctor was pressing on my belly from above, everyone was watching, shouting something, giving me different instructions, it was really chaotic. And the problem was that I, under all that anaesthesia, I felt nothing. I was like trying to push, I was trying, but I had no idea... (...) With my second birth I had the urge, I also felt the stitching of the episiotomy a lot more because obviously they had reduced the epidural dose, but I also felt in control of the whole process." (from a recent interview with a woman who gave birth in a central maternity hospital in Belgrade)*[41]

Therefore, epidural anaesthesia might help women preserve their integrity by allowing them a kind of re-embodiment, but it might also deny them a sense of agency by deepening the already existing process of dys-embodiment. This analysis has implications for our understanding of the relationship between embodiment and agency, as it suggests that appropriate embodiment (in the sense of a body-self relationship) is crucial for a sense of agency. This issue will be revisited in the concluding chapter.

Childbirth, especially in institutional settings where interventions occur, can seriously threaten crucial dimensions of women's subjectivity—their capacity to integrate the experience and their ability to act. However, I argue that it is not the context (e.g. hospital or home) or the type of birth (physiological birth or caesarean section) that determines the outcomes of childbirth. There is no specific list of actors that must be present in the situation or their predetermined arrangement that guarantees that women's embodied subjectivity and agency will be supported or promoted. What is crucial is the establishment of an intersubjective setting in which a woman together with others, including medical practitioners, can jointly engage in the process of examining her body or intervening on it, with the mediation of different techniques and tools—including medical technology.

[41] This quote comes from an interview that my colleagues and I conducted as part of a recent research project on women's birth experiences and the (dis)respectful maternal care in Serbian maternity hospitals during the Covid-19 pandemic (Pantović et al., 2024, p. 63).

References

Akrich, M., & Pasveer, B. (1998). We deliver our children—In pain? In B. Brenna & J. Law (Eds.), *Machines, agency and desire* (pp. 109–123). TMV Report Series.

Akrich, M., & Pasveer, B. (2004). Embodiment and disembodiment in childbirth narratives. *Body and Society, 10*(2–3), 63–84. https://doi.org/10.1177/1357034X04042935

Andersen, L., Melvaer, L., Videbech, P., & Lamont, R. (2012). Risk factors for developing post-traumatic stress disorder following childbirth: A systematic review. *Acta Obstetricia et Gynecologica Scandinavica, 91*(11), 1261–1272. https://doi.org/10.1111/j.1600-0412.2012.01476.x

Arsenijevic, J., Pavlova, M., & Groot, W. (2014). Shortcomings of maternity care in Serbia. *Birth, 41*(1), 14–25.

Baker, S., Choi, P., Henshaw, C., & Tree, J. (2005). "I felt as though I'd been in jail": Women's experiences of maternity care during labour, delivery, and the immediate postpartum. *Feminism & Psychology, 15*(3), 315–342.

Beckett, K. (2005). Choosing cesarean: Feminism and the politics of childbirth in the United States. *Feminist Theory, 6*(3), 251–275. https://doi.org/10.1177/1464700105057363

Birth Incentive Strategy. (2018). *Official Gazette-Republic of Serbia, 25/2018–16.*

Bordo, S. (1993). *Unbearable weight: Feminism, Western culture, and the body.* University of California Press.

Bowser, D., & Hill, K. (2010). *Exploring evidence for disrespect and abuse in facility-based childbirth.* USAID-TRAction Project. Harvard School of Public Health.

Chadwick, R. (2018). *Bodies that birth: Vitalizing birth politics.* Routledge.

Chadwick, R., Cooper, D., & Harries, J. (2014). Narratives of distress about birth in South African public maternity settings: A qualitative study. *Midwifery, 30*(7), 862–868.

Creedy, D., Shochet, I., & Horsfall, J. (2000). Childbirth and the development of acute trauma symptoms: Incidence and contributing factors. *Birth, 27*(2), 104–111.

Cunningham, G. F., Leveno, K. J., Bloom, S. L., Hauth, J. C., Rouse, D. J., & Spong, C. Y. (2010). *Williams obstetrics* (23rd ed.). McGraw-Hill Medical.

Čutura, N. (2005). Porođajni faktori. In D. Plećaš, B. Stanimirović, A. Stanković, & M. Vasiljević (Eds.), *Ginekologija i akušerstvo: Udžbenik za studente medicine.* Medicinski fakultet Univerziteta u Beogradu.

Czarnocka, J., & Slade, P. (2000). Prevalence and predictors of post-traumatic stress symptoms following childbirth. *British Journal of Clinical Psychology, 39*, 35–51.

D'Oliveira, A., Diniz, S., & Schraiber, L. (2002). Violence against women in health-care institutions: An emerging problem. *The Lancet, 359*, 1681–1685.

Elmir, R., Schmied, V., Wilkes, L., & Jackson, D. (2010). Women's perceptions and experiences of a traumatic birth: A meta-ethnography. *Journal of Advanced Nursing, 66*(10), 2142–2153.

Esposito, N. (1999). Marginalized women's comparisons of their hospital and freestanding birth center experiences: A contrast of inner-city birthing systems. *Health Care for Women International, 20*(2), 111–126.

Foucault, M. (1995). *Discipline and punish: The birth of the prison*. Vintage Books.

Foucault, M. (2006). *Psychiatric power: Lectures at the Collège de France, 1973–1974*. Palgrave Macmillan.

Gadow, S. (1984). Touch and technology: Two paradigms of patient care. *Journal of Religion and Health, 23*(1), 63–69. https://doi.org/10.1007/BF00999900

Green, J., & Baston, H. (2003). Feeling in control during labor: Concepts, correlates, and consequences. *Birth, 30*(4), 235–247.

Griffin, S. (2001). Feminism and motherhood. In M. Davey (Ed.), *Mother reader: Essential literature on motherhood* (pp. 33–45). Seven Stories Press. (Original work published 1974).

Hallam, J. L., Howard, C. D., Locke, A., & Thomas, M. (2016). Communicating choice: An exploration of mothers' experiences of birth. *Journal of Reproductive and Infant Psychology, 34*(3), 257–269. https://doi.org/10.1080/02646838.2015.1119260

Harris, R., & Ayers, S. (2012). What makes labour and birth traumatic? A survey of intrapartum "hotspots". *Psychology & Health, 27*(10), 1166–1177.

Hauck, Y., Fenwick, J., Downie, J., & Butt, J. (2007). The influence of childbirth expectations on Western Australian women's perceptions of their birth experience. *Midwifery, 23*(3), 235–247. https://doi.org/10.1016/j.midw.2006.02.002

Hodnett, E. (2002). Pain and women's satisfaction with the experience of childbirth: A systematic review. *American Journal of Obstetrics & Gynecology, 186*(5), S160–S172.

Larkin, P., Begley, C. M., & Devane, D. (2012). 'Not enough people to look after you': An exploration of women's experiences of childbirth in the Republic of Ireland. *Midwifery, 28*(1), 98–105. https://doi.org/10.1016/j.midw.2010.11.007

Law on Patients' Rights. (2013). *Official Gazette-Republic of Serbia, 45*.
Lazarus, E. (1994). What do women want? Issues of choice, control, and class in pregnancy and childbirth. *Medical Anthropology Quarterly, 8*(1), 25–46.
Learly, A. D. (2006). Shame, gender, birth. *Hypatia, 21*(1), 101–118.
Leder, D. (1990). *The absent body*. University of Chicago Press.
Lundgren, I., Karlsdottir, S. I., & Bondas, T. (2009). Long-term memories and experiences of childbirth in a Nordic context: A secondary analysis. *International Journal of Qualitative Studies on Health and Well-being, 4*(2), 115–128.
Maher, J. (2007). *The painful truth about birth?: Contemporary discourses of caesareans, risk and the realities of pain*. Presented at the Australian Sociological Association (TASA) 2007 Conference. Retrieved from http://www.tasa.org.au/conferences/conferencepapers07/papers/19.pdf
Martin, K. A. (2003). Giving birth like a girl. *Gender & Society, 17*(1), 54–72. https://doi.org/10.1177/0891243202238978
Mathews, R., & Callister, L. (2004). Childbearing women's perceptions of nursing care that promotes dignity. *Journal of Obstetric, Gynecologic & Neonatal Nursing, 33*(4), 498–507.
Milošević, B., & Prica, R. (1968). *Bezbolni porođaj*. Medicinska knjiga.
Mladenović, D., Mladenović-Bogdanović, Z., & Mladenović-Mihailović, A. (2008). *Ginekologija i akušerstvo*. Zavod za udžbenike.
Mol, A. (2002). *The body multiple: Ontology in medical practice*. Duke University Press.
Momčilov, P. (2005). Normalni porođaj. In D. Plećaš, B. Stanimirović, A. Stanković, & M. Vasiljević (Eds.), *Ginekologija i akušerstvo: Udžbenik za studente medicine*. Medicinski fakultet Univerziteta u Beogradu.
Nilsson, C., Bondas, T., & Lundgren, I. (2010). Previous birth experience in women with intense fear of childbirth. *Journal of Obstetric, Gynecologic & Neonatal Nursing, 39*(3), 298–309. https://doi.org/10.1111/j.1552-6909.2010.01139.x
O'Driscoll, K., Stronge, J. M., & Minogue, M. (1973). Active management of labour. *British Medical Journal, 3*(5872), 135–137. https://doi.org/10.1136/bmj.3.5872.135
Olde, E., van der Hart, O., Kleber, R. J., van Son, M., Wijnen, H., & Pop, V. (2005). Posttraumatic dissociation and emotions as predictors of PTSD symptoms following childbirth. *Journal of Trauma & Dissociation, 6*(3), 125–142.

Pantović, L. (2016). Buying a connection: Private practice in public health care—The case of a Serbian maternity hospital. *Anthropology of East Europe Review, 34*(1).
Pantović, L. (2022). Providing a service or seeking a favor? The role of private prenatal care on the continuity of care in Serbian public maternity hospitals. *Birth, 49*(3), 506–513.
Pantović, L., Stanković, B., & Ćeriman, J. (2024). *Iskustva žena u porodilištima u Srbiji tokom i nakon pandemije kovida-19.* UNFPA.
Physiological Childbirth: The guide for doctors and midwives. (2009). Ministry of Health of Republic of Serbia.
Plath, S. (2006). *The bell jar*. Harper Perennial Modern Classics.
Rich, A. (1986b). *Of woman born: Motherhood as experience and institution.* W. W. Norton & Company.
Ristić, L. (2001). *Praktično porodiljstvo*. Freemental.
Scarry, E. (1985). *The body in pain: The making and unmaking of the world.* Oxford University Press.
Schroll, A. M., Kjaergaard, H., & Midtgaard, J. (2013). Encountering abuse in health care: Lifetime experiences in postnatal women—A qualitative study. *BMC Pregnancy and Childbirth, 13*, 74.
Skočajić, M., & Stanković, B. (2020). Uloga socijalne podrške u iskustvu abortusa: Kvalitativna analiza ličnih izveštaja žena. *Sociologija, LXII*(2), 171–192. https://doi.org/10.2298/SOC2002171S
Stanković, B., Skočajić, M., & Đorđević, A. (2017). Upravljanje porođajem u Srbiji: Medicinske intervencije i porođajna iskustva. *Limes Plus: Journal of Social Science and Humanities, 14*(2), 197–225.
Swahnberg, K., Thapar-Björkert, S., & Berterö, C. (2007). Nullified: Women's perceptions of being abused in health care. *Journal of Psychosomatic Obstetrics & Gynecology, 28*(3), 161–167.
Thompson, C. (2005). *Making parents: The ontological choreography of reproductive technologies*. MIT Press.
Thomson, G., & Downe, S. (2008). Widening the trauma discourse: The link between childbirth and experiences of abuse. *Journal of Psychosomatic Obstetrics & Gynecology, 29*(4), 268–273.
van der Gucht, N., & Lewis, K. (2015). Women's experiences of coping with pain during childbirth: A critical review of qualitative research. *Midwifery, 31*, 349–358.

Vidić, J., Stanković, B., & Džamonja Ignjatović, T. (2022). Iskustva medicinske tranzicije transrodnih osoba u Srbiji: Od afirmacije identiteta do institucionalnog nasilja. *Sociologija, LXIV*(3), 401–427. https://doi.org/10.2298/SOC2203401V

Waldenström, U., Hildingsson, I., Rubertsson, C., & Rådestad, I. (2004). A negative birth experience: Prevalence and risk factors in a national sample. *Birth, 31*(1), 17–27.

World Health Organization (WHO). (2018). *WHO recommendations: Intrapartum care for a positive childbirth experience*. World Health Organization.

5

Conclusion

The focus of theoretical and empirical analysis in this book has been on the process of shaping and transformation of women's subjectivity during pregnancy and childbirth as significant stages in the transition to motherhood, especially considering the dramatic bodily changes that occur and the ways in which medical knowledge, practices and techniques mediate this process. By examining this, in many ways specific phenomenon, the book explores a long-standing concern of the cultural-historical tradition—the relationship between human subjects and technology/mediators. However, it also aims at expanding and enriching the sociocultural perspective by incorporating theoretical resources from contemporary science and technology studies and feminism to account for a changed understanding of subject and technology, as well as resources from phenomenology to account for the embodied aspects of experience.

The empirical sections of the book follow women on their journeys through pregnancy and childbirth as they negotiate their changing position, learn to live in their continuously transforming bodies, enter medical contexts and develop ways of coping with new, exciting, but sometimes also challenging and overwhelming experiences. To address the fact that these experiences are situated and embedded in the concrete and local

B. Stanković, *Giving Birth To A Subject*, Sociocultural Psychology of the Lifecourse,
https://doi.org/10.1007/978-3-031-77236-8_5

context, the empirical parts also closely examined the Serbian maternity care system—from the official documents regulating the normative aspect to the concrete practices assessed through both field research and women's testimonies, and taking into account the role of ideological and cultural specificities of a post-socialist society.

Close attention to context and cultural-historical particularities served as a safeguard against treating motherhood as "a static, 'natural' experience" since "the myth of eternally changeless motherhood is a central pillar upholding patriarchal privilege" (Bowers, 1996, p. 19). What is special about mothers is not what they feel—for their emotions are diverse, possibly ambivalent and constantly changing—and definitely cannot be reduced to a single emotion such as love for their children. Motherhood is also not simply a prescribed social role, although, as we have seen, culturally and historically shaped norms (often masquerading as universal and timeless) play an important role in the experience and conduct of mothers. Thus, instead of a transition from one life role and identity (that of a childless woman) to another (that of a mother), I have attempted to trace the beginnings of a mothering process that is understood as a kind of "caring labour" (Ruddick, 1989) and encompasses many experiences and practices. As shown earlier, from the moment a woman learns that she is pregnant, and especially from the moment she "sees" her baby on the ultrasound scan and later feels the baby's movements, her actions and decisions, thoughts and preferences are shaped by its (imagined) needs and demands, and she is oriented towards nurturing and protecting it. So I have tried to approach the process of the early transition to motherhood as "a moving plurality of potential behaviours always undergoing supervision, revision, and contest, constructed in particularity" (Bowers, 1996, p. 19).

The empirical analysis in the previous chapters has attempted to preserve the complexity and variability of women's trajectories and life contexts situated in the specific institutional and cultural setting of contemporary Serbia. It has highlighted developmental continuities, but also various ruptures in the way women experience themselves, their bodies and their surroundings, as well as in the way they act and interact with others. This concluding chapter will try to elaborate and connect the theoretical and ethical-political insights and implications laid out in the previous parts of the book by revisiting the concepts already recognised as crucial dimensions of subjectivity—*embodiment*, *mediatedness* and *embeddedness*.

5.1 Maternal Embodiment

The concept of embodiment occupies a central place in this book. By relying on it, I have tried to move away from the understanding of the body as "a nongendered, prediscursive phenomenon that plays a central role in perception, cognition, action" and focus on exploring "a way of living or inhabiting the world through one's acculturated body" (Weiss & Haber, 1999, p. xiii). My aim was to explore both the cultural-historical specificities of this process of acculturation of the body and the particularities of inhabiting the world through a pregnant and birthing body. During the early transition to motherhood, I explored the woman's body—and thus her embodied subjectivity—as *double mutable*: "it is mutable in the obvious sense that it undergoes continuous physiological (and sometimes pathological) change, and mutable culturally, in that it is viewed through constantly shifting interpretive frameworks (...) constructed through the interrelation of medicine and culture" (Hanson, 2004, p. 3).

In the usual course of life, we become acutely aware of our own body mainly when we are confronted with a dysfunction in one of its parts. Drew Leder (1990, p. 89) suggests that "when my embodiment radically diverges from the habitual, dys-appearance is likely to result". However, a radical deviation from the *normal* is not only characteristic of cases of bodily failure or dysfunction. It also occurs in some quite ordinary phases of life, such as puberty, old age or the menopause. The tendency to view major changes in the usual structure, functionality or appearance of the body as something that deviates from the normal, rather than just the habitual, is a matter of cultural prejudice. In the second chapter it was discussed that this is due to specific patriarchal prejudices surrounding pregnancy, which take the middle-aged man as the standard of normality, whose experience of health is the experience of an unchanging body and for whom any transformation in the usual bodily condition is a sign that something is wrong (Leder, 1990, p. 89; Young, 2005b, p. 57).

Nevertheless, the *unusual* functioning of the body and the significant change in its shape and size during pregnancy and childbirth make these experiences somewhat similar to the experiences we have when the body becomes dysfunctional. The similarity lies in the increased presence of the body for the woman, which becomes the centre of her thoughts and activities. The prominent and continuous changes both inside the body and on its surface cause the woman's attention to turn from the environment, to which it is directed in the ordinary course of life, to the body itself. These adaptations are partly due to anatomical and physiological changes but, as suggested earlier, are also significantly influenced by contemporary society's ethical obligation to "take care" of oneself. Women are expected to (and thus often feel the need to) eat healthier than usual, avoid activities that require a lot of energy, refrain from making "risky" movements with their bodies and so on. Thus, turning to the body becomes an entirely new project around which their existing field of existential projects is organised. Life *towards* the body, which consists of various bodily treatments—altered diet, sleeping positions, exercise routines, etc.—pushes the previous life *from* the body to the periphery (Leder, 1990).

What facilitates this shift is certainly the fact that there is another being inside a woman's body, whose presence becomes increasingly noticeable and evident. And yet this being remains hidden and elusive, and the woman learns about it only indirectly. There is a complex dynamic of symbiosis and separation, utter dependence and emerging autonomy at play. Thus, her body functions on the one hand as a mediator through which the woman gets to know the baby and forms an increasingly complex and differentiated image of it, and on the other hand as an environment that keeps the baby alive and developing. In other words, the baby is what the woman is implicitly focused on and what she takes care of by explicitly focusing on and taking care of her own body. Kristeva gives a vivid description of this ambivalent and liminal phenomenological situation inherent in pregnancy: "Cells fuse, split, and proliferate; volumes grow, tissues stretch, and body fluids change rhythm, speeding up or slowing down. Within the body, growing as a graft, indomitable, there is another. And no one is present within that simultaneously dual and alien space to signify what is going on. 'It happens, but I'm not there.' 'I cannot realise it, but it goes on.' Motherhood's impossible syllogism" (Kristeva, 1990, p. 441). Despite its captivating poetics, which appeals to our imagination, I believe that this depiction unjustifiably mystifies the embodied process of becoming a mother. Sharing one's body with another being is a genuine challenge, a process that is inherently spontaneous and beyond the woman's control, but at the same time, this process is carefully monitored and regulated by the woman herself. She is often actively involved in it, which is crucial to how she experiences herself and her (future) baby. So it is misleading to say that she is "not there". In fact, she strives to resolve this "impossible syllogism" in various ways throughout the pregnancy (and after), drawing on a multitude of discursive-material mediators.

The discussions in this book have tried to problematise the assumption that maternal embodiment is something "given, organic, necessary" and inherently and unproblematically related to female embodiment that has traditionally been identified with the "skill in mothering and its metaphoric extensions" (Haraway, 1991a, p. 180). While some aspects of women's embodied experience might seem less mutable than others,[1] the perception and interpretation of the body during pregnancy are largely dependent on cultural representations that are historically relative, as—"pregnancy is experienced through the cultural sense making of its day" (Riley et al., 2019, p. 98). As already asserted, the increased attention and sensitivity to the processes of the reproductive body that characterise modern women can be linked to the fact that these processes are now treated as medical phenomena. The result of the change taking place in recent decades, discussed in detail in previous chapters, is not only the subordination of pregnancy and childbirth to the jurisdiction of medicine, but also the fact that medical discourse and technology have become important mediators and resources in women's everyday thinking and functioning. As a result, a woman's understanding and actions are often guided by the representation of pregnancy as a risky condition and the pregnant body as fragile, in need of special care and protection. However,

[1] In the Chap. 3, I discussed the conservative nature of the body schema, which reflects the fact that our proprioception takes a long time to adapt to the changing size and boundaries of the body.

despite the almost hegemonic presence of medical discourse, this is not the only framework through which individual experiences are refracted.

The fact that "the body is pregnant with symbolic meanings, deep, intensely charged and often highly contradictory" (Porter, 2002, p. 53) implies that women are talked into or nudged towards certain representations and normative standards that shape the way they feel, interpret and use their bodies. However, it is important to keep in mind that besides being culturally shaped and mediated, our bodies are also sites of resistance and protest, because "there is a tension between women's lived bodily experiences and the cultural meanings inscribed on the female body that always mediate those experiences" (Conboy et al., 1997, p. 1). Our embodied experiences clearly point to the occasionally oppressive nature of the dominant practices and representations that shape us as women in a (patriarchal neoliberal) society. Nevertheless, the dominant representations and norms are regularly supported and promoted by rigid socio-material networks imbued with power and authority, so that resistance to them often proves futile (Halfon, 2010). Women then frequently turn to another coping strategy—*re-embodiment*. When confronted with intense bodily sensations and/or oppressive institutional practices, especially during and after childbirth, a woman alters the relationship she has to her body as an embodied self—radically objectifying her body (so it becomes "just a body") or distancing and dissociating herself from it (and positioning it as something other and opposed to the self). Even after the baby is born, maternal embodiment continues to be challenged. The postpartum body has very unstable boundaries—blood and milk leak out, the uterus contracts and the breasts swell. And again, this process does not take place in a vacuum—a woman's body becomes a public object within the medical setting, but also outside of it. This poses a challenge to her embodied subjectivity, so the shift in her relationship to her own body is an adaptive response to the enormous changes it undergoes during this dynamic and challenging period of early motherhood.

When the challenges she faces are very intense and disruptive—as in some extremely problematic constellations of institutionalised birth—re-embodiment as a coping strategy is unavailable to women. The resulting effect is *dys-embodiment*—a radical disruption of women's integrity and agency, in other words, their embodied subjectivity. I have tried to show through analysis that this outcome only occurs in very specific circumstances when the internal challenges (e.g. overwhelming pain or loss of sensation from one's own body and complete numbness) are combined with the external challenges (disrespectful and oppressive institutional practices inside the maternity hospital). In evaluating the effects of medical procedures and technologies, it is important to remember that objectification resulting from medical treatment in many cases follows objectification that was already present before and independent of any kind of treatment or observation. This is especially evident in cases of severe pain accompanying labour or non-transparent processes during pregnancy and childbirth, which are both pervasive and deemed indicative. Problematic medical interventions routinely performed in local maternity hospitals (such as labour augmentation and administration of sedatives) often deepen and exacerbate the process of dissociation and alienation that has already occurred independently of entering the hospital.

Outside of these situations, and in relatively ordinary circumstances, the body during pregnancy and childbirth does pose a challenge to women's embodied subjectivity due to the spontaneous physiological changes and cultural meanings associated with these changes, but without disembodying effects. Nevertheless, the resulting crisis and its resolution can lead to radically different outcomes for women's subjectivity, i.e. to very different ways of experiencing and reacting.

The dominance of the discourse of risk, reflected in the very cautious way in which most women treat their own bodies during pregnancy, and the heightened anxiety that accompanies the entire process of becoming a mother, could lead us to assume that the pregnant and birthing body appears to the woman exclusively as fragile and vulnerable. In fact, pregnancy can also be an *empowering* experience during which a woman can develop a peculiar intimacy with her body and begin to attribute special value to it. According to Iris Marion Young (2005b, p. 52), pregnancy represents a paradigmatic case of what Sally Gadow (1980) calls an *aesthetic* relationship between a person and their body. An aesthetic relationship is characterised by "a complex balance of form and freedom, in which both subject and object reciprocally affect and develop one another" (Gadow, 1980, p. 183). It involves an emotional attachment to the object and an intellectual focus on it, resting on the subject ascribing *intrinsic* rather than instrumental value to the object.[2]

During pregnancy, the numerous bodily transformations are sometimes a source of wonder, concern and even anxiety, but often also cause astonishment and joy. Some women are fascinated by the many changes that pregnancy brings with it, by the processes that take place in the body, by its abilities and its strength.[3] A woman is not simply identified with her body—she does not experience that *she is doing* the things that are happening to her. The body *itself*, its hidden capacities, are responsible for these changes. But this body does not appear as something alienated, as something that stands opposite the subject and is foreign to her. She admires it, is proud of it and finds in it a source of pleasure and strength. The crisis of embodiment during pregnancy, which necessarily entails a certain duality between the subject and the body, or at least the explicit appearance of the body as object, can thus provide a woman with the opportunity for a new form of intimacy with her body and offer her a fulfilling embodied experience. In this sense, pregnancy can be empowering for a woman.

The fact is, however, that not many of the women studied were able to articulate such a relationship with their bodies, possibly indicating that this aesthetic modality of experiencing one's own body remains somewhat unrealised potential due to the dominance of worry and insecurity resulting from the prevailing cultural representation of the reproductive body as risky. It seems that this modality was primarily available to those women who had developed confidence in the abilities and strengths of their bodies during earlier bodily socialisation processes (some of them

[2] This is not only typical of pregnancy. While ordinary functioning involves an implicit attribution of instrumental value to one's body, Gadow suggests that in old age we develop an aesthetic relationship with our bodies and that the failure to recognise this is the reason we treat old age as less valuable than other stages of life: "From the point of view solely of the body as object of mastery, we must say that in aging the body withers, loses its vitality and its capacity to respond. From the point of view of the body as aesthetic object, however, the aging body can be experienced as the richest reality of forms and meanings that can be imagined" (Gadow, 1980, p. 183).

[3] Here is a vivid example: "*And then I was fascinated when I found out I was pregnant. I mean, almost like a child learning to walk and looking at its feet. Then I looked at my nails, looked at my skin, everything was amazing. I examined my belly. I examined every little sign. It was really interesting to me. And I really enjoyed it all. (…) I was so full of energy. I mean, you really feel a kind of strength…*" (Una).

referred to the body as their "safe zone") and viewed its changes with interest and pleasure rather than concern and fear. However, most women did report at least individual situations, i.e. particular embodied experiences, when their bodies were not only explicitly thematised (and objectified) in a non-threatening way, but when they experienced them as a source of fascination and enjoyment.

Still, for some of them their bodies appeared not only as distanced in a neutral or positive way, but also as something unknown and carrying negative connotations. Women who are concerned about the course of their pregnancy experience their body as extremely vulnerable and easily susceptible to negative influences from the environment that pose a danger to the baby. They listen attentively and anxiously to even the slightest bodily sign and interpret it as an indication of something potentially threatening going on. This attitude towards one's own body during pregnancy is certainly due to the prevailing medical representation of pregnancy as a risky and potentially pathological process. In such a situation of pregnancy, the body is experienced as foreign and alienated and becomes a source of anxiety for the woman.

These two ways in which their body appears in their experience during pregnancy have very different consequences for how women will treat not only the body itself but also all their other life projects—whether they will continue working, whether they will travel or use public transport, to what extent they will be physically active, what food, drinks, supplements and medication they will consume. If they experience their body as strong and competent, women will continue to behave as unproblematically embodied subjects and participate in various activities, perhaps only with increased attention to bodily signs. They will be considerate of their condition—many of them report, for example, that they refrain from physical exertion and carrying heavy things, even though they "have the strength and feel they could". However, this consideration will not limit them in a broader sense. If, on the other hand, they experience their body as distant and a source of anxiety, then everything they do (or not do) will be determined by concern for the pregnancy and consideration for the fragility and vulnerability of their own body. The choice of food, sleeping position, clothing and activities will be entirely subordinated to concern for their body and indirectly, but crucially, for the health and well-being of their baby. Of course, the first group of women also care about the well-being of their baby, but they do not perceive their body as something that can be easily threatened and injured, and that is fragile and unpredictable.

These two modalities of the relationship a woman can have to her pregnant and birthing body reflect the dissociative representation of the female and maternal body vividly articulated by Adrienne Rich and Rebecca Kukla and discussed at the beginning of Chap. 2. Empirical analysis of women's experiences of pregnancy and birth shows that this dissociative representation of the reproductive body is deeply internalised by women themselves, as Adrienne Rich says (1986b, p. 34), "even in the most independent of us". It is also important to remember that neither of these representations, i.e. regulatory ideals, is a priori associated with empowering women and supporting their subjectivity. The situation is more complex because these two representations and ways of treating the female reproductive body meet, collide and diverge in real-life circumstances. For example, when a woman who "fetishises" her pregnant and birthing body encounters a medical institution whose practices are aimed at regulating it driven by the idea that this body is unstable and unpredictable, she is likely to feel threatened and disempowered. But the same applies to the reverse situation—a woman who experiences her changing body as a source of anxiety and feels the need to be monitored and to entrust the care of her body to an external authority, will feel threatened and overwhelmed if she is expected to follow her intuition and get through pregnancy and childbirth without any external intervention. Therefore, I believe that the specific constellation of a woman's embodied subjectivity with which she enters transition to motherhood, and which is formed through a lifelong process of bodily socialisation, is crucial to the concrete role medical practitioners and technologies can play in her experience and agency.

5.2 Technological Mediatedness

5.2.1 Hermeneutic Role of Medical Knowledge and Technology

The opacity of the reproductive processes and their withdrawal from the phenomenological field determine the way in which it is (im)possible to understand and act upon them. Insofar as the reproductive body is not *within our sight*, it is not *within our reach*—"self-knowledge and self-command are thus achieved through technological mediation; what was depth is artificially made to surface" (Leder, 1990, p. 53). Therefore, the process of "reading" and influencing the body, performed both by ourselves and by others, as argued throughout the book, is never an unmediated one.[4] Donna Haraway asserts that since "we are not immediately present to ourselves" we need "a semiotic-material technology linking meanings and bodies" in order to acquire self-knowledge (Haraway, 1991b, p. 192). This general epistemological claim, which argues for the mediated nature of all knowledge, including self-knowledge, actually implies two important assertions. One entails that the subject is always already dissociated, "partial in all its guises, never finished, whole, simply there and original" (Haraway, 1991b, p. 193), not unified, stable or transparent to herself. I will return to this understanding of subjectivity at the end of this chapter. The other claim points to a dual and ambiguous nature of mediating technology, which is both discursive and material, enabling a discursive rendering of the material/bodily sphere of our existence. For example, a variety of diagnostic technologies, from thermometers to MRIs, could be understood as a set of hermeneutic tools that, in an age of technological progress significantly increase the interpretive power of both medical professionals and laypeople: "Since technology makes the body readable, we can speak legitimately of the

[4] Under regular circumstances and in our adult lives, this may sound like an overstatement. But it is obvious when we observe small children who need the practical and symbolic mediation of others in order to learn and be able to interpret their own embodied feelings. It also becomes evident when our usual embodied functioning is challenged, as in situations of illness or pregnancy.

hermeneutic function which scientific instruments perform for us" (Daniel, 1986, p. 204).

In the contemporary context, medicine thus regularly provides answers to hermeneutical questions that women are not in a position to answer by themselves. Due to widespread and easily accessible medical knowledge, women's bodies are often considerably "unblackboxed" even before they enter a medical institution. So today, prior to any direct intervention by medical professionals, medical knowledge acquired through books, magazines, websites, preparatory courses, lay discussions, etc., is often actively shaping women's perceptions, behaviours, ways of expression and modes of experience. Medical knowledge makes women today more attentive than in the past and enables them to attribute appropriate meaning and significance to various bodily events. For instance, the knowledge about the relatively reliable signs of the onset of labour or the fact that the baby's movements can be felt from the fourth month of pregnancy makes a woman particularly sensitive to corresponding stimuli from within her body. It enables her to recognise, connect and interpret them correctly when they occur. In this sense, medicine enables the reproductive body to emerge from the hermetic depths in which it resides and allows its processes to gain a clear place in the woman's experience. Medical explanations can also lead to a bodily process, which initially attracts the woman's attention due to its unusual nature, receding into the background of her awareness once it is recognised as irrelevant. The early onset of contractions, which is initially unsettling for the woman, can be dismissed if it is identified as "false" or preparatory and subsequently moved to the background. Medical knowledge thus not only provides a framework for the *interpretation* of the body but also mediates the *experiential* emergence and disappearance of the body for the woman herself.

The unfounded assumption that people possess an authentic insight into their own bodies, which is immediately accessible to them, leads to medical knowledge being regarded as external and as suppressing that authentic and immediate knowledge. However, it is not the case that people are readily capable of adequate insight into the state of their own bodies unless they are silenced by medicine. In some areas, medicine is even striving to raise persons' awareness of their own bodies through the use of measuring devices to increase sensitivity (e.g. in people with diabetes, see Mol & Law, 2004). This certainly calls into question the relationship between internal and external knowledge.

There is an additional hermeneutic role that medical knowledge and technology fulfil. As this research focused on the analysis of verbalised experiences, participants had the task of constructing coherent narratives. Attempting to impose structure and continuity to a sequence of events was relatively straightforward in the case of pregnancy. However, the attempts to impose a narrative structure to childbirth experience were often frustrating and uncertain, as it was not always easy to connect and chronologically organise the experiences that were chaotic, intensely dramatic and occasionally dissociative in real-life circumstances. Arthur Frank (1997, p. 98) highlighted the chaotic and incoherent narrative pattern associated with overwhelming, painful and traumatic experiences that resist verbalisation: "The story traces the edges of a wound that can only be told around. Words suggest its rawness, but that wound is so much of the body, its insults, agonies and losses, that words necessarily fail". A person faces the problem of integrating the experience and the difficulty of putting it into words and connecting it in a way that makes sense to both the listener and to herself. The narratives of women, especially those who have undergone psychophysical preparation, reveal that the medical framework of childbirth (number of centimetres dilated, frequency of contractions, stages of labour, etc.) often plays a significant role in organising their birth experience and serves as an important resource for managing the situation, preventing it from becoming overwhelming or threatening.

Some feminist authors (Chadwick, 2009; Martin, 2003) argue that the medical scenario of childbirth imposes an external perspective on women's own experiences. They point out that this schematic narrative pattern typically omits subjective experiences, bodily sensations and any inappropriate details that indicate disorder, messiness or the extremely corporeal aspects of childbirth. This dominant medical, technocratic discourse is, as Rachelle Chadwick argues, suppressing and "silencing the potentially paradoxical, split and often indeterminate subjectivity" of the birthing woman (Chadwick, 2009, p. 119).

This assertion is partially accurate—referring to established norms and markers shared by members of the community makes it easier for a woman to explain and share what she has experienced. It should be clear that a dilation of five centimetres indicates approximately mid-labour and fairly severe pain. However, even when encouraged in the interviews to describe and elaborate on specific moments of their birth and aspects of their experience in detail, the women found it difficult to represent their embodied experiences during birth without relying on a medical framework. Particularly when it came to painful and overwhelming aspects, the women in the interviews often struggled to find and create their discourse. Nevertheless, it seems unjustified to draw the above conclusion from this. The fact that women are frequently spontaneously invested in trying to fit their childbirth experience into the medical scenario pertains precisely to their difficulty in tolerating a "potentially paradoxical, split, and often indeterminate subjectivity" (Chadwick, 2009, p. 119). They use medical knowledge to have an interpretive framework for understanding the chaotic and overwhelming process of birth, and this framework makes the experience—especially the unfamiliar and intense bodily sensations—more comprehensible and manageable. What feminist authors, who unequivocally reject the medical narrative framework as external and alienating, seem to overlook is the fact that when labour begins, many women enter the institution already feeling somewhat threatened and not safe enough to "surrender" to their embodied experience. The normative ideal of subjectivity they identify with due to living in contemporary Western culture compels them to strive to integrate their experiences, develop a sense of agency and thus achieve a basic psychological well-being. Moreover, recourse to medical knowledge is extremely functional and practically useful in the institutional context in which they find themselves. It enables them to anticipate and understand not only what is happening inside their bodies, but also what is happening in their environment.

So when the embodied experience in a hospital context resists and disrupts the usual medical narrative of birth because it cannot fit the timeline, alternative (chaotic) narrative emerges that features vivid descriptions of bodily sensations and a representation of subjectivity "in crisis, torn between order and chaos, life and death, body and self, me and it, inside and outside, here and there, sense and non-sense" (Chadwick, 2009, p. 123). This narrative seems to indicate a loss of control, overwhelming negative bodily sensations and an inability to maintain an appropriate form of embodiment. Therefore, I do not consider it as an expression of some authentic, "paradoxical" birthing subjectivity, silenced and obscured by the externally imposed coherence of the medical framework, but rather as an expression of the subject's vulnerability, the disruption of her sense of coherence, her embodiment, her ability to symbolise experiences. However, the concrete role and impact of medical knowledge and narrative patterns should be assessed in concrete terms, i.e. empirically, and here I agree with Rachelle Chadwick's assertion that "women can be empowered or disempowered by biomedical information and scripts, depending on particular corpomaterial configurations" (2018, p. 71). I will come back to this issue later on.

It is also important to emphasise that in the destabilising circumstances of childbirth, women not only readily embrace medical *discourse* as a mediator to facilitate the integration of their experience and its incorporation into the rest of their life narrative, but they also rely on medical *technology* to intervene in a way that enables them to achieve re-embodiment, i.e. a more appropriate form of embodiment, and to restore their sense of agency.

5.2.2 Relationship Between Embodiment and Agency: The Intervening Role of Medical Technology

Intense, painful, disturbing and overwhelming physical sensations during childbirth fill the woman's experiential space and the world recedes into the background of her consciousness. The body (or its individual parts and organs) becomes the focus of her experience—not as an intimate aspect of herself, but as the presence of something foreign and threatening. She experiences her body as alienated. This alleged split between her body and her (embodied) self is not only initiated by the pain in these moments—it is also an adaptive response to it (Leder, 1990, p. 77). The painful body part is positioned opposite to the self in the phenomenological space and becomes something external to the subject's embodied experience, thereby enabling her to preserve her integrity at least to some extent in the face of the internal threat she suffers. The feeling of pain or physical discomfort is therefore not only experienced as "an attack on my instrumental body *(Körper)* but as a radical intrusion into my embodied selfhood" (Turner, 1992, p. 167). The subject, who until recently and during everyday functioning was directly and easily identified with her corporeality, is now confronted with problems of integration, of overcoming the challenges of an altered state and of establishing agency.

While under normal circumstances the subject is (unproblematically) embodied—meaning that the body is not perceived or mentioned at all—it is important to emphasise that in situations when embodied subjectivity is challenged the subject doesn't become disembodied—through dissociation between the mental self on the one hand and the body on the other—but some part of the subject's bodily experience is objectified and positioned opposite to the (challenged) *embodied* self (Akrich & Pasveer, 2004). The "object" that emerges from the process of objectification in the above sense is neither an object obtained through theoretical abstraction, nor is it the "body which the anatomist dissects and classifies", but "the existential otherness of the self, the phenomena of sheer heaviness and recalcitrance which it experiences within itself as interrupting its projects" (Gadow, 1980, p. 176).

Medical technology can play a role not only in the integration and interpretation of experience, but also in the literal moulding of that experience. Epidural anaesthesia is a paradigmatic example of a medical technology that enables an intervention in the flow of embodied experience and alters the relationship between the body and the embodied self (Akrich & Pasveer, 2004). It can allow an active dichotomy and an appropriate distance to be maintained between the body and the embodied self, so that women are not overwhelmed by the pain and can preserve the integrity that enables them to assume an active role at the end of childbirth. However, we have also seen that epidural anaesthesia does not always lead to such a positive outcome for the woman as a subject. When the epidural deprives the woman of the ability to feel the sensations from the lower half of her body, it leads to an alienating experience of birth and denies her any sense of agency. This scenario is comparable to the another one analysed, in which women are unable to actively participate in the final stage of their labour due to their severely compromised integrity resulting from the overwhelming pain caused by chemically intensified contractions. Both represent extremes of impaired embodiment—being completely disconnected from bodily sensations and being overwhelmed by them are both associated with the inability to be an agent in one's own childbirth (Akrich & Pasveer, 2004). Thus, while medical technology may lead to a continuation and deepening of the process of dissociation and alienation that women are already experiencing, it may also enable them to retain some form of integrity and agency, which explains why they sometimes utilise medical technology themselves and appropriate some aspects of the institutional context.

From this analysis of the birth situation we can draw some more general conclusions about the relationship between embodiment and agency. Agency is only experienced when there is an adequate relationship between the (embodied) self and the body. At one pole of an imaginary continuum there is a complete fusion of body and self—when the woman is overwhelmed by pain—and at the other pole there is a complete separation of body and self—when the anaesthesia prevents the woman from feeling the sensations from her body. Neither of these two extreme modes of embodiment (or, more precisely, dys-embodiment) enables agency, which indicates that an *adequate embodiment* of the subject is a *condition of possibility for agency*. In most regular situations, our embodiment is not compromised, so the connection between these two modalities of subjectivity is not obvious, and it seems to us that agency can be manifested independently of embodiment.

This insight also has practical implications, for example, with regard to the regulation of pain during childbirth. It seems that neither the proponents of the medical model of childbirth nor the proponents of the natural model reckon with this relationship between agency and embodiment. The question is not whether to provide women with a painless childbirth via the use of anaesthesia or insist on a natural birth without medication, but rather what level of pain/sensation corresponds to an adequate body-embodied self-dynamic that allows a woman to be an agent during her childbirth. What seems to be crucial for a woman's integrity and well-being is that she feels neither overwhelmed and powerless nor numb and dissociated.

5.2.3 Complex Empirical Realities: Embodied vs. Technologically Mediated Modes of Experience

I have argued so far that medical knowledge and technology play varied and significant roles in how women experience, understand and treat their changing bodies during pregnancy and birth. There are at least two important aspects that determine this—the relationship that women have to their changing bodily experience and the organisation of medical practice in which the technology is situated. The first aspect has already been discussed in the section on maternal embodiment. The second aspect concerns the institutional embeddedness of technology and socio-material networks that produce various effects on women's embodiment and agency, and I will turn to this topic in the next section. Now I want to look more closely at how embodied and technologically mediated modes of experience are related to each other.

Although the differentiation between these two modes of experience is analytically useful, it is necessarily artificial and simplistic. Technologically mediated experience is always embodied, while embodied experience is often mediated by knowledge and technology—the difference is primarily one of emphasis, it is by no means absolute. Embodiment is a prerequisite for the experience of what technology provides, and once our experience is mentalised (especially when it is verbalised), we rely on a representation that is certainly culturally mediated and, in modern times, often technologically mediated as well. Although the analytical separation of two modalities of experience led to a certain simplification, it enabled us to examine their dynamics and interaction in greater detail and precision. Sometimes the technologically mediated experience is an incentive for the embodied one, and sometimes the situation is reversed. Technological knowledge also appears as an extension and supplement to embodied knowledge, and sometimes as its confirmation or correction. On the other hand, in many situations, technologically mediated information is called into question because it deviates from the embodied experience. So instead of a dichotomy that implies an opposing or even exclusionary relationship between them, or at least a priori privileging one or the other, they involve in complex and variable relationships—interacting, coordinating, complementing, but also challenging and correcting each other, thus jointly shaping the experience of pregnancy and an evolving baby that are mutually co-constitutive. Regardless of whether a direct connection and interaction between technologically mediated and embodied experience has been established in the situation, almost all the cases considered in this book indicate that there is a seeming coordination of these two modalities, rather than their mutual exclusion.

We have seen in the previous chapters that the dynamic interplay of embodied and technologically mediated experience is present throughout the early transition to motherhood, but it is especially prominent during the complex process of individuation of the baby for the mother-to-be. On the one hand, women's experience of pregnancy and the baby is mediated by medical knowledge/technology, and ultrasound occupies an important place in this respect. On the other hand, the woman has privileged epistemological access to the baby through the embodied experience of its position and movements, recognises patterns of activity and even interactions. In some situations embodied knowledge dominates, such as in the experience of the baby's movements, while in other situations it is mainly technologically mediated, as in the experience of an ultrasound examination. But, as already indicated, the experience of movement also involves how the woman imagines the baby based on the ultrasound image, and the experience of the medical examination involves how the woman feels the baby's movements and position. The joint unfolding of these processes leads the pregnant woman to perceive the baby as increasingly more specific and elaborate, and eventually to begin to regard it as an independent being. The baby thus enters the symbolic and imaginary universe of the mother-to-be and the future family, as the expectant parents give it a personalised nickname, and later discuss a personal name as well as the habits, preferences and character of their not-yet-born child. At the same time, the woman undergoes profound changes in the way she experiences herself and her own body, but also other people and various everyday situations in a complex process of becoming a mother.

Not all authors agree with this depiction. The critical stance towards medical technology is an important part of feminist literature, especially among second-wave and phenomenologically oriented authors, because it devalues and deprivileges female embodied knowledge and experience by introducing objective, technologically mediated information (Bergum, 1994; Duden, 1993; Rich, 1986b; Young, 2005b). It is suggested that prenatal diagnostic techniques, such as ultrasound, place other people in an analogous epistemic position to the pregnant woman, who previously held a privileged position due to her access to the embodied experience of the foetus. At the same time, what the ultrasound technology delivers becomes more real than what the woman feels, acquiring the status of authoritative knowledge: "the conversion of this subjective experience into objective entities that can be observed by anyone with the proper instruments. These objectified observables come to be defined as the authoritative knowledge of the process of gestation and the state of the fetus, and thereby the pregnant woman's privileged insider knowledge comes to be devalued" (Young, 2005b, p. 61). Young also points out that the visual representation of the foetus is favoured over the tactile, reflecting the prevailing trend of privileging the visual in modern culture. It is assumed that by shifting the emphasis to the visual sensory modality, modern medicine makes the mother's kinaesthetic and tactile knowledge less exclusive and valuable.[5] Barbara Katz Rothman also points out that women no longer rely on the experience of movement to perceive the baby as real and independent, but on the ultrasound image on the screen: "It is no longer quickening that marks the first realisation of the baby as a separate being within: it is now the moment it is first seen on the screen. Women report that in that moment of seeing the fetus on the ultrasound screen, it suddenly becomes real to them: *real* is probably the most often used word to describe the fetus on the screen" (Rothman, 1993, p. 125). According to Rothman, ultrasound is a technological means that enables the perception of the foetus "as a separate patient essentially trapped within the woman", making "the woman

[5] It is sometimes noted that even women themselves become "voyeurs of the foetus" and feel excluded if they are not allowed to see the screen during an ultrasound examination (Sandelowski & Black, 1994, p. 608).

erased from the image on our screens and increasingly in our minds" (Rothman, 2007a, p. XXI–XXII). By placing the foetus in the foreground, the woman is necessarily repositioned during pregnancy and childbirth and her role is altered, primarily by being displaced from the situation (Ginsburg & Rapp, 1991; Squier, 1996).

While some of these criticisms sound convincing, they are based on a number of arguments that I consider problematic and unfounded, leading to an overly one-sided understanding of the role of medical technology in the embodied experience of women: firstly, the temporal character of the baby's individuation process is neglected by overemphasising the importance of prenatal technology only at one particular stage; secondly, the woman's privileged and unique position in relation to the baby is reduced to the specificity of the sensory modality or the relationship of proximity; and finally, the complexity of the medical encounter is unjustifiably reduced. I will now address all three arguments in more detail.

By making some inaccessible parts of the body visible and potentially manipulable, ultrasound technology introduces new actors onto the stage (Thompson, 2005). In the case of pregnancy, this is the foetus, whose contours appear on the screen (and possibly in a photograph that the woman can take with her) and whose characteristics are noted in the specialist's report. This constructed foetus relates in various ways to the "experienced" foetus, and both types of experiences and representations enable the process we have referred to as the individuation of the baby. As the pregnancy progresses, the baby takes on a more defined form and becomes a distinct being with certain physical characteristics known from the ultrasound (e.g., sex) and certain activity rhythms, behaviours and even character inferred from embodied insights. It has already been discussed in detail how women move from barely perceptible sensations in mid-pregnancy to a fully differentiated representation of the baby by drawing on different types of insights.[6]

[6] It should not be forgotten that their embodied experience is not immediate, even if it seems so—a woman learns to recognise vague sensations as the baby's movements by relying on medical knowledge of when they should occur or on the image on the screen showing the foetus' movements and activity. The experience of movements in the later course of pregnancy is also conveyed through the representation of the baby's position (which women usually know from the ultrasound scan) and

The relative importance and contribution of these two modes of experience change over the course of the pregnancy, depending on the presence and richness of embodied knowledge about the baby. Therefore, it does not make much sense to ask about the role of ultrasound technology in pregnancy in general.[7] At the beginning of pregnancy, when the woman does not yet feel the movements of the foetus, the ultrasound image makes the pregnancy "more real" for many women and promotes identification with it (and thus also changes in their daily behaviour). It is the first situation in which their future baby appears to them to be defined and real in some way (see also Clement et al., 1998). However, it should not be forgotten that there are various milestones in the baby's individuation and that most of the participants in this study experienced the baby as "real" in a more specific and meaningful way after they began to feel the movements. Thus, although the moment when the foetus becomes "real" for the woman is presented as a single event in the above critical evaluation, it is in fact a process, and what is meant by the experience of the "real baby" changes during pregnancy. The final outcome for most women involves a very specific and concrete conception of an autonomous being that they feel as their own, almost in contrast to the ultrasound representation of the generic, "canonical" foetus that technology provides (Kukla, 2005, p. 109). What the advent of ultrasound technology has probably changed regarding the experience of modern women is that the process of the baby's individuation or "becoming real" begins earlier than it used to.

Furthermore, on what basis can we claim that a pregnant woman has a special and privileged relationship with her baby compared to all other people who may also have some experience of the baby in her womb?

---

through the medical representation of the interior of their own body. This specific mediation enables the woman, for example, to interpret a sudden dull pain in her lower abdomen as "the baby kicking my cervix" (Sonja).

[7] Most studies ask this general question but are actually concerned with the specific role of ultrasound, focusing only on a particular period of pregnancy—ultrasound is considered primarily or even exclusively as a means of *seeing* the baby, and its use in the second trimester, when the woman can already feel the baby's movements, is being investigated. The main question that arises, then, is whether this technologically mediated knowledge about the baby, which is available to different people, disregards the privileged embodied access that the pregnant woman herself has.

Does the fundamental difference lie in the modality of sensory experience—while the pregnant woman has tactile and kinaesthetic experiences of her baby, the doctor only has a visual experience through the ultrasound? Furthermore, it can be argued that the woman has an *internal* experience of the baby, whereas all other people only have an *external* experience—for example, they can feel the baby's movements by placing their hand on her belly, but only from the outside. These two characteristics are both emphasised in the literature when it comes to the specific and privileged immediate experience of the mother in contrast to the (technologically) mediated experience of the baby that other people can have. Moreover, the criticism of medical technology points out that it devalues the woman's *immediate* embodied knowledge and replaces it with *mediated* visual knowledge, thus placing other people on an equal footing with the woman and jeopardising her privileged position.[8]

I believe that this critique of medical technology actually reduces the complex and unique relationship that the mother has with her unborn baby to the characteristics of sensory modality (visual vs. tactile/kinaesthetic) or to the position in relation to the epistemic object (external vs. internal). What makes the relationship between a woman and a foetus exclusive is the day-long experience of carrying a baby in the belly, recognising the baby's activity patterns and developing an interaction with it. Women very often associate the baby's movements with their own rhythm or actions and interpret the baby's activity as a response to which they often try to adapt. They also imagine the pauses between the perceived

[8] It is often pointed out that ultrasound diagnostics place the expectant father in an analogous position to the mother. How do men experience the ultrasound scan? Some authors claim that the opportunity to participate in ultrasound examinations and to see the foetus on the screen contributes significantly to the expectant fathers' perception of the baby as real and as an independent being. During pregnancy, visual knowledge is their most important form of knowledge about the baby (Draper, 2002). I have not explored this topic in my research, but based on the limited insight I have gained from what women have said about their partners' experiences with ultrasound (I only have information from a few interviewees who have had private ultrasound exams, as men are prohibited from attending them in public practice), it seems that men rely more on the reactions of the women themselves than what they see on the screen, or even what the doctor tells and shows them. The expectant fathers about whom I have received some indirect information, thus do not seem to have an autonomous relationship to the technologically mediated insight and appear to favour the woman's perspective. Of course, detailed study on this topic is needed to draw reliable conclusions.

movements as sleep, rest or as the baby "calming down and waiting". This process of (proto-)interaction and (proto-)communication leads to the individuation of the baby, which is transformed from a generic foetus on the screen into a being with autonomy, habits, activity patterns and even preferences and certain character traits (stubbornness, naughtiness, shyness, etc.). If we understand the specificity of the relationship between a woman and a foetus in this more complex way, then the existence of ultrasound information or the possibility that other people can see or feel the baby does not appear as an alternative or something that can jeopardise or replace a woman's embodied experience of her future child. It may complement it, provide an occasion for further individuation or some specific representations, but in any case it is not a relation of opposition between two modalities of experience or the exclusion of embodied experience, but a complex interaction.

Since they begin to feel the baby's movements, most women prefer the embodied mode of knowing and interacting with their baby, which calls into question the thesis that technologically mediated knowledge is the authoritative knowledge about the foetus. Based on the analysis, I would argue that this is only the case in one very specific sense—in relation to the baby's health.[9] In terms of identification with the pregnancy and the relationship with the baby—which are actually the key aspects of the transition to motherhood—the embodied experience plays a more significant role. Women often do not relate to ultrasound differently than to diagnostic techniques applied to them independently of pregnancy. Just as our bodies sometimes send no clear signals even when we are ill (and there are many pathological conditions that cause no subjectively perceived symptoms for a long time), the baby's perceived movements also say nothing about the health of its kidneys or heart.

There is another unwarranted simplification that often appears in criticism of ultrasound technology and features prominently in the work of both Iris Marion Young (2005b) and Barbara Duden (1993). Optical technologies—telescope, microscope, ultrasound—provide visual access

[9] It turns out that this even applies to 4D ultrasound, which is advertised as a way for prospective parents to get to know their unborn child.

to remote or inaccessible environments. They are often assumed to neglect all senses other than sight (Dolezal, 2009), reflecting the habit of Western societies to privilege the visual as the sense most relevant to cognition and the one on whose authority scientific knowledge rests (Ihde, 2002). It is believed that this has consequences for the status of embodied experience in the situation of pregnancy, which is primarily tactile and kinaesthetic in nature. Although this qualification of ultrasound technology contains true elements, it is overly simplified. Barbara Duden, for example, draws a distinction between the embodied experience of women from the past and the *disembodied* experience that characterises modern women, taking the ultrasound as a paradigmatic example and claiming that "the Enlightenment has removed from our bellies, as from our minds, any reality that is not perceived by the eye" (Duden, 1993, p. 8). She contrasts the eighteenth century encounter between a doctor and a woman, who reports a wide range of sensory experiences and perceptions, with today's encounter, which is "sensory deprived" and relies exclusively on visual representations provided by instruments. This clear-cut dichotomy of two mutually exclusive options is questionable because it oversimplifies the whole situation of the ultrasound examination, which in reality is never reduced to a single sensory modality (Martin, 1996). The very experience of an ultrasound examination for a woman involves other sensory modalities (touch, sound, the experience of inner space), and these are sometimes crucial to the role that the ultrasound image will play for her. A close examination of the women's narratives presented in the previous chapters indicates that it is difficult to establish a simple relationship of opposition or mutual exclusion between the visual (technologically mediated) and the tactile-kinaesthetic (embodied) experience. These two modalities of experience often refer to different objects (or subjects), and when they interact, their relationship needs to be understood and described in a much more complex and dynamic way.

Indeed, the dystopian account of technology outlined in the feminist critique is in many ways similar to that derived from the classical theory of technology influenced by Karl Jaspers and Martin Heidegger. This theoretical position is dominated by the alienation thesis, which sees technology as "a radically transformative power that estranges human beings from themselves, from each other, and from reality itself. Technological culture is seen as transforming human beings into cogs in a social machine, and as transforming reality into raw material that can only be approached via domination and control" (Verbeek, 2005, p. 3). The conceptualisation of technology that underlies this critical approach implies that technology has some built-in properties that make it inherently "bad" for people, because its nature is reduced solely to non-technological elements (such as social organisation and power structures).[10]

As we have seen, crucially important resources for reconceptualising technology came from science and technology studies and the relatively recent developments in the philosophy of technology known as postphenomenology. These stances sought to "avoid the extremes of both utopian and dystopian interpretations of technology, which have too often captured the field" (Ihde, 1990, p. X), by examining the different roles that technologies play in human experience and existence. This led to the recognition that both our experience of the world and our actions towards it, at least in our contemporary society, are (almost) always technologically mediated. The further development of this position resulted in a more radical perspective, according to which "subject and object are not merely intertwined with each other but constitute each other" (Verbeek, 2005, p. 112). This thesis poses a radical challenge to the modernist understanding of both subjects and objects and their relationships.

Technology should therefore be understood as being inextricably linked to practice and thus relative to the context and activity in which it is used. While it has no fixed set of essential properties, it facilitates some courses of action or interpretation, and at the same time discourages some others. While technology is certainly the product of some social relations and fields of practice, it simultaneously shapes and co-produces these relations and practices. Thus, the specific materiality of technology

[10] An alternative view of technology assumes that technological artefacts are merely neutral means to achieve certain human goals, so that their influence depends solely on how they are used. Therefore, it is either assumed that "technologies are 'merely' instrumental and thus implicitly neutral", or that they are "fully determinative and thus uncontrollable" (Ihde, 1990, p. 140). Both positions are, however, too simplistic and problematic, which is in line with Kranzberg's first law of technology (1986): "Technology is neither good nor bad; nor is it neutral".

should not be ignored, even if it should not be conceptualised in essential, but in relational terms.

5.3 Socio-material Embeddedness

Understanding the various forms of technological mediation and their consequences for embodied subjectivity requires an assessment of the concrete empirical reality of technology, which can only arise within specific practical contexts of its use. A situated and contextualised approach to *medical* technology therefore entails not examining it as something that has a fixed, medically defined meaning that is stable over time and across different contexts. Instead, it is investigated as embedded in medical practice in particular circumstances—including procedures, doctor-patient relationships, protocols and norms, as well as material characteristics of an institutional setting. Thus, medical practice is seen as complex, heterogeneous and context-specific (Kontopodis et al., 2011), involving a variety of interpretations of numbers and images, styles of interaction with patients, criteria for decision making, intervention practices and different technologies in diverse institutional contexts with various regional variations (Berg & Mol, 1998).[11] What becomes the aim of empirical research is to identify all relevant actors involved in medical practice and to determine their relationships, as well as the various outcomes resulting from these diverse patterns of entanglements. The role of medical technology depends not only on the individuals to whom it is applied or the specificities of their bodies (which I have already discussed),

[11] In medical books and clinical guides, the various objects of medical practice are usually arranged to form a coherent whole, but the same does not apply to everyday medical practice: "Where in textbooks the various versions of a disease tend to be neatly aligned to form a coherent overall picture, in practice there are gaps, fissures and frictions between different performances of any 'one' disease (…) even if they go under the same name, the 'diseases' diagnosed in different sites, do not necessarily coincide" (Mol, 2000, p. 96). If incoherence between different medical performances occurs in practice, some will be privileged over the others. A hierarchy established in this way is not inherent in any system of medical knowledge. Rather, it is a product of hospital protocols, conventions, the organisation of the health care system and other both policy-level and individual-level decisions.

but also on the *role and agency of medical practitioners* (Lock et al., 2000, p. 12).

Medical professionals play a significant role in facilitating the process of women's self-exploration, primarily by mediating between women and medical technology, which is often not sufficiently comprehensible and directly accessible to them:[12] "Through the mediation of another, we come to see our body in a series of technologically and conceptually extended ways that otherwise would be unavailable" (Leder, 1990, p. 78). The fact that women turn to medical professionals should not necessarily be seen as something that leads to alienation, but as an extension of a woman's self-examination using means that she cannot control herself and that are only accessible to her when used by another person. However, it is only by acting as *mediators*[13] between women and technology that medical practitioners manage to establish and maintain a genuine mutual triadic relationship (Reiser, 1984).[14] In real-life conditions, this triadic

[12] Either because they lack an interpretative and normative framework or because it is not accessible to them due to the way the examination is staged.

[13] In the framework of Latour's theory, medical practitioners are not neutral "intermediaries", but full-fledged "mediators" (Latour, 2005, p. 39). There is a crucial difference between mediators and intermediaries in ANT that should be kept in mind when analysing the role of medical practitioners. Intermediaries are described by Latour (2005, p. 39) as something that "transports meaning or force without transformation: defining its inputs is enough to define its outputs", which implies that they can be treated as black boxes without fear of overlooking an important aspect of the situation. Mediators, on the other hand, should not be treated as "black boxes" because "their input is never a good predictor of their output; their specificity has to be taken into account every time" (Latour, 2005, p. 59). Mediators transform and modify the situation and lead to diverse outcomes. Only mediators understood in this sense are actually fully-fledged actors and must be taken into account when analysing a network. Medical professionals are mediators in this strong sense and their activity should always be examined when analysing a medical encounter in contemporary technologised institutional contexts.

[14] It should be noted that the image of a triadic relationship is a very simplified one. In reality, we are dealing with a complex network consisting of a multitude of human and non-human actors. The complex, situated and multidimensional nature of both patients and medical technology has been discussed previously. When it comes to medical professionals, the situation becomes even more complicated—in addition to nurses, general practitioners and numerous medical specialists (obstetricians, gynaecologists, surgeons, endocrinologists), laboratory technicians, radiologists, pathologists, epidemiologists, physiologists, etc., also play an important role (for a detailed empirical analysis, see Mol, 2002). Of course, we could also consider a "broader" network that includes health insurance companies, pharmaceutical companies, health policy organisations, etc. However, when conducting a concrete analysis, it is necessary to have a certain analytical focus (specific to a particular research project), so that the "network character" of many actors has to be omitted from the picture—it is acknowledged but not analysed in detail, because it is impossible to "unblackbox" the whole world at once and track all the mediators.

relationship sometimes fails to be neither triadic nor a relationship, if the mediating roles of both professionals and medical technology are missing, thus leaving the subjectivity of women out of the medical encounter.

In case medical practitioners are exclusively focused on a woman's body (or more commonly only a part of it) while completely ignoring her embodied subjectivity, she is not included in any way in the process of medical examination or intervention. As a consequence, she cannot co-participate in the objectification of her body, so she is prevented from connecting her embodied experience with the technologically mediated one. Under these conditions, technology fails to act as a mediator and be anything for a woman herself, because a mediating role of healthcare practitioners is missing. It is just something medical professionals use amongst themselves for their own purposes (even if the procedure can be clearly beneficial for the woman). Furthermore, the objectified part of the woman's body can lose the connection to her embodied subjectivity, leading to alienation and dys-embodiment.[15] This is a paradigmatic case of an objectifying and alienating practice that has a number of negative outcomes for a woman because she is excluded from the socio-material constellation of medical practice as a relevant actor.

It is obvious that these consequences are not due to some inherent properties of medical technology. They result from the entire network of institutionally bound relationships, norms and practices in which the medical practitioners play a decisive role. As already mentioned earlier, the (in)ability of medical professionals to act as mediators between women and technology is crucial. What is needed is the creation of an intersubjective constellation of the medical encounter in which a doctor or nurse and a woman can be jointly involved in examining her body or even intervening on it, by relying on medical technology. Under such circumstances, the relationship with the other ceases to be alienating and the objectified body part appears to a woman as a non-alienated aspect of her own experience. In this way, technologically mediated care during pregnancy and childbirth could be transformed into a collaborative

[15] We can recognise this situation as a *social* cause of dys-embodiment—which can be triggered by the "incorporated gaze of the Other" in circumstances when another person looks at us with an "objectifying gaze that refuses cotranscendence" (Leder, 1990, p. 96).

project that should serve as a model for woman-centred or, more generally, person-centred care.[16]

A paradigmatic example of "blaming" technology—without acknowledging the entire network in which it is embedded—is the criticism of the use of advanced technologies in the contemporary medical contexts that is said to contribute to the loss of intimate contact between pregnant women and medical staff (Davis-Floyd, 2001; Duden, 1993). It is implied that the older technology mostly involved the direct sensory contact and conversation with the patient, whereas the newer technology usually only involves a machine being in direct contact with the patient and the diagnostic procedure that is based on the reading of electronic data. The following quote is very illustrative of this attitude: "When a doctor uses a 'low-tech' tool like a stethoscope, he touches the patient, speaks to her, listens with his own ears to hers or the baby's heartbeats, interprets the sounds through his own bodily perceptions, and arrives at a diagnosis that depends in large part on his physical senses. When the same doctor uses a computerized axial tomography (CAT) scanner or an electronic fetal monitor (EFM), only the machine touches or interacts with the patient during the procedure. Thc physician's role is to interpret the mechanically mediated results" (Davis-Floyd, 2001, p. 4). Davis-Floyd argues that the advent of sophisticated contemporary technology has led to a distancing between doctors and patients and the disappearance of some of the more intimate modalities of their relationship.[17] Except, what if an MRI is not "guilty" of preventing doctors from touching patients and talking to them, but a stethoscope was "guilty" of compelling them to do so? Touch was never a part of the medical model, but a historically contingent practical necessity. This became clear when it disappeared along with the cessation of that necessity.

[16] In the last chapter we saw that this collaborative project or a functioning socio-material network of birth can be achieved with the participation of very different actors and in different contexts, even in those that we usually consider as literally opposite options on an imaginary spectrum—a home birth and a caesarean section.

[17] There is also an obvious privileging, almost a fetishisation, of immediacy in Davis-Floyd's account, which acknowledges the advantage of sensory over technologically mediated experience, based on a simplified account of their dichotomy and mutual exclusivity, as discussed previously.

Technology, therefore, is not the one to blame. It has merely highlighted the relational and ethical problem of "attending to the 'objectness' of persons without reducing them to the moral status of objects" that has been "inherent in health care in any era" (Gadow, 1984, p. 63), and that is a consequence of the dominant scientific paradigm that conceptualises the body exclusively as a scientific object devoid of subjectivity.[18] The Cartesian foundations of modern medicine led to the separation between mind and body, which was followed by the mechanistic reduction of the body into a set of individual parts (Leder, 1984) and which further enabled the problems of the body to be understood as technical problems requiring technical solutions. This historical trend not only typically led to a practical desubjectification of women during medical treatment, but also radically altered the practice of care, since medical practitioners were only responsible for the body and not for the person whose body it is (Davis-Floyd, 1994).[19] These phenomena were at the heart of the dystopian depiction of medical technology in reproductive healthcare that was prevalent in feminist literature. Contemporary medical environment in which the treatment of reproductive processes takes place was criticised by authors belonging to second-wave feminism as having multiple alienating consequences for women (Beckett, 2005; Martin, 1984; Young, 2005b). It is suggested that the alienation women experience in the institutional context permeates the most relevant spheres of their existence.

---

[18] Sally Gadow (1984, p. 63) even argues that "it is ethically naive to imagine that the issue of regarding patients as objects originated with the introduction of apparatus into the practice of health care". The appropriate strategy aimed at the provision of better medical care should therefore not focus on *de-technologisation* (and not only because there will always be cases that require the use of sophisticated technologies), but on the promotion of non-technological aspects of care together with the *rational* and sensitive use of existing technologies adapted to each context and acknowledging the specificities of the embodied subjectivity of the individual. I emphasise rational use—that is based on a critical reflection of medical practice and an empirical study of its effects—since it has turned out that the aspects that are most alienating and threatening to women in the local institutional setting are in fact those that have been rejected in other medical systems precisely because of their empirically confirmed ineffectiveness, even harmfulness (e.g., the routine administration of induction or episiotomy). This means that Serbian medical institutions, where outdated practices and conservative patterns of thinking and behaviour prevail, paradoxically need more, not less, science and technology.

[19] Part of medical training is to develop the ability to avoid emotional involvement (Davis-Floyd, 1987). Therefore, in the treatment of pregnancy and childbirth, as well as in the medical treatment of other conditions, no physical contact or expression of caring beyond what is necessary for medical treatment is expected.

Women are separated from their life projects, from significant others, and even from their own bodies, because on repeated occasions during pregnancy and almost during the whole process of labour they are subjected to a series of standardised institutional procedures and hooked up to sophisticated technological systems of supervision and care. While empirical reality often corresponded to this dystopian depiction (and certainly still does in Serbia), the problem with feminist critique is that it only recognises necessary (or universal) causes, rather than merely historically contingent ones.

I believe this is a consequence of the established network of hospital care, which makes the situation appear universal and permanent. The dualistic metaphysics of modern medicine is embodied and materialised through a long historical process in the way hospitals are built and arranged, in the set of rules, protocols and conventions, in the medical university textbooks and the norms of professional socialisation of obstetricians, in the way medical technology is designed, handled and applied. This complex constellation is relatively rigid and operates according to its own sturdy choreography, because "it is a system with a well organized, internal logic, supported by experience and training, language, hospital rules and insurance needs, specific technologies, and a profound logic of risk and a focus on 'the baby'—you do want a healthy baby, don't you?" (Halfon, 2010, p. 64). However, we should understand this rigid and complex network constitutive of medical practice in relational rather than essential terms, which prevents us from ascribing to both medical technology and women and their bodies a set of inherent properties that make them incompatible with each other.

What is at the basis of this changed approach to technology that calls for empirical investigation of its relationship with subjectivity is a different theory of both subject and technology than the one implicit in the criticism discussed above. They are no longer considered as given, coherent and well-individualised wholes, but as complex constellations that are locally situated and can only be described empirically. This shift in perspective, stemming from STS and contemporary feminism, has enabled me to focus on the discursive-material aspects of the social environment and institutional and technological practice when exploring the subjectivity of women going through this peculiar stage of development. In closing the book, I will outline a number of ethical and practical consequences of this altered model of subjectivity and argue that it should be recognised as an important resource for a revision of a mainstream psychological theory of the subject.

5.4 A Revised Theory of Subjectivity and Ethical-Political Consequences

Traditional political projects were mainly concerned with preserving integrity and agency of individuals, as these qualities were recognised as *essential* aspects of human subjects. Criticism of modern medicine often refers to the fact that it threatens the unity of the patient, divides her into isolated body parts and reduces her to particular organs or bodily functions. As an expression of this general critical attitude towards medical technology, the medicalisation, institutionalisation and technologisation of pregnancy and birth have been recognised as necessary leading to the alienation and desubjectification of women.[20] As already suggested, this critical stance often goes hand in hand with the promotion of an alternative model that is centred on the idea of naturalness, spontaneity and non-interference (exemplified in practices such as natural pregnancy and birth or exclusive breastfeeding). What many authors from second-wave feminism and proponents of the natural model share is the modernist representation of (female) subjectivity as singular, unified, transparent to itself, clearly separated from others and the world of objects, with stable mental and physical boundaries, and with the capacity for agency conceptualised as an inherent property (Hatgis, 2001; Venn, 1998). Women's embodied experience is considered authentic only insofar as it is *unmediated* and they are regarded as having natural and intuitive competencies to guide them through pregnancy and childbirth. Another significant feature of this modernist account is the belief that women can only be

[20] While this critique has been a powerful political strategy for feminists in their struggle for women's reproductive rights, authors such as Donna Haraway warn that the postulate of wholeness and integrity of both bodies and subjects is highly problematic, as it rests on the assumption that these are universal, ahistorical categories, which seriously calls into question any political projects that might be centred on them (Berg & Akrich, 2004).

agents if they have *sole authority* over their reproductive processes. Consequently, any interference or intervention is considered as something that inevitably undermines women's authority and threatens their agency. Medical technology is thus seen only as an aggressor—an objectifying and disciplinary instance, which leads to a plethora of negative consequences for the subject. It is claimed that if the subject is to remain whole and autonomous, it must be clearly separated from the institutional and technological domain. No possibility is left for the women to delegate their authority to medical professionals or to actively appropriate medical technology, use it as a resource and adapt it to their needs.

The recognition of medical technology as inherently alienating can, therefore, be attributed to the modernist conception (or misconception) of subjectivity. We have seen that the subjectivity of a woman going through the early transition to motherhood clearly and in various respects defies the criteria of this conception outlined above. Her bodily boundaries are literally shifting as her body radically alters its shape and size—both its interior and its surface are changing and becoming permeable in a way she did not know before this phase of her life.[21]

But more importantly, this life stage problematises the distinction between outer and inner spaces, here and there, me and the other. Within her body resides another being that is increasingly gaining autonomy and which she primarily cares for by relating to her body, and thus to herself, in a particular manner. This situation has specific *ethical* implications: "A pregnant woman is in the midst of transforming from one being into two beings, who are themselves not morally independent from one another but deeply and intimately bound to one another in complex, ethically subtle ways. Our fetuses are not independent agents, but they are not simply more of us either" (Kukla, 2005, p. 137). The internal presence of the foetus, which in a certain sense is an independent agent, places the woman in a unique psychological and phenomenological situation. The

[21] Rebecca Kukla's assertion (2005, p. 3) illustrates this in a striking manner: "Female bodies, and especially pregnant and newly maternal bodies, leap, drip, squirt, expand, contract, crave, divide, sag, dilate, and expel. It is hard not to see why such bodies have long seemed to have dubious, hard to fix, permeable boundaries. And to the extent that we take the integrity and boundaries of the body as integrally intertwined with the integrity and boundaries of the self—and we have done so, at least throughout the history of Western culture and probably beyond—these dubious boundaries have been the source of various species of intellectual and visceral anxiety".

baby is affected by what transpires in the most intimate space of her thoughts and feelings—due to the responsibility towards the baby, it becomes a "luxury" for her to be angry or sad. In short, a pregnant woman's subjectivity does not begin where her skin begins. But, her subjectivity does not end where her skin ends either. She is not the sole source of her knowledge or her actions. When agency is reified as an inherent attribute of individuals, it is decontextualised, detached from the sociocultural and material nexus that enables or limits it. Contrary to the traditional understanding, the appropriate reliance on "external" resources actually enhances, rather than diminishes, her agency, since "emancipation (...) does not mean 'freed from bonds' but well-attached" (Latour, 2005, p. 218).

The encounter with medical examinations and interventions inevitably entails a form of objectification that regularly takes place under the authority and expertise of others (e.g. during a gynaecological examination, an ultrasound scan or a surgical procedure). Nevertheless, on the basis of this altered understanding of subjectivity, I have argued that this does not necessarily lead to negative consequences for women as subjects. We have seen that women themselves often initiate and participate in the objectification of their own bodies during the early transition to motherhood, and without any alienating effects. The phenomenological analysis of pregnancy and childbirth has shown us that before a woman enters a medical institution (and independently of it) she goes through a series of changes. Her own body appears to her as objectified in various ways due to the heightened awareness of its processes. The presence of intense bodily sensations she cannot control or even adequately integrate (as is the case in childbirth) is experienced as essentially destabilising to the woman's sense of self. Medical knowledge, technology, procedures and practitioners, when adequately arranged and interconnected, can serve as relevant mediators and be used as resources that allow her to overcome situations of uncertainty or, in more dramatic cases, "dys-embodiment". Similarly, the sharing of responsibility and delegation of authority, which are very common in the medical context, do not automatically lead to reduced agency of the woman.

Using reproductive technologies and drawing on the expertise of others can even lead to empowerment, as women can act in ways that were unavailable to them before technological advances in the field. In many situations, women are willing to accept the role of the object of a medical examination and even actively participate (through self-monitoring and preparation), in order to realise their life projects (e.g. getting pregnant, giving birth safely). In these circumstances, situated medical technology takes on the task of monitoring, repairing and supporting the life project of the woman as subject (Thompson, 2005). On the other hand, as we have seen, medical technologies and procedures sometimes fail in this mediating role and only initiate or perpetuate the process of objectification and alienation. Throughout the book, I have tried to move beyond both utopian and dystopian representations of technology in reproductive healthcare and to avoid advocating either a medical or a natural model of pregnancy and childbirth—that is, I have not wanted to position myself on either side of the cultural and ideological divide. Instead, drawing on critical theoretical resources and empirical findings, I aimed to explore how concrete medical practices and techniques situated in local institutional contexts are involved in the experience and agency of women. I believe that a different approach would essentialise both the woman undergoing reproductive processes and the medical environment in which these processes predominantly take place today.

There is a widespread stereotypical representation of women in the biomedical paradigm that involves women as passive recipients of care and medical technology and medical professionals as agents who enable them to achieve something that would not be possible outside the institution—an uncomplicated pregnancy, a healthy baby, a safe birth. This is the official narrative of progress and risk reduction that represents medical technology in a strictly utopian light. On the other hand, opponents of reproductive technology and medical approach view medical practitioners and procedures as primarily objectifying and threatening to women and therefore only portray them in a dystopian light.[22] Charis

[22] The affirmation of natural childbirth as the only model that grants women a central role during pregnancy and birth implies that under artificial conditions women cannot have a central role in their experience. A critical approach from the 1970s and 1980s suggested that women are inevitably positioned as weak and passive before the technocratic and patriarchal institution of biomedicine, and that the only way for them to emerge as agents is to remove them from this context. Since the 1990s, the research approach to the problem of women's relationship to the medical model and the use of technology in reproduction has changed significantly. Studies have appeared showing

Thompson (2005) argues that both representations position a woman as *passive*—regardless of whether she is someone who is saved or someone who is victimised. We often get a different picture when we follow the narratives of women themselves, who experience encounters with technology as neither rescued nor victimised—except in particular circumstances that should be addressed empirically.

Criticising or promoting medical technology a priori therefore entails separating subjects and technology and their opposing essential characteristics. This is precisely the notion that I have tried to critically re-examine in this book by distancing myself from the understanding of agency and embodiment as self-relying on unmediated insights and competences. I have argued instead that the subject is not a priori separated from other subjects and objects from the environment. Nor are her wholeness and integrity a priori guaranteed—so they could be jeopardised by the use of technology. Rather, a unified and integrated subject can only be seen as a normative standard, a theoretical and ethical-political model of the subject that simply belongs to a particular, albeit dominant, image of human nature (Berg & Mol, 1998) that is culturally and historically specific: "[t]he Western conception of the person as a bounded, unique, more or less integrated motivational and cognitive universe, a dynamic center of awareness, emotion, judgement and action, organized into a distinctive whole and set contrastively against other such wholes and against a social and natural background is, however incorrigible it may seem to us, a rather peculiar idea within the context of the world's cultures" (Geertz, 1979, p. 222, quoted in Rose, 1996, p. 225). Moreover, this model deviates considerably from empirical reality, especially when we look at a person entering the medical context or going through certain developmental transitions, as the previous phenomenologically grounded analysis has shown.

At the same time, while the traditional model of subjectivity is clearly normative, we should not hastily dismiss these norms as something that

that a certain, rather large number of women experience highly medicalised and technologised childbirth as an empowering experience (Davis-Floyd, 1994). To claim that this is only possible under the assumption that a woman views birth from a male perspective means to essentialise the female perspective (Beckett, 2005), which is heavily criticised in contemporary feminism, and for good reasons.

is arbitrary or easily changeable and thus "less real". This normative account of the subject is deeply rooted in a range of social institutions (from the legal system to the nuclear family) and is reproduced through a variety of discursive-material arrangements and everyday practices. Consequently, it is also deeply rooted in how people feel about themselves, what guides their behaviour, their imagination and their relationships with others. This implies that we should consider embodied subjects as culturally and historically constituted, but also as relatively historically stable and rooted in socio-material practices that are not easily changeable. This is in line with Kukla's assertion (2005, p. 218) that "while the maternal body is a historical entity, the history of the maternal body is mostly one of robust continuities and endurance".

In recent decades, primarily owing to Foucault's work, the idea that a person, an individual, is a given ahistorical category has become highly problematic. Regimes of power and institutional practices are seen as productive, they constitute what we recognise as a subject (Foucault, 2006).[23] This view has considerable political implications, for it problematises the approach that criticises and rejects power regimes and institutional structures on the grounds that they threaten some inherent properties and guaranteed rights of the subject—who is actually constituted by them in the first place.[24] What applies to the subject applies to the body too, which is also only constituted through regimes and practices within different institutional and disciplinary frameworks: "(...) bodies only appear, only endure, only live within the productive constraints of certain highly gendered regulatory schemas" (Butler, 1993, p. xi).

[23] The productivity of the political power is explained as follows: "What we may call the individual is not what political power latches on to; what we should call the individual is the effect produced on the somatic singularity, the result of this pinning, by the techniques of political power I have indicated" (Foucault, 2006, p. 56).

[24] Foucault (2006, p. 56) articulates this perfectly: "There is no point then in wanting to dismantle hierarchies, constraints, and prohibitions so that the individual can appear, as if the individual was something existing beneath all relationships of power, preexisting relationships of power, and unduly weighed down by them. In fact, the individual is the result of something that is prior to it: this mechanism, these procedures, which pin political power on the body. It is because the body has been 'subjectified,' that is to say, that the subject-function has been fixed on it, because it has been psychologized and normalized, it is because of all this that something like the individual appeared, about which one can speak, hold discourses, and attempt to found sciences".

Many contemporary authors following Foucault focus on the productive side of the discursive and institutional practices that constitute bodies and subjects, but they supplement this perspective with some new elements (Lock et al., 2000, p. 11–12). First, they aim to include the experiences of those who are subjected to the practices and techniques, seeing them not as passive recipients but as those who can actively relate to the medical technology and the institutional framework (Akrich & Pasveer, 2000; Thompson, 2005). Therefore, individual agency is emphasised over the technological manipulation of subjects—even though this agency is not understood as an inherent property of the individual—and it is assumed that the plane of individual experience and behaviour is not a simple replica of discursive patterns and practices. The political implication of this is that possibilities for resistance and subversion are sought at the lowest micro-social level.[25] The second novelty is the recognition of the fact that objects or non-human actors can be seen as agentic, since they participate in the production of knowledge and practices (Latour, 1991, 1994, 1999). This changed perspective in theorising and research allows for the reconceptualisation of both technology and subjects, as well as their complex and situated interactions that can lead to different, context-dependent outcomes.

The embodied subject is thus conceptualised as having no fixed properties that exist independently of encounters with medical, or more broadly social, practices and technologies, but neither are her properties merely a product of these encounters. Subjective experience is shaped and transformed through interaction with other actors (both human and non-human), so the individual subject does not have to be reduced or threatened by the encounter with technology—a woman can even acquire new aspects of embodied experience and opportunities for agency through this

[25] Bruno Latour, for example, points out that concepts that are commonly believed to have the greatest critical and political potential (power, structure, Empire) actually prevent any real political action because they refer to something inherently vague, unattainable and omnipresent: "if you have to fight against a force that is invisible, untraceable, ubiquitous, and total, you will be powerless and roundly defeated. It's only if forces are made of smaller ties, whose resistance can be tested one by one, that you might have a chance to modify a given state of affairs" (Latour, 2005, p. 250). An alternative approach is therefore advantageous because it operates within a local framework and attempts to delineate the concrete connections that lead to certain outcomes, thus making the situation accessible for transformation.

encounter that would be unavailable to her otherwise. Therefore, we should not "pronounce any reproductive technology to be intrinsically bad for women or necessarily eugenic because choices present themselves differently under different circumstances. The complexities that animate technology as it operates in different times and places, with different reagents, and with different professional staff become intertwined with different political and personal stories. Ambivalence about reproductive technologies has grown into a respect for the people and the objects who participate in a complex mutual choreography that allows unexpected agencies and political configurations to emerge" (Thompson, 2005, p. 23). Accordingly, there can be different patterns and modalities of the relationship between subjectivity and technology. If we abandon the a priori premise that medical technology and subjectivity are at odds with each other, and acknowledge the complexity, variability and ambiguity of both women as embodied subjects and situated medical technology, we open up a space for the empirical investigation of their relationship.

In the preceding chapters, I have attempted to do just that, in the hope that the analysis will demonstrate an alternative account of subjectivity as embodied, multiply mediated by both symbolic and material means, and with the capacity for agency performed through the coordination of manifold situated actors. The early transition to motherhood is a dynamic process that involves numerous social and technological mediations and cannot be considered in isolation, as something happening within the individual. I believe that this is also true of other life transitions and phases—particularly those associated with both profound bodily changes and a significant role of technological and/or institutional mediation, such as adolescence and old age, but also those experienced by adult men, whose subjectivity has traditionally been seen in psychology as a paradigm for subjectivity in general. Instead of viewing pregnant and birthing subjectivity as a special case or a deviation, it should serve as instructive when formulating psychological theories even of those subjects whose processuality and distributedness are not so evident.

Therefore, the conceptualisation of subjectivity that I propose on the basis of the theoretical and empirical analysis in this book may offer a number of relevant implications for the sociocultural psychology of development across the lifecourse. The focus on embodiment as a crucial aspect of subjectivity suggests that any account of human development must include the body as a central site where cultural and social mediators operate. It is also a call for developmental psychology to pay particular attention to the complex and lifelong process of bodily socialisation and the transformation of our embodied experiences, shaped by a range of normative symbolic and material practices. The focus on the specifically technological mediation of subjectivity draws on the central sociocultural thesis of the centrality of the processes of semiotic mediation, but also underscores the need to pay attention to the material aspects of tools that serve as relevant mediators and resources in our experience and behaviour. The sociocultural psychology of the lifecourse should specifically consider how particular technological tools and practices, as well as the respective institutional contexts, shape developmental trajectories across the lifespan—e.g. in the transition to school, the workplace, the military, the retirement home. Furthermore, the notion of distributed agency reflects the sociocultural perspective that development is co-constructed within a network of social relations and cultural practices. By challenging the notion of the individual as a bounded and autonomous agent, it emphasises the interconnectedness of social and material influences on development. Situating my analysis within the specific cultural-historical context of a post-socialist society and also considering the broader cultural and historical influences of patriarchal and neoliberal society underscores the importance of truly contextualised research in sociocultural and developmental psychology. At the same time, I critically examined normative frameworks and dominant discourses and practices while following the complex ways in which individuals navigate these influences in their everyday lives in order to argue for a more nuanced, interdisciplinary and context-sensitive approach to developmental transitions. By focusing on embodiment, technological mediation, distributed agency and the cultural and historical specificity of life transitions, I have sought to provide a robust framework for exploring different stages of the human lifecourse and to emphasise the complexity and contextuality of developmental processes.

Besides theoretical, the reconceptualisation of subjectivity I am proposing also has important ethical and political implications, as it may inform contemporary debates on the role of medicine and technology in human health and well-being in general and in female reproduction in particular. My position in this book is consistent with a shift in feminist thinking over the last two decades towards theorising that, while not advocating technological optimism, is certainly not technophobic, but involves a greater appreciation of the complexity and situatedness of scientific-technological practices, particular interests and social relations, as well as a more nuanced approach to theoretical, ethical and political questions of agency and resistance in relation to reproductive issues (Akrich & Pasveer, 2004; Dolezal, 2009; Haraway, 1991a; Lam, 2015; Lock et al., 2000; Thompson, 2005). My analysis also aligns with the suggestion that we should move beyond the traditional critique of the medicalisation of pregnancy and birth, for it has been shown that positive and even empowering experiences are possible in a range of institutional circumstances and environments (Davis-Floyd, 1994; Learly, 2006; Thomson & Downe, 2008). The complex and hybrid character of subjects is already recognised in the literature as a way of bridging the seeming polarity between person-centred and technologised medical care (Lapum et al., 2012). Only a critical reexamination of our own technologically mediated (Ihde), hybrid (Latour) or cyborg (Haraway) ontology will open the space for recognising the possibilities for truly person-centred care in today's technologised medical environments.[26]

Recognising the possibility that technology, when adequately situated, can play a productive and empowering role for a woman during pregnancy and childbirth is an indispensable starting point in the struggle to improve the conditions under which female reproduction takes place today. I believe that the adaptation of the model of reproductive care should not focus on the concept of naturalness and the protection of mothers from external interventions, around which the model of natural pregnancy and birth revolves. Contrary to the inclination of natural model proponents to see technology and interventions as a threat to the

[26] Furthermore, the changed perspective on the nature of technology and its role in human subjectivity allows us not to see technology as something external to medical care, as an outsider that should be integrated in some way. Since it is recognised as an important part not only of our everyday lives (which is a trivial fact), but also of our bodily and psycho-social functioning and experience, the important question is not how person-centred care "can be fully actualized in these [technologized] environments, but also how technology is a part and shapes person-centered practice" (Lapum et al., 2012, p. 278).

authentic female reproductive experience, one should not assume "that something as simple as an epidural needle could corrupt her maternality" (Kukla, 2005, p. 223).[27] Instead of this strategy, which implies a rejection of the entire medical framework—and thus its undoubtedly beneficial aspects—we should look for the possibilities of resistance and positive change that exist in the current situation. I believe that only a complex, subtle, contextualised and thus empirically grounded account of the reproductive reality of contemporary women that takes their embodied experience as its central starting point will lead to this. Hopefully, the analysis presented in this book is at least a small step in this direction.

Finally, while embodiment is the crucial aspect of women's subjectivity during their transition to motherhood—and certainly beyond that, "the reduction of motherhood to an embodied relation, and the reduction of this embodied relation to one of proximity, misrepresents not just metaphysical but ethical and political reality" (Kukla, 2005, p. 158), for our embodied subjectivity is mediated and extended in manifold ways. The model of distributed subjectivity that can be performed collectively through the interactions between multiple actors challenges the traditional understanding of subjectivity as something purely internal and individual and emphasises its dynamic and relational character, as well as its interconnectedness and interdependence with social, cultural and technological aspects of the context. This model also emphasises the historical ontology of subjectivity, since "human beings are the kinds of creatures who have no universal ontology, no essence whether this be spiritual or genetic. Our ontology is historical: it is both temporal and spatial. What humans are—perhaps better, what human beings are capable of, what we can do—is variable, historical, situational—not an originary 'being' but a mobile 'becoming'" (Rose, 1996, p. 234). Based on the extensive theoretical and empirical analysis in this book, I wish to argue that this model of subjectivity is the one that psychology should endorse if it aspires to understand subjectivity in a culturally and historically sensitive, ethically informed and empirically grounded way.

[27] Ultimately, a truly natural transition to motherhood may seem an impossible ideal because, as explained in the Chap. 2, in all social communities and throughout history, almost every aspect of pregnancy, birth and the care of the baby is culturally regulated, monitored and controlled.

References

Akrich, M., & Pasveer, B. (2000). Multiplying obstetrics: Techniques of surveillance and forms of coordination. *Theoretical Medicine and Bioethics, 21*(1), 63–83. https://doi.org/10.1023/A:1009943017769

Akrich, M., & Pasveer, B. (2004). Embodiment and disembodiment in childbirth narratives. *Body and Society, 10*(2–3), 63–84. https://doi.org/10.1177/1357034X04042935

Beckett, K. (2005). Choosing cesarean: Feminism and the politics of childbirth in the United States. *Feminist Theory, 6*(3), 251–275. https://doi.org/10.1177/1464700105057363

Berg, M., & Akrich, M. (2004). Bodies on trial: Performances and politics in medicine and biology. *Body and Society, 10*(2–3), 1–12. https://doi.org/10.1177/1357034X04042929

Berg, M., & Mol, A. (1998). *Differences in medicine: Unraveling practices, techniques, and bodies*. Duke University Press.

Bergum, V. (1994). Commentary on the epistemology of expectant parenthood. *Western Journal of Nursing Research, 16*(6), 616–618.

Bowers, T. (1996). *The politics of motherhood: British writing and culture, 1680–1760*. Cambridge University Press.

Butler, J. (1993). *Bodies that matter: On the discursive limits of "sex"*. Routledge.

Chadwick, R. (2009). Between bodies, cultural scripts and power: The reproduction of birthing subjectivities in home-birth narratives. *Subjectivity, 27*, 109–133. https://doi.org/10.1057/sub.2009.1

Chadwick, R. (2018). *Bodies that birth: Vitalizing birth politics*. Routledge.

Clement, S., Wilson, J., & Sikorski, J. (1998). Woman's experiences of antenatal ultrasound scans. In S. Clement (Ed.), *Psychological perspectives on pregnancy and childbirth* (pp. 7–24). Elsevier Science.

Conboy, K., Medina, N., & Stanbury, S. (1997). Introduction. In K. Conboy, N. Medina, & S. Stanbury (Eds.), *Writing on the body: Female embodiment and feminist theory* (pp. 1–12). Columbia University Press.

Daniel, S. L. (1986). The patient as text: A model of clinical hermeneutics. *Theoretical Medicine, 7*(2), 195–210. https://doi.org/10.1007/BF00489230

Davis-Floyd, R. (1987). Obstetric training as a rite of passage. *Medical Anthropology Quarterly, 1*(3), 288–318. https://doi.org/10.1525/maq.1987.1.3.02a00050

Davis-Floyd, R. (1994). The technocratic body: American childbirth as cultural expression. *Social Science and Medicine, 38*(8), 1125–1140. https://doi.org/10.1016/0277-9536(94)90228-3

Davis-Floyd, R. (2001). The technocratic, humanistic, and holistic paradigms of childbirth. *International Journal of Gynecology and Obstetrics, 75*(1), S5–S23. https://doi.org/10.1016/S0020-7292(01)00510-0

Dolezal, L. (2009). The remote body: The phenomenology of telepresence and re-embodiment. *Human Technology, 5*(2), 208–226.

Draper, J. (2002). 'It was a real good show': The ultrasound scan, fathers and the power of visual knowledge. *Sociology of Health & Illness, 24*(6), 771–795. https://doi.org/10.1111/1467-9566.00318

Duden, B. (1993). *Disembodying women: Perspectives on pregnancy and the unborn*. Harvard University Press.

Foucault, M. (2006). *Psychiatric power: Lectures at the Collège de France, 1973–1974*. Palgrave Macmillan.

Frank, A. W. (1997). *The wounded storyteller: Body, illness, and ethics*. University of Chicago Press.

Gadow, S. (1980). Body and self: A dialectic. *Journal of Medicine and Philosophy, 5*(3), 172–185. https://doi.org/10.1093/jmp/5.3.172

Gadow, S. (1984). Touch and technology: Two paradigms of patient care. *Journal of Religion and Health, 23*(1), 63–69. https://doi.org/10.1007/BF00999900

Ginsburg, F., & Rapp, R. (1991). The politics of reproduction. *Annual Review of Anthropology, 20*(1), 311–343. https://doi.org/10.1146/annurev.an.20.100191.001523

Halfon, S. (2010). Encountering birth: Negotiating expertise, networks, and my STS self. *Science as Culture, 19*(1), 61–77. https://doi.org/10.1080/09505430903558062

Hanson, C. (2004). *A cultural history of pregnancy: Pregnancy, medicine and culture, 1750–2000*. Palgrave Macmillan.

Haraway, D. (1991a). A cyborg manifesto: Science, technology, and socialist-feminism in the late twentieth century. In *Simians, cyborgs and women: The reinvention of nature* (pp. 149–181). Routledge.

Haraway, D. (1991b). Situated knowledges: The science question in feminism and the privilege of partial perspective. In *Simians, cyborgs and women: The reinvention of nature* (pp. 183–202). Routledge.

Hatgis, C. (2001). Agency and the deconstructed subject. In N. Stephenson, H. L. Radtke, R. Jorna, & H. J. Stam (Eds.), *Theoretical psychology: Critical contributions* (pp. 129–140). Captus University Publications.

Ihde, D. (1990). *Technology and the lifeworld: From garden to earth*. Indiana University Press.

Ihde, D. (2002). *Bodies in technology*. University of Minnesota Press.

Kontopodis, M., Beck, S., & Niewöhner, J. (2011). Investigating emerging biomedical practices: Zones of awkward engagement on different scales. *Science Technology Human Values, 36*(5), 599–615. https://doi.org/10.1177/0162243910392798

Kranzberg, M. (1986). Technology and history: Kranzberg's laws. *Technology and Culture, 27*(3), 544–560.

Kristeva, J. (1990). Motherhood according to Giovanni Bellini. In J. M. Thompson (Ed.), *Twentieth century theories of art* (pp. 441–467). Carleton University Press.

Kukla, R. (2005). *Mass hysteria: Medicine, culture and mothers' bodies*. Rowman & Littlefield Publishers.

Lam, C. (2015). *New reproductive technologies and disembodiment: Feminist and material resolutions*. Ashgate.

Lapum, J., Fredericks, S., Beanlands, H., McCay, E., Schwind, J., & Romaniuk, D. (2012). A cyborg ontology in health care: Traversing into the liminal space between technology and person-centred practice. *Nursing Philosophy, 13*, 276–288.

Latour, B. (1991). Technology is society made durable. In J. Law (Ed.), *A sociology of monsters: Essays on power, technology, and domination* (pp. 103–131). Routledge.

Latour, B. (1994). On technical mediation—philosophy, sociology, genealogy. *Common Knowledge, 3*(2), 29–64.

Latour, B. (1999). On recalling ANT. In J. Law & J. Hassard (Eds.), *Actor-network theory and after* (pp. 15–25). Blackwell Publishing.

Latour, B. (2005). *Reassembling the social: An introduction to actor-network theory*. Oxford University Press.

Learly, A. D. (2006). Shame, gender, birth. *Hypatia, 21*(1), 101–118.

Leder, D. (1984). Medicine and paradigms of embodiment. *Journal of Medicine and Philosophy, 9*(1), 29–44.

Leder, D. (1990). *The absent body*. University of Chicago Press.

Lock, M., Young, A., & Cambrosio, A. (2000). *Living and working with the new medical technologies: Intersections of inquiry*. Cambridge University Press.

Martin, E. (1984). Pregnancy, labor and body image in the United States. *Social Science & Medicine, 19*(11), 1201–1206. https://doi.org/10.1016/0277-9536(84)90371-X
Martin, E. (1996). Disembodying women: Perspectives on pregnancy and the unborn. *Medical Anthropology Quarterly, 10*(2), 307–309. https://doi.org/10.1525/maq.1996.10.2.02a00150
Martin, K. A. (2003). Giving birth like a girl. *Gender & Society, 17*(1), 54–72. https://doi.org/10.1177/0891243202238978
Mol, A. (2000). Pathology and the clinic: An ethnographic presentation of two atheroscleroses. In M. Lock, A. Young, & A. Cambrosio (Eds.), *Living and working with the new medical technologies: Intersections of inquiry* (pp. 82–102). Cambridge University Press.
Mol, A. (2002). *The body multiple: Ontology in medical practice.* Duke University Press.
Mol, A., & Law, J. (2004). Embodied action, enacted bodies: The example of hypoglycaemia. *Body & Society, 10*(2–3), 43–62. https://doi.org/10.1177/1357034X04042932
Porter, R. (2002). *Blood and guts: A short history of medicine.* Allen Lane.
Reiser, S. J. (1984). The machine at the bedside: Technological transformations of practices and values. In S. J. Reiser & M. Anbar (Eds.), *The machine at the bedside: Strategies for using technology in patient care* (pp. 3–19). Cambridge University Press.
Rich, A. (1986b). *Of woman born: Motherhood as experience and institution.* W. W. Norton & Company.
Riley, S., Evans, A., & Robson, M. (2019). *Postfeminism and health: Critical psychology and media perspectives.* Routledge.
Rose, N. (1996). Assembling the modern self. In R. Porter (Ed.), *Rewriting the self: Histories from the Renaissance to the present* (pp. 224–248). Routledge.
Rothman, B. K. (1993). Recreating motherhood: American lessons for the Netherlands. *Nemesis, 9*(4), 123–130.
Rothman, B. K. (2007a). Introduction: A lifetime's labor: Women and power in the birthplace. In W. Simonds, B. K. Rothman, & B. M. Norman (Eds.), *Laboring on: Birth in transition in the United States* (pp. xi–xxii). Routledge.
Ruddick, S. (1989). *Maternal thinking: Toward a politics of peace.* Beacon Press.
Sandelowski, M., & Black, B. P. (1994). The epistemology of expectant parenthood. *Western Journal of Nursing Research, 16*(6), 601–614. https://doi.org/10.1177/019394599401600602

Squier, S. (1996). Fetal subjects and maternal objects: Reproductive technology and the new fetal/maternal relation. *Journal of Medicine and Philosophy, 21*, 515–535. https://doi.org/10.1093/jmp/21.5.515

Thompson, C. (2005). *Making parents: The ontological choreography of reproductive technologies*. MIT Press.

Thomson, G., & Downe, S. (2008). Widening the trauma discourse: The link between childbirth and experiences of abuse. *Journal of Psychosomatic Obstetrics & Gynecology, 29*(4), 268–273.

Turner, B. S. (1992). *Regulating bodies: Essays in medical sociology*. Routledge.

Venn, C. (1998). The subject of psychology. In J. Henriques, W. Hollway, C. Urwin, C. Venn, & V. Walkerdine (Eds.), *Changing the subject: Psychology, social regulation and subjectivity* (pp. 115–147).

Verbeek, P. (2005). *What things do: Philosophical reflections on technology, agency, and design*. The Pennsylvania State University Press.

Weiss, G., & Haber, H. F. (1999). Introduction. In G. Weiss & H. F. Haber (Eds.), *Perspectives on embodiment: The intersections of nature and culture* (pp. xiii–xvii).

Young, I. M. (2005b). Pregnant embodiment: Subjectivity and alienation. In *On female body experience: 'Throwing like a girl' and other essays* (pp. 46–61). Oxford University Press.

References

Ainsworth, M. D. S., Bell, S. M., & Stayton, D. (1974). Infant-mother attachment and social development. In M. P. Richards (Ed.), *The introduction of the child into a social world* (pp. 99–135). Cambridge University Press.

Akrich, M., & Pasveer, B. (1998). We deliver our children—In pain? In B. Brenna & J. Law (Eds.), *Machines, agency and desire* (pp. 109–123). TMV Report Series.

Akrich, M., & Pasveer, B. (2000). Multiplying obstetrics: Techniques of surveillance and forms of coordination. *Theoretical Medicine and Bioethics, 21*(1), 63–83. https://doi.org/10.1023/A:1009943017769

Akrich, M., & Pasveer, B. (2004). Embodiment and disembodiment in childbirth narratives. *Body and Society, 10*(2–3), 63–84. https://doi.org/10.1177/1357034X04042935

Alhusen, J. L. (2008). A literature update on maternal-fetal attachment. *Journal of Obstetric, Gynecologic, and Neonatal Nursing, 37*(3), 315–328.

Andersen, L., Melvaer, L., Videbech, P., & Lamont, R. (2012). Risk factors for developing post-traumatic stress disorder following childbirth: A systematic review. *Acta Obstetricia et Gynecologica Scandinavica, 91*(11), 1261–1272. https://doi.org/10.1111/j.1600-0412.2012.01476.x

B. Stanković, *Giving Birth To A Subject*, Sociocultural Psychology of the Lifecourse,
https://doi.org/10.1007/978-3-031-77236-8

Arendell, T. (2000). Conceiving and investigating motherhood: The decade's scholarship. *Journal of Marriage and Family, 62*(4), 1192–1207. Retrieved from http://www.jstor.org/stable/1566731

Arijes, F. (1989). *Eseji o istoriji smrti na Zapadu od srednjeg veka do današnjih dana*. Rad.

Arsenijevic, J., Pavlova, M., & Groot, W. (2014). Shortcomings of maternity care in Serbia. *Birth, 41*(1), 14–25.

Ayers, S., & Pickering, A. D. (2005). Women's expectations and experience of birth. *Psychology and Health, 20*(1), 79–92.

Bailham, D., & Joseph, S. (2003). Post-traumatic stress following childbirth: A review of the emerging literature and directions for research and practice. *Psychology, Health & Medicine, 8*(2), 159–168. https://doi.org/10.1080/1354850031000087537

Baker, S., Choi, P., Henshaw, C., & Tree, J. (2005). "I felt as though I'd been in jail": Women's experiences of maternity care during labour, delivery, and the immediate postpartum. *Feminism & Psychology, 15*(3), 315–342.

Barad, K. (2003). Posthumanist performativity: Toward an understanding of how matter comes to matter. *Signs, 28*(3), 801–831.

Barad, K. (2007). *Meeting the universe halfway: Quantum physics and the entanglement of matter and meaning*. Duke University Press.

Baraitser, L. (2009). *Maternal encounters: The ethics of interruption*. Routledge.

Barber, C. C. (2012). Prelude to parenthood: The impact of anxiety and depression during pregnancy. In M. G. R. Castillo (Ed.), *Perinatal depression* (pp. 19–38). InTech. https://doi.org/10.5772/32076

Beckett, K. (2005). Choosing cesarean: Feminism and the politics of childbirth in the United States. *Feminist Theory, 6*(3), 251–275. https://doi.org/10.1177/1464700105057363

Benn, P. A., Ying, J., Beazoglou, T., & Egan, J. F. (2001). Estimates for the sensitivity and false-positive rates for second trimester serum screening for Down syndrome and trisomy 18 with adjustment for cross-identification and double-positive results. *Prenatal Diagnosis, 21*(1), 46–51.

Benson, C. (2001). *The cultural psychology of self: Place, morality and art in human worlds*. Routledge.

Berg, M., & Akrich, M. (2004). Bodies on trial: Performances and politics in medicine and biology. *Body and Society, 10*(2–3), 1–12. https://doi.org/10.1177/1357034X04042929

Berg, M., & Mol, A. (1998). *Differences in medicine: Unraveling practices, techniques, and bodies*. Duke University Press.

Bergum, V. (1994). Commentary on the epistemology of expectant parenthood. *Western Journal of Nursing Research, 16*(6), 616–618.

Bielinski-Blattmann, D., Gürber, S., Lavallee, K., Grob, A., Surbek, D., & Stadlmayr, W. (2016). Labour experience and postpartum stress and depression: A quantitative and qualitative examination. *Journal of Reproductive and Infant Psychology, 34*(2), 162–174.

Birth Incentive Strategy. (2018). *Official Gazette-Republic of Serbia, 25/2018–16.*

Blagojević, M. (1997). *Roditeljstvo i fertilitet: Srbija devedesetih.* ISIFF.

Blagojević-Hjuson, M. (2014). Transformation of parenthood: The semiperipheral perspective. *Sociologija, 56*(4), 383–402.

Boesch, E. E. (2001). Symbolic action theory in cultural psychology. *Culture & Psychology, 7*(4), 479–483.

Bordo, S. (1993). *Unbearable weight: Feminism, Western culture, and the body.* University of California Press.

Bowers, T. (1996). *The politics of motherhood: British writing and culture, 1680–1760.* Cambridge University Press.

Bowser, D., & Hill, K. (2010). *Exploring evidence for disrespect and abuse in facility-based childbirth.* USAID-TRAction Project. Harvard School of Public Health.

Bracewell, W. (1996). Women, motherhood, and contemporary Serbian nationalism. *Women's Studies International Forum, 19*(1/2), 25–33.

Brković, Č. (2012). The pursuit of relations as a constitutive part of biological citizenship in a Bosnian border town. *Antropologija, 12*(2).

Bruner, J. (1991). The narrative construction of reality. *Critical Inquiry, 18*(1), 1–21. https://doi.org/10.1086/448619

Buchanan, L. (2013). *Rhetorics of motherhood.* Southern Illinois University Press.

Butler, J. (1993). *Bodies that matter: On the discursive limits of "sex".* Routledge.

Butler, J. (2004). *Undoing gender.* Routledge.

Cabell, K. R., Marsico, G., Cornejo, C., & Valsiner, J. (Eds.). (2015). *Making meaning, making motherhood.* Information Age Publishing.

Camberis, A. L., McMahon, C. A., Gibson, F. L., & Boivin, J. (2014). Age, psychological maturity, and the transition to motherhood among English-speaking Australian women in a metropolitan area. *Developmental Psychology, 50*(8), 2154–2164. https://doi.org/10.1037/a0037301

Camic, P. M., Rhodes, J. E., & Yardley, L. (2003). Naming the stars: Integrating qualitative methods into psychological research. In P. M. Camic, J. E. Rhodes, & L. Yardley (Eds.), *Qualitative research in psychology: Expanding perspectives in methodology and design* (pp. 3–15). American Psychological Association.

Cannella, B. L. (2005). Maternal-fetal attachment: An integrative review. *Journal of Advanced Nursing, 50*, 60–68.
Caton, D. (1999). *What a blessing she had chloroform: The medical and social response to the pain of childbirth from 1800 to the present*. Yale University Press.
Chadwick, R. (2006). Pathological wombs and raging hormones: Psychology, reproduction and the female body. In T. Shefer, F. Boonzaaier, & P. Kiguwa (Eds.), *The gender of psychology*. UCT Press.
Chadwick, R. (2009). Between bodies, cultural scripts and power: The reproduction of birthing subjectivities in home-birth narratives. *Subjectivity, 27*, 109–133. https://doi.org/10.1057/sub.2009.1
Chadwick, R. (2018). *Bodies that birth: Vitalizing birth politics*. Routledge.
Chadwick, R., Cooper, D., & Harries, J. (2014). Narratives of distress about birth in South African public maternity settings: A qualitative study. *Midwifery, 30*(7), 862–868.
Charmaz, K. (1995). Grounded theory. In A. J. Smith, R. Harre, & L. van Langenhove (Eds.), *Rethinking methods in psychology* (pp. 27–65). Sage.
Clark, A., Skouteris, H., Wertheim, E. H., Paxton, S. J., & Milgrom, J. (2009). My baby body: A qualitative insight into women's body-related experiences and mood during pregnancy and the postpartum. *Journal of Reproductive and Infant Psychology, 27*(4), 330–345. https://doi.org/10.1080/02646830903190904
Clement, S., Wilson, J., & Sikorski, J. (1998). Woman's experiences of antenatal ultrasound scans. In S. Clement (Ed.), *Psychological perspectives on pregnancy and childbirth* (pp. 7–24). Elsevier Science.
Cole, M. (1996). *Cultural psychology: A once and future discipline*. Harvard University Press.
Conboy, K., Medina, N., & Stanbury, S. (1997). Introduction. In K. Conboy, N. Medina, & S. Stanbury (Eds.), *Writing on the body: Female embodiment and feminist theory* (pp. 1–12). Columbia University Press.
Coole, D., & Frost, S. (2010). Introducing the new materialisms. In D. Coole & S. Frost (Eds.), *New materialisms: Ontology, agency, and politics* (pp. 1–43). Duke University Press.
Creedy, D., Shochet, I., & Horsfall, J. (2000). Childbirth and the development of acute trauma symptoms: Incidence and contributing factors. *Birth, 27*(2), 104–111.
Csordas, T. J. (1994). *Embodiment and experience*. Cambridge University Press.
Cunningham, G. F., Leveno, K. J., Bloom, S. L., Hauth, J. C., Rouse, D. J., & Spong, C. Y. (2010). *Williams obstetrics* (23rd ed.). McGraw-Hill Medical.

Cussins, C. (1996). Ontological choreography: Agency through objectification in infertility clinics. *Social Studies of Science, 26*(3), 575–610. https://doi.org/10.1177/030631296026003004

Čutura, N. (2005). Porođajni faktori. In D. Plećaš, B. Stanimirović, A. Stanković, & M. Vasiljević (Eds.), *Ginekologija i akušerstvo: Udžbenik za studente medicine*. Medicinski fakultet Univerziteta u Beogradu.

Czarnocka, J., & Slade, P. (2000). Prevalence and predictors of post-traumatic stress symptoms following childbirth. *British Journal of Clinical Psychology, 39*, 35–51.

D'Oliveira, A., Diniz, S., & Schraiber, L. (2002). Violence against women in health-care institutions: An emerging problem. *The Lancet, 359*, 1681–1685.

Daniel, S. L. (1986). The patient as text: A model of clinical hermeneutics. *Theoretical Medicine, 7*(2), 195–210. https://doi.org/10.1007/BF00489230

Darvill, R., Skirton, H., & Farrand, P. (2010). Psychological factors that impact on women's experiences of first-time motherhood: A qualitative study of the transition. *Midwifery, 26*(3), 357–366. https://doi.org/10.1016/j.midw.2008.07.006

Davis-Floyd, R. (1987). Obstetric training as a rite of passage. *Medical Anthropology Quarterly, 1*(3), 288–318. https://doi.org/10.1525/maq.1987.1.3.02a00050

Davis-Floyd, R. (1993). The technocratic model of birth. In S. T. Hollis, L. Pershing, & M. J. Young (Eds.), *Feminist theory and the study of folklore* (pp. 297–326). University of Illinois Press.

Davis-Floyd, R. (1994). The technocratic body: American childbirth as cultural expression. *Social Science and Medicine, 38*(8), 1125–1140. https://doi.org/10.1016/0277-9536(94)90228-3

Davis-Floyd, R. (2001). The technocratic, humanistic, and holistic paradigms of childbirth. *International Journal of Gynecology and Obstetrics, 75*(1), S5–S23. https://doi.org/10.1016/S0020-7292(01)00510-0

de Beauvoir, S. (2011). *The second sex* (C. Borde & S. Malovany-Chevallier, Trans.). Vintage Books. (Original work published 1949).

Declercq, E. R., Paine, L., & Winter, M. R. (1995). Home birth in the United States, 1989–1992: A longitudinal descriptive report of national birth certificate data. *Journal of Nurse-Midwifery, 40*(6), 474–482. https://doi.org/10.1016/0091-2182(95)00061-5

Denmark, F. L., Klara, M., Baron, E., & Cambareri-Fernandez, L. (2008). Historical development of the psychology of women. In F. L. Denmark & M. A. Paludi (Eds.), *Psychology of women: A handbook of issues and theories* (pp. 3–39). Praeger.

DiPietro, J. A. (2010). Psychological and psychophysiological considerations regarding the maternal-fetal relationship. *Infant and Child Development, 19*(1), 27–38. https://doi.org/10.1002/icd.651

DiQuinzio, P. (1999). *The impossibility of motherhood: Feminism, individualism, and the problem of mothering*. Routledge.

Djanogly, T., Nicholls, J., Whitten, M., & Lanceley, A. (2022). Choice in episiotomy—Fact or fantasy: A qualitative study of women's experiences of the consent process. *BMC Pregnancy and Childbirth, 22*, 139. https://doi.org/10.1186/s12884-022-04475-8

Djoric, G., & Gavrilovic, D. (2006). Between pronatalist population policy and women's reproductive rights: The analysis of exposure of the two discourses in press media after 2000. *Sociologija, 48*(1), 73–95.

Dolezal, L. (2009). The remote body: The phenomenology of telepresence and re-embodiment. *Human Technology, 5*(2), 208–226.

Draper, J. (2002). 'It was a real good show': The ultrasound scan, fathers and the power of visual knowledge. *Sociology of Health & Illness, 24*(6), 771–795. https://doi.org/10.1111/1467-9566.00318

Drezgić, R. (2004). *(Re)Producing the nation: The politics of reproduction in Serbia in the 1980s and 1990s* [Unpublished PhD thesis]. University of Pittsburgh.

Duby, G., & Perrot, M. (Eds.). (1992). *A history of women in the west*. Harvard University Press.

Duden, B. (1991). *The woman beneath the skin: A doctor's patients in eighteenth-century Germany*. Harvard University Press.

Duden, B. (1993). *Disembodying women: Perspectives on pregnancy and the unborn*. Harvard University Press.

Dunn, P. M. (1998). Henrick van Deventer (1651–1724) and the pelvic birth canal. *Archives of Disease in Childhood—Fetal and Neonatal Edition, 79*(2), F157–F158. https://doi.org/10.1136/fn.79.2.F157

Eatough, V., & Smith, J. A. (2008). Interpretative phenomenological analysis. In C. Willig & W. Stainton Rogers (Eds.), *The Sage handbook of qualitative research in psychology* (pp. 179–194). Sage.

Edmonds, D., & Warburton, N. (Hosts). (2013, April 2). Ann Oakley on women's experience of childbirth [Audio podcast episode]. In *Social science bites*. Sage. Retrieved from https://www.socialsciencespace.com/2013/04/podcast-ann-oakley-on-womens experience-of-childbirth/

Ehrenreich, B., & English, D. (2010). *Witches, midwives and nurses: A history of women healers*. The Feminist Press.

Elliott, A. (2002). Identity politics and privatisation: Modern fantasies, post-modern after-effects. In V. Walkerdine (Ed.), *Challenging subjects: Critical psychology for a new millennium* (pp. 11–22). Palgrave Macmillan.

Elmir, R., Schmied, V., Wilkes, L., & Jackson, D. (2010). Women's perceptions and experiences of a traumatic birth: A meta-ethnography. *Journal of Advanced Nursing, 66*(10), 2142–2153.

Endžier, N. (2010). *Žena: Intimna geografija*. NNK Internacional.

Engel, G. L. (1977). The need for a new medical model: A challenge for biomedicine. *Science, 196*(4286), 129–136. https://doi.org/10.1126/science.847460

Engeström, Y. (1987). *Learning by expanding: An activity-theoretical approach to developmental research*. Orienta-Konsultit.

Ennis, L. R. (Ed.). (2014). *Intensive mothering: The cultural contradictions of modern motherhood*. Demeter Press. Retrieved from http://www.jstor.org/stable/j.ctt1rrd8rb

Esposito, N. (1999). Marginalized women's comparisons of their hospital and freestanding birth center experiences: A contrast of inner-city birthing systems. *Health Care for Women International, 20*(2), 111–126.

Everett, C. (1997). Incidence and outcome of bleeding before the 20th week of pregnancy: Prospective study from general practice. *British Medical Journal, 315*(7099), 32–34. https://doi.org/10.1136/bmj.315.7099.32

Flick, U. (1992). Triangulation revisited: Strategy of validation or alternative? *Journal for the Theory of Social Behaviour, 22*(2), 175–197. https://doi.org/10.1111/j.1468-5914.1992.tb00215.x

Foucault, M. (1982). The subject and power. *Critical Inquiry, 8*(4), 777–795. Retrieved from https://www.jstor.org/stable/1343197

Foucault, M. (1988). Technologies of the self. In L. H. Martin, H. Gutman, & P. H. Hutton (Eds.), *Technologies of the self: A seminar with Michel Foucault* (pp. 16–49). University of Massachusetts Press.

Foucault, M. (1995). *Discipline and punish: The birth of the prison*. Vintage Books.

Foucault, M. (2003). *The birth of the clinic: An archaeology of medical perception*. Routledge.

Foucault, M. (2006). *Psychiatric power: Lectures at the Collège de France, 1973–1974*. Palgrave Macmillan.

Frank, A. W. (1997). *The wounded storyteller: Body, illness, and ethics*. University of Chicago Press.

Frazier, K. E., Jackson, T. E., & Mangione, H. (2015). Commentary: Beyond stigma: Critical approaches to violations of the motherhood narrative. In K. R. Cabell, G. Marsico, C. Cornejo, & J. Valsiner (Eds.), *Making meaning, making motherhood* (pp. 133–150). Information Age Publishing.

Fricker, M. (2007). *Epistemic injustice: Power and the ethics of knowing*. Oxford University Press.

Gadow, S. (1980). Body and self: A dialectic. *Journal of Medicine and Philosophy, 5*(3), 172–185. https://doi.org/10.1093/jmp/5.3.172

Gadow, S. (1984). Touch and technology: Two paradigms of patient care. *Journal of Religion and Health, 23*(1), 63–69. https://doi.org/10.1007/BF00999900

Gallagher, S. (2005). *How the body shapes the mind*. Clarendon Press.

Gallagher, S., & Zahavi, D. (2008). *The phenomenological mind: An introduction to philosophy of mind and cognitive science*. Routledge.

Gannon, L. (1998). The impact of medical and sexual politics on women's health. *Feminism & Psychology, 8*(3), 285–302. https://doi.org/10.1177/0959353598083004

Gergen, K. (2009). *Relational being: Beyond self and community*. Oxford University Press.

Gerson, M., Alpert, J. L., & Richardson, M. S. (1984). Mothering: The view from psychological research. *Signs, 9*(3), 434–453. https://doi.org/10.1086/494070

Ginsburg, F., & Rapp, R. (1991). The politics of reproduction. *Annual Review of Anthropology, 20*(1), 311–343. https://doi.org/10.1146/annurev.an.20.100191.001523

Gloger-Tippelt, G. (1983). A process model of the pregnancy course. *Human Development, 26*(3), 134–148. https://doi.org/10.1159/000272877

Goer, H. (1995). *Obstetric myths versus research realities*. Greenwood Publishing Group.

Gornall, J. (2009). The dangers of listening to the fetal heart at home. *BMJ*. Retrieved from https://www.bmj.com/bmj/sectionpdf/186393?path=/bmj/339/7730/Feature.full.pdf

Gracia, C. R., Sammel, M. D., Chittams, J., Hummel, A. C., Shaunik, A., & Barnhart, K. T. (2005). Risk factors for spontaneous abortion in early symptomatic first-trimester pregnancies. *Obstetrics & Gynecology, 106*(5/1), 993–999. https://doi.org/10.1097/01.AOG.0000183604.09922.e0

Graham, I. D., Carroli, G., Davies, C., & Medves, J. M. (2005). Episiotomy rates around the world: An update. *Birth, 32*(3), 219–223. https://doi.org/10.1111/j.0730-7659.2005.00373.x

Green, H. M. (2008a). *Making women's medicine masculine: The rise of male authority in pre-modern gynaecology*. Oxford University Press.
Green, H. M. (2008b). Gendering the history of women's healthcare. *Gender & History, 20*(3), 487–518. https://doi.org/10.1111/j.1468-0424.2008.00534.x
Green, J., & Baston, H. (2003). Feeling in control during labor: Concepts, correlates, and consequences. *Birth, 30*(4), 235–247.
Griffin, S. (2001). Feminism and motherhood. In M. Davey (Ed.), *Mother reader: Essential literature on motherhood* (pp. 33–45). Seven Stories Press. (Original work published 1974).
Gross, H., & Pattison, H. (2007). *Sanctioning pregnancy: A psychological perspective*. Routledge.
Gudović, M. (2013). Crtica—Epiziotomija. In A. Vilenica (Ed.), *Postajanje majkom u vreme neoliberalnog kapitalizma* (pp. 250–253). uz)bu))na))).
Halfon, S. (2010). Encountering birth: Negotiating expertise, networks, and my STS self. *Science as Culture, 19*(1), 61–77. https://doi.org/10.1080/09505430903558062
Hall, G. S. (1904). *Adolescence: Its psychology and its relations to physiology, anthropology, sociology, crime, religion and education* (Vol. 2). Retrieved from https://psychclassics.yorku.ca/Hall/Adolescence/chap17.htm
Hallam, J. L., Howard, C. D., Locke, A., & Thomas, M. (2016). Communicating choice: An exploration of mothers' experiences of birth. *Journal of Reproductive and Infant Psychology, 34*(3), 257–269. https://doi.org/10.1080/02646838.2015.1119260
Hanson, C. (2004). *A cultural history of pregnancy: Pregnancy, medicine and culture, 1750–2000*. Palgrave Macmillan.
Haraway, D. (1991a). A cyborg manifesto: Science, technology, and socialist-feminism in the late twentieth century. In *Simians, cyborgs and women: The reinvention of nature* (pp. 149–181). Routledge.
Haraway, D. (1991b). Situated knowledges: The science question in feminism and the privilege of partial perspective. In *Simians, cyborgs and women: The reinvention of nature* (pp. 183–202). Routledge.
Haraway, D. (1991c). The biopolitics of postmodern bodies: Constitutions of self in immune system discourse. In *Simians, cyborgs and women: The reinvention of nature* (pp. 203–230). Routledge.
Harré, R. (2001). Metaphysics and narrative: Singularities and multiplicities of self. In J. Brockmeier & D. Carbaugh (Eds.), *Narrative and identity: Studies in autobiography, self and culture* (pp. 59–73). John Benjamins Publishing.
Harris, R., & Ayers, S. (2012). What makes labour and birth traumatic? A survey of intrapartum "hotspots". *Psychology & Health, 27*(10), 1166–1177.

Hatgis, C. (2001). Agency and the deconstructed subject. In N. Stephenson, H. L. Radtke, R. Jorna, & H. J. Stam (Eds.), *Theoretical psychology: Critical contributions* (pp. 129–140). Captus University Publications.

Hauck, Y., Fenwick, J., Downie, J., & Butt, J. (2007). The influence of childbirth expectations on Western Australian women's perceptions of their birth experience. *Midwifery, 23*(3), 235–247. https://doi.org/10.1016/j.midw.2006.02.002

Hays, S. (1998). *The cultural contradictions of motherhood.* Yale University Press.

Healthcare for women during pregnancy: National guidelines for doctors. (2005). Serbian Medical Society.

Healthcare Law. (2019). *Official Gazette-Republic of Serbia, 25.*

Hegel, G. W. F. (2018). *The phenomenology of spirit: Translation with introduction and commentary.* Oxford University Press.

Heron, J., O'Connor, T. G., Evans, J., Golding, J., & Glover, V. (2004). Course of anxiety and depression through pregnancy and the puerperium in a community sample. *Journal of Affective Disorders, 80*(1–2), 65–73.

Hider, N. (1978). *Radikalne perspektive u psihologiji.* Nolit.

Hodnett, E. (2002). Pain and women's satisfaction with the experience of childbirth: A systematic review. *American Journal of Obstetrics & Gynecology, 186*(5), S160–S172.

Holland, S. E. (1951). The Princess Charlotte of Wales: A triple obstetric tragedy. *BJOG: An International Journal of Obstetrics & Gynaecology, 58*(6), 905–919.

Hubbard, R. (1997). *The politics of women's biology*. Rutgers University Press.

Ihde, D. (1990). *Technology and the lifeworld: From garden to earth.* Indiana University Press.

Ihde, D. (2002). *Bodies in technology*. University of Minnesota Press.

Institute for Mother and Child Healthcare. (2010). *Guidelines for the implementation of the national program of healthcare for women, children, and youth.*

Institute of Public Health "Dr Milan Jovanović Batut". (2012). *Selected health indicators.*

Janevic, T., Sripad, P., Bradley, E., & Dimitrievska, V. (2011). "There's no kind of respect here". A qualitative study of racism and access to maternal health care among Romani women in the Balkans. *International Journal for Equity in Health, 10*(1), 53. https://doi.org/10.1186/1475-9276-10-53

Jenkinson, C., Coulter, A., Bruster, S., Richards, N., & Chandola, T. (2002). Patients' experiences and satisfaction with health care: Results of a questionnaire study of specific aspects of care. *Quality and Safety in Health Care, 11*(4), 335–339. https://doi.org/10.1136/qhc.11.4.335

Juarez, L. (2015). Motherhood and becoming: The construction of motherhood through pregnancy and birth. In K. R. Cabell, G. Marsico, C. Cornejo, & J. Valsiner (Eds.), *Making meaning, making motherhood* (pp. 21–40). Information Age Publishing.

Kaptelinin, V., & Nardi, B. A. (2006). *Acting with technology: Activity theory and interaction design*. The MIT Press.

Kastratović-Kotlica, B. (2005). Dijagnoza trudnoće, nadzor trudnice i metode praćenja stanja ploda. In D. Plećaš, B. Stanimirović, A. Stanković, & M. Vasiljević (Eds.), *Ginekologija i akušerstvo: Udžbenik za studente medicine*. Medicinski fakultet Univerziteta u Beogradu.

King, H. (1998). *Hippocrates' woman: Reading the female body in Ancient Greece*. Routledge.

King, H. (2007). *Midwifery, obstetrics and the rise of gynaecology: The uses of sixteenth-century compendium*. Ashgate Publishing.

Kitzinger, S. (2006). *Birth crisis*. Routledge.

Klassen, P. E. (2001). Sacred maternities and postbiomedical bodies: Religion and nature in contemporary home birth. *Signs, 26*(3), 775–809. Retrieved from http://www.jstor.org/stable/3175539

Klein, L. (Director). (1998). *Body story: The takeover* [Documentary series, S1 E5]. Discovery Channel.

Kontopodis, M. (2012). How things matter in everyday lives of preschool age children: Material-semiotic investigations in psychology and education. *Journal für Psychologie, 20*(1), 1–14.

Kontopodis, M., Beck, S., & Niewöhner, J. (2011). Investigating emerging biomedical practices: Zones of awkward engagement on different scales. *Science Technology Human Values, 36*(5), 599–615. https://doi.org/10.1177/0162243910392798

Køster, A. (2017). Narrative and embodiment—A scalar approach. *Phenomenology and the Cognitive Sciences, 16*(5), 893–908. https://doi.org/10.1007/s11097-016-9485-8

Køster, A., & Winther-Lindqvist, D. A. (2018). Personal history and historical selfhood: The embodied and pre-reflective dimension. In A. Rosa & J. Valsiner (Eds.), *The Cambridge handbook of sociocultural psychology* (pp. 538–555). Cambridge University Press.

Kranzberg, M. (1986). Technology and history: Kranzberg's laws. *Technology and Culture, 27*(3), 544–560.

Kristeva, J. (1990). Motherhood according to Giovanni Bellini. In J. M. Thompson (Ed.), *Twentieth century theories of art* (pp. 441–467). Carleton University Press.

Kristeva, J. (2009). *This incredible need to believe*. Columbia University Press.

Kukla, R. (2005). *Mass hysteria: Medicine, culture and mothers' bodies*. Rowman & Littlefield Publishers.

Kukla, R. (2008). Measuring mothering. *International Journal of Feminist Approaches to Bioethics, 1*(1), 67–90. https://doi.org/10.2979/FAB.2008.1.1.67

Kuriyama, S. (1999). *The expressiveness of the body and the divergence of Greek and Chinese medicine*. Zone Books.

Lam, C. (2015). *New reproductive technologies and disembodiment: Feminist and material resolutions*. Ashgate.

Laney, E. K., Hall, M. E. L., Anderson, T. L., & Willingham, M. M. (2015). Becoming a mother: The influence of motherhood on women's identity development. *Identity, 15*(2), 126–145. https://doi.org/10.1080/15283488.2015.1023440

Lapum, J., Fredericks, S., Beanlands, H., McCay, E., Schwind, J., & Romaniuk, D. (2012). A cyborg ontology in health care: Traversing into the liminal space between technology and person-centred practice. *Nursing Philosophy, 13*, 276–288.

Laqueur, T. W. (1990). *Making sex: Body and gender from the Greeks to Freud*. Harvard University Press.

Larkin, M., Watts, S., & Clifton, E. (2006). Giving voice and making sense in interpretative phenomenological analysis. *Qualitative Research in Psychology, 3*(2), 102–120.

Larkin, P., Begley, C. M., & Devane, D. (2012). 'Not enough people to look after you': An exploration of women's experiences of childbirth in the Republic of Ireland. *Midwifery, 28*(1), 98–105. https://doi.org/10.1016/j.midw.2010.11.007

Latour, B. (1991). Technology is society made durable. In J. Law (Ed.), *A sociology of monsters: Essays on power, technology, and domination* (pp. 103–131). Routledge.

Latour, B. (1993). *We have never been modern*. Harvard University Press.

Latour, B. (1994). On technical mediation—philosophy, sociology, genealogy. *Common Knowledge, 3*(2), 29–64.

Latour, B. (1999). On recalling ANT. In J. Law & J. Hassard (Eds.), *Actor-network theory and after* (pp. 15–25). Blackwell Publishing.

Latour, B. (2005). *Reassembling the social: An introduction to actor-network theory*. Oxford University Press.

Law, J. (1992). Notes on the theory of the actor-network: Ordering, strategy and heterogeneity. *Systemic Practice and Action Research, 5*(4), 379–393. https://doi.org/10.1007/BF01059830

Law, J. (1999). After ANT: Complexity, naming and topology. In J. Law & J. Hassard (Eds.), *Actor network theory and after* (pp. 1–14). Blackwell Publishing.

Law, J. (2002). *Aircraft stories: Decentering the object in technoscience*. Duke University Press.

Law on Patients' Rights. (2013). *Official Gazette-Republic of Serbia, 45*.

Lawrence, J. A., & Valsiner, J. (2003). Making personal sense: An account of basic internalization and externalization processes. *Theory & Psychology, 13*(6), 723–752.

Lazarus, E. (1994). What do women want? Issues of choice, control, and class in pregnancy and childbirth. *Medical Anthropology Quarterly, 8*(1), 25–46.

Learly, A. D. (2006). Shame, gender, birth. *Hypatia, 21*(1), 101–118.

Leder, D. (1984). Medicine and paradigms of embodiment. *Journal of Medicine and Philosophy, 9*(1), 29–44.

Leder, D. (1990). *The absent body*. University of Chicago Press.

Leder, D. (1992). A tale of two bodies: The Cartesian corpse and the lived body. In D. Leder (Ed.), *The body in medical thought and practice* (pp. 17–36). Kluwer Academic Publishers.

Lehoux, P. (2006). *The problem of health technology: Policy implications for modern health care systems*. Routledge.

Leifer, M. (1977). Psychological changes accompanying pregnancy and motherhood. *Genetic Psychology Monographs, 95*, 55–96.

Leifer, M. (1980). Pregnancy. *Signs, 5*(4), 754–765.

Lemieux, K. L. (2006). 13 short pieces, but not the whole [t]ruth. *Hypatia, 21*(1), 74–79. https://doi.org/10.1353/hyp.2005.0144

Leont'ev, A. N. (1981). *Problems of the development of the mind*. Progress.

Leontyev, A. N. (1978). *Activity, consciousness, and personality*. Marxist Internet Archive. Retrieved from http://www.marxists.org/archive/leontev/works/1978/index.htm

Lock, M., Young, A., & Cambrosio, A. (2000). *Living and working with the new medical technologies: Intersections of inquiry*. Cambridge University Press.

Locke, A. (2015). Agency, 'good motherhood' and 'a load of mush': Constructions of baby-led weaning in the press. *Women's Studies International Forum, 53*, 139–146. https://doi.org/10.1016/j.wsif.2014.10.018

Lorentzen, J. M. (2008). 'I know my own body': Power and resistance in women's experiences of medical interactions. *Body & Society, 14*(3), 49–79. https://doi.org/10.1177/1357034X08093572

Lowis, G. W., & McCaffery, P. (2004). Sociological factors affecting the medicalization of midwifery. In E. R. Van Teijlingen, G. W. Lowis, P. McCaffery, & M. Porter (Eds.), *Midwifery and the medicalization of childbirth: Comparative perspectives* (pp. 5–42). Nova Science Publishers.

Lundgren, I., Karlsdottir, S. I., & Bondas, T. (2009). Long-term memories and experiences of childbirth in a Nordic context: A secondary analysis. *International Journal of Qualitative Studies on Health and Well-being, 4*(2), 115–128.

Lyerly, A. D., Armstrong, E. M., Harris, L. H., Kukla, R., Kuppermann, M., Little, M. O., & Mitchell, L. M. (2007). Risks, values, and decision making surrounding pregnancy. *Obstetrics & Gynecology, 109*(4), 979–984. https://doi.org/10.1097/AOG.0b013e3181888fd8

Lyerly, A. D., Mitchell, L. M., Armstrong, E. M., Harris, L. H., Kukla, R., Kuppermann, M., & Little, M. O. (2009). Risk and the pregnant body. *Hastings Center Report, 39*(6), 34–42. https://doi.org/10.1353/hcr.0.0211

Lyons, S. (1998). A prospective study of post-traumatic stress symptoms 1 month following childbirth in a group of 42 first-time mothers. *Journal of Reproductive and Infant Psychology, 16*(2–3), 91–106. https://doi.org/10.1080/02646839808404562

Mack, A. (2018). Critical approaches to motherhood. In *Oxford research encyclopedia of communication*. Retrieved July 15, 2023, from https://oxfordre.com/communication/view/10.1093/acrefore/9780190228613.001.0001/acrefore-9780190228613-e-579

Maher, J. (2007). *The painful truth about birth?: Contemporary discourses of caesareans, risk and the realities of pain*. Presented at the Australian Sociological Association (TASA) 2007 Conference. Retrieved from http://www.tasa.org.au/conferences/conferencepapers07/papers/19.pdf

Marecek, J., Kimmel, E. B., Crawford, M., & Hare-Mustin, R. (2003). Psychology of women and gender. In D. K. Freedheim & I. B. Weiner (Eds.), *Handbook of psychology, vol. 1: History of psychology* (pp. 249–266). Wiley.

Markus, H. R., & Hamedani, M. G. (2007). Sociocultural psychology: The dynamic interdependence among self systems and social systems. In S. Kitayama & D. Cohen (Eds.), *Handbook of cultural psychology* (pp. 3–40). Guilford Press.

Martin, E. (1984). Pregnancy, labor and body image in the United States. *Social Science & Medicine, 19*(11), 1201–1206. https://doi.org/10.1016/0277-9536(84)90371-X

Martin, E. (1992). *The woman in the body: A cultural analysis of reproduction*. Beacon Press.

Martin, E. (1996). Disembodying women: Perspectives on pregnancy and the unborn. *Medical Anthropology Quarterly, 10*(2), 307–309. https://doi.org/10.1525/maq.1996.10.2.02a00150

Martin, K. A. (2003). Giving birth like a girl. *Gender & Society, 17*(1), 54–72. https://doi.org/10.1177/0891243202238978

Matejić, B., Milićević, M. S., Vasić, V., & Djikanović, B. (2014). Maternal satisfaction with organized perinatal care in Serbian public hospitals. *BMC Pregnancy and Childbirth, 14*, 14. https://doi.org/10.1186/1471-2393-14-14

Mathews, R., & Callister, L. (2004). Childbearing women's perceptions of nursing care that promotes dignity. *Journal of Obstetric, Gynecologic & Neonatal Nursing, 33*(4), 498–507.

McClive, C. (2002). The hidden truths of the belly: The uncertainties of pregnancy in early modern Europe. *Social History of Medicine, 15*(2), 209–227. https://doi.org/10.1093/shm/15.2.209

McGrath, R. (2002). *Seeing her sex: Medical archives and the female body*. Manchester University Press.

McLaren, A. (1999). *Twentieth-century sexuality: A history*. Blackwell Publishing.

McTavish, L. (2005). *Childbirth and the display of authority in early modern France*. Ashgate Publishing.

Merleau-Ponty, M. (2005). *Phenomenology of perception* (C. Smith, Trans.). Routledge. (Original work published 1945).

Miettinen, R. (1999). The riddle of things: Activity theory and actor-network theory as approaches to studying innovations. *Mind, Culture, and Activity, 6*(3), 170–195. https://doi.org/10.1080/10749039909524725

Miller, S., Abalos, E., Chamillard, M., Ciapponi, A., Colaci, D., Comandé, D., Diaz, V., Geller, S., Hanson, C., Langer, A., Manuelli, V., Millar, K., Morhason-Bello, I., Castro, C. P., Pileggi, V. N., Robinson, N., Skaer, M., Souza, J. P., Vogel, J. P., & Althabe, F. (2016). Beyond too little, too late and too much, too soon: A pathway towards evidence-based, respectful maternity care worldwide. *Lancet (London, England), 388*(10056), 2176–2192. https://doi.org/10.1016/S0140-6736(16)31472-6

Milošević, B., & Prica, R. (1968). *Bezbolni porođaj*. Medicinska knjiga.

Milošević, B., Rajhvajn, B., & Berić, B. (1988). *Porodiljstvo: Udžbenik za studente medicine*. Medicinska knjiga.

Ministry of Health of Republic of Serbia. (2011). *Standards of health care adapted to the needs of mothers and children*.

Ministry of Labour and Social Policy of Republic of Serbia. (2008). *National strategy for advancing the status of women and promoting gender equality.*

Mladenović, D., Mladenović-Bogdanović, Z., & Mladenović-Mihailović, A. (2008). *Ginekologija i akušerstvo.* Zavod za udžbenike.

Mol, A. (2000). Pathology and the clinic: An ethnographic presentation of two atheroscleroses. In M. Lock, A. Young, & A. Cambrosio (Eds.), *Living and working with the new medical technologies: Intersections of inquiry* (pp. 82–102). Cambridge University Press.

Mol, A. (2002). *The body multiple: Ontology in medical practice.* Duke University Press.

Mol, A., & Law, J. (2004). Embodied action, enacted bodies: The example of hypoglycaemia. *Body & Society, 10*(2–3), 43–62. https://doi.org/10.1177/1357034X04042932

Momčilov, P. (2005). Normalni porođaj. In D. Plećaš, B. Stanimirović, A. Stanković, & M. Vasiljević (Eds.), *Ginekologija i akušerstvo: Udžbenik za studente medicine.* Medicinski fakultet Univerziteta u Beogradu.

Moscucci, O. (1990). *The science of woman: Gynaecology and gender in England 1800–1929.* Cambridge University Press.

Mujezinovic, F., & Alfirevic, Z. (2007). Procedure-related complications of amniocentesis and chorionic villous sampling: A systematic review. *Obstetrics & Gynecology, 110*(3), 687–694.

Mullin, A. (2005). *Reconceiving pregnancy and childcare: Ethics, experience, and reproductive labor.* Cambridge University Press.

Myers-Helfgott, M. G., & Helfgott, A. W. (1999). Routine use of episiotomy in modern obstetrics. Should it be performed? *Obstetrics and Gynecology Clinics of North America, 26*(2), 305–325. https://doi.org/10.1016/s0889-8545(05)70077-2

National Millennium Development Goals. (2006). Government of Republic of Serbia.

National Program of Health Care for Women, Children and Youth. (2009). *Official Gazette-Republic of Serbia, 28.*

Nicolson, P. (1998). *Post-natal depression: Psychology, science and the transition to motherhood.* Routledge.

Nicolson, P. (2010). What is 'psychological' about 'normal' pregnancy? *The Psychologist, 23*(3), 190–193.

Nilsson, C., Bondas, T., & Lundgren, I. (2010). Previous birth experience in women with intense fear of childbirth. *Journal of Obstetric, Gynecologic & Neonatal Nursing, 39*(3), 298–309. https://doi.org/10.1111/j.1552-6909.2010.01139.x

Ninković, M., Ilić, S., & Damnjanović, K. (2024). Women's trust in the healthcare system in Serbia: Validation of the Women's Trust and Confidence in Healthcare System scale. *Women's Health, 20*. https://doi.org/10.1177/17455057241249866

O'Dowd, M. J., & Philipp, E. E. (1994). *The history of obstetrics & gynaecology*. The Parthenon Publishing Group.

O'Driscoll, K., Stronge, J. M., & Minogue, M. (1973). Active management of labour. *British Medical Journal, 3*(5872), 135–137. https://doi.org/10.1136/bmj.3.5872.135

O'Reilly, A. (2004). *From motherhood to mothering: The legacy of Adrienne Rich's "Of Woman Born"*. State University of New York Press.

Oakley, A. (1979). A case of maternity: Paradigms of women as maternity cases. *Signs, 4*(4), 607–631.

Oakley, A. (1981). Interviewing women: A contradiction in terms. In H. Roberts (Ed.), *Doing feminist research* (pp. 30–61). Routledge & Kegan Paul.

Ochs, E., & Capps, L. (1996). Narrating the self. *Annual Review of Anthropology, 25*(1), 19–43. https://doi.org/10.1146/annurev.anthro.25.1.19

Olde, E., van der Hart, O., Kleber, R. J., van Son, M., Wijnen, H., & Pop, V. (2005). Posttraumatic dissociation and emotions as predictors of PTSD symptoms following childbirth. *Journal of Trauma & Dissociation, 6*(3), 125–142.

Pantović, L. (2016). Buying a connection: Private practice in public health care—The case of a Serbian maternity hospital. *Anthropology of East Europe Review, 34*(1).

Pantović, L. (2021). Somebodies or nobody's patient: The importance of social positioning and informal relations during childbirth in Serbia. *Glasnik Etnografskog instituta SANU, 69*(1), 205–225. https://doi.org/10.2298/GEI2101205P

Pantović, L. (2022). Providing a service or seeking a favor? The role of private prenatal care on the continuity of care in Serbian public maternity hospitals. *Birth, 49*(3), 506–513.

Pantović, L., Stanković, B., & Ćeriman, J. (2024). *Iskustva žena u porodilištima u Srbiji tokom i nakon pandemije kovida-19*. UNFPA.

Pelling, M., & Webster, C. (1979). Medical practitioners. In C. Webster (Ed.), *Health, medicine and mortality in the sixteenth century* (pp. 164–235). Cambridge University Press.

Philipp, D. A., & Carr, M. L. (2001). Normal and medically complicated pregnancies. In N. Stotland & D. E. Stewart (Eds.), *Psychological aspects of women's health care: The interface between psychiatry and obstetrics and gynecology* (pp. 13–32). American Psychiatric Press.

Physiological Childbirth: The guide for doctors and midwives. (2009). Ministry of Health of Republic of Serbia.

Pittrof, R., Campbell, O. M. R., & Filippi, V. G. A. (2002). What is quality in maternity care? An international perspective. *Acta Obstetricia et Gynecologica Scandinavica, 81*(4), 277–283.

Plath, S. (2006). *The bell jar*. Harper Perennial Modern Classics.

Platon. (1995). *Timaj*. Eidos.

Plećaš, D., Stanimirović, B., Stanković, A., & Vasiljević, M. (2005). *Ginekologija i akušerstvo: Udžbenik za studente medicine*. Medicinski fakultet Univerziteta u Beogradu.

Porter, R. (2002). *Blood and guts: A short history of medicine*. Allen Lane.

Porter, R. (2003). *Flesh in the age of reason*. W.W. Norton & Company.

Ratner, C. (1999). Three approaches to cultural psychology: A critique. *Cultural Dynamics, 11*(1), 7–31.

Regulation on Healthcare Quality Indicators and Quality Assurance of Professional Work. (2021). *Official Gazette-Republic of Serbia, 123/2021.*

Reis, L. P. C., & Santos, J. E. F. (2015). The experiences of mothers from the railroad suburb of Salvador-Bahia: Conceptualizing a semiotic theory of protection and empowerment in adverse conditions. In K. R. Cabell, G. Marsico, C. Cornejo, & J. Valsiner (Eds.), *Making meaning, making motherhood* (pp. 107–132). Information Age Publishing.

Reiser, S. J. (1984). The machine at the bedside: Technological transformations of practices and values. In S. J. Reiser & M. Anbar (Eds.), *The machine at the bedside: Strategies for using technology in patient care* (pp. 3–19). Cambridge University Press.

Rich, A. (1986a). Notes toward a politics of location. In *Blood, bread, and poetry: Selected prose 1979–1985* (pp. 210–231). W. W. Norton & Company.

Rich, A. (1986b). *Of woman born: Motherhood as experience and institution*. W. W. Norton & Company.

Rich, A. (1995). Motherhood: The contemporary emergency and the quantum leap. In *On lies, secrets, and silence: Selected prose 1966–1978* (pp. 259–273). W. W. Norton & Company. (Original work published 1978).

Riggs, D. W., & Bartholomaeus, C. (2023). *First-time parenting journeys: Expectations and realities*. Cambridge University Press.

Riley, S., Evans, A., & Robson, M. (2019). *Postfeminism and health: Critical psychology and media perspectives*. Routledge.

Ristić, L. (2001). *Praktično porodiljstvo*. Freemental.

Rivkin-Fish, M. (2005). *Women's health in post-Soviet Russia: The politics of intervention*. Indiana University Press.

Rose, N. (1996). Assembling the modern self. In R. Porter (Ed.), *Rewriting the self: Histories from the Renaissance to the present* (pp. 224–248). Routledge.

Rosenberg, K., & Trevathan, W. (2002). Birth, obstetrics and human evolution. *BJOG: An International Journal of Obstetrics & Gynaecology, 109*(11), 1199–1206. https://doi.org/10.1046/j.1471-0528.2002.00010.x

Rothman, B. K. (1993). Recreating motherhood: American lessons for the Netherlands. *Nemesis, 9*(4), 123–130.

Rothman, B. K. (2007a). Introduction: A lifetime's labor: Women and power in the birthplace. In W. Simonds, B. K. Rothman, & B. M. Norman (Eds.), *Laboring on: Birth in transition in the United States* (pp. xi–xxii). Routledge.

Rothman, B. K. (2007b). Laboring then: The political history of maternity care in the United States. In W. Simonds, B. K. Rothman, & B. M. Norman (Eds.), *Laboring on: Birth in transition in the United States* (pp. 3–28). Routledge.

Ruddick, S. (1989). *Maternal thinking: Toward a politics of peace*. Beacon Press.

Sandelowski, M., & Black, B. P. (1994). The epistemology of expectant parenthood. *Western Journal of Nursing Research, 16*(6), 601–614. https://doi.org/10.1177/019394599401600602

Sartre, J. P. (2003). *Being and nothingness: An essay on phenomenological ontology* (H. E. Barnes, Trans.). Routledge. (Original work published 1943).

Savage, W. (2003). Professional control or women's choice in childbirth? Is either possible? In G. Boswell & F. Poland (Eds.), *Women's minds, women's bodies: Interdisciplinary approaches to women's health* (pp. 103–115). Palgrave Macmillan.

Scarry, E. (1985). *The body in pain: The making and unmaking of the world*. Oxford University Press.

Schroll, A. M., Kjaergaard, H., & Midtgaard, J. (2013). Encountering abuse in health care: Lifetime experiences in postnatal women—A qualitative study. *BMC Pregnancy and Childbirth, 13*, 74.

Sekulić, N. (2014). Social status of motherhood with special reference to Serbia today. *Sociologija, 56*(4), 402–426.

Sekulić, N. (2016). *Kultura rađanja: Istraživanje o seksualnoj i reproduktivnoj socijalizaciji žena*. Institut za sociološka istraživanja Filozofskog fakulteta u Beogradu.

Shaw, J. (2012). The birth of the clinic and the advent of reproduction: Pregnancy, pathology and the medical gaze in modernity. *Body & Society, 18*(2), 110–138. https://doi.org/10.1177/1357034X10394666

Shiffman, J., Skrabalo, M., & Subotic, J. (2002). Reproductive rights and the state in Serbia and Croatia. *Social Science & Medicine, 54*(5), 625–642.

Shorter, E. (1991). *Women's bodies: A social history of women's encounter with health, ill-health and medicine*. Transaction Publishers.

Shweder, R. A., Goodnow, J. J., Hatano, G., LeVine, R. A., Markus, H. R., & Miller, P. J. (2006). The cultural psychology of development: One mind, many mentalities. In R. M. Lerner (Ed.), *Handbook of child psychology* (Vol. 1, pp. 716–793). Wiley.

Simić, J., & Jerinić, J. (2014). Pravo na porođaj kod kuće—Izbor, a ne slučajnost i neke pravne posledice. *Pravni zapisi, 5*(1), 120–161. https://doi.org/10.5937/pravzap0-6103

Sims-Schouten, W., Riley, S. C. E., & Willig, C. (2007). Critical realism in discourse analysis: A presentation of a systematic method of analysis using women's talk of motherhood, childcare and female employment as an example. *Theory & Psychology, 17*(1), 101–124. https://doi.org/10.1177/0959354307073153

Skočajić, M., & Stanković, B. (2020). Uloga socijalne podrške u iskustvu abortusa: Kvalitativna analiza ličnih izveštaja žena. *Sociologija, LXII*(2), 171–192. https://doi.org/10.2298/SOC2002171S

Slade, P., & Cree, M. (2010). A psychological plan for perinatal care. *The Psychologist, 23*(3), 194–197.

Smit, D. K. (2005). Hermeneutika i kvalitativno istraživanje. *Pedagogija, 3*, 315–330.

Smith, J. A. (1994). Reconstructing selves: An analysis of discrepancies between women's contemporaneous and retrospective accounts of the transition to motherhood. *British Journal of Psychology, 85*, 371–392. https://doi.org/10.1111/j.2044-8295.1994.tb02530.x

Smith, J. A. (1995). Semi-structured interviewing and qualitative analysis. In J. A. Smith, R. Harré, & L. van Langenhove (Eds.), *Rethinking methods in psychology* (pp. 9–26). Sage.

Smith, J. A. (1999). Identity development during the transition to motherhood: An interpretative phenomenological analysis. *Journal of Reproductive and Infant Psychology, 17*(3), 281–299. https://doi.org/10.1080/02646839908404595

Soet, J., Brack, G., & Dilorio, C. (2003). Prevalence and predictors of women's experience of psychological trauma during childbirth. *Birth, 30*(1), 36–46. https://doi.org/10.1046/j.1523-536X.2003.00215.x

Spencer, H. R. (1927). *The history of British midwifery from 1650 to 1800*. John Bale, Sons & Danielsson.

Spinuzzi, C. (2008). *Network: Theorizing knowledge work in telecommunications*. Cambridge University Press.

Squier, S. (1996). Fetal subjects and maternal objects: Reproductive technology and the new fetal/maternal relation. *Journal of Medicine and Philosophy, 21*, 515–535. https://doi.org/10.1093/jmp/21.5.515

Stam, H. J. (2000). Theorizing health and illness: Functionalism, subjectivity and reflexivity. *Journal of Health Psychology, 5*(3), 273–283. https://doi.org/10.1177/135910530000500309

Stanković, B. (2013). Medical practice in transition: The case of Serbian maternity care services and their users. In L. Popovic, M. Vidakovic, & D. Kostic (Eds.), *Resources of Danubian Region: The possibility of cooperation and utilization*. Humboldt-Club Serbien.

Stanković, B. (2014). Woman as a subject of childbirth: Physical, technological and institutional aspects. *Sociologija, 56*(4), 524–544. https://doi.org/10.2298/SOC1404524S

Stanković, B. (2016). Kritički prikaz istorije medikalizacije i maskulinizacije staranja o ženskom reproduktivnom telu. In N. Sekulić & M. Radoman (Eds.), *Izabrani radovi iz studija roda* (pp. 82–109). Institut za sociološka istraživanja Filozofskog fakulteta u Beogradu.

Stankovic, B. (2017a). Women's experiences of childbirth in Serbian public healthcare institutions: A qualitative study. *International Journal of Behavioral Medicine, 24*(6), 803–814. https://doi.org/10.1007/s12529-017-9672-1

Stankovic, B. (2017b). Situated technology in reproductive health care: Do we need a new theory of the subject to promote person-centred care? *Nursing Philosophy, 18*(1), e12159. https://doi.org/10.1111/nup.12159

Stanković, B. (2020). Qualitative approach to social trauma research. In A. Hamburger, V. D. Volkan, & C. Hancheva (Eds.), *Social trauma—An interdisciplinary textbook* (pp. 335–342). Springer.

Stanković, B., Skočajić, M., & Đorđević, A. (2017). Upravljanje porođajem u Srbiji: Medicinske intervencije i porođajna iskustva. *Limes Plus: Journal of Social Science and Humanities, 14*(2), 197–225.

Stanojević, D. (2005). Epiziotomija. In D. Plećaš, B. Stanimirović, A. Stanković, & M. Vasiljević (Eds.), *Ginekologija i akušerstvo: Udžbenik za studente medicine*. Medicinski fakultet Univerziteta u Beogradu.

Stanton, A., Lobel, M., Sears, S., & DeLuca, R. (2002). Psychosocial aspects of selected issues in women's reproductive health: Current status and future directions. *Journal of Consulting and Clinical Psychology, 70*, 751–770.

Stern, D., Bruschweiler-Stern, N., & Freeland, A. (1998). *The birth of a mother: How the motherhood experience changes you forever*. Basic Books.

Stewart, M. (2004). *Pregnancy, birth, and maternity care: Feminist perspectives*. Elsevier Science.

Strauss, A., & Corbin, J. (1998). *Basics of qualitative research: Techniques and procedures for developing grounded theory*. Sage.

Swahnberg, K., Thapar-Björkert, S., & Berterö, C. (2007). Nullified: Women's perceptions of being abused in health care. *Journal of Psychosomatic Obstetrics & Gynecology, 28*(3), 161–167.

Taylor, J. S. (2008). *The public life of the fetal sonogram: Technology, consumption, and the politics of reproduction*. Rutgers University Press.

Thompson, C. (2005). *Making parents: The ontological choreography of reproductive technologies*. MIT Press.

Thomson, G., & Downe, S. (2008). Widening the trauma discourse: The link between childbirth and experiences of abuse. *Journal of Psychosomatic Obstetrics & Gynecology, 29*(4), 268–273.

Tone, A. (2012). Medicalizing reproduction: The pill and home pregnancy tests. *Journal of Sex Research, 49*(4), 319–327. https://doi.org/10.1080/00224499.2012.688226

Treichler, P. (1990). Feminism, medicine and the meaning of childbirth. In M. Jacobus, E. F. Keller, & S. Shuttleworth (Eds.), *Body/politics: Women and the discourses of science* (pp. 113–138). Routledge.

Turkel, K. D. (1995). *Women, power, and childbirth: A case study of a free-standing birth center*. Greenwood Publishing Group.

Turner, B. S. (1992). *Regulating bodies: Essays in medical sociology*. Routledge.

U.S. Food and Drug Administration (FDA). (2014). Avoid fetal "keepsake" images, heartbeat monitors. *FDA Consumer Health Information*. Retrieved from https://shorturl.at/msCQZ

Unger, R. K. (2001). Women as subjects, actors, and agents in the history of psychology. In R. K. Unger (Ed.), *Handbook of the psychology of women and gender* (pp. 3–16). Wiley.

Ussher, J. (1990). Choosing psychology or not throwing the baby out with the bathwater. In E. Burman (Ed.), *Feminists and psychological practice* (pp. 47–61). Sage.

Ussher, J. (2006). *Managing the monstrous feminine: Regulating the reproductive body*. Routledge.

Ussher, J. (2008). Reclaiming embodiment within critical psychology: A material-discursive analysis of the menopausal body. *Social and Personality Psychology Compass, 2*(5), 1781–1798. https://doi.org/10.1111/j.1751-9004.2008.00151.x

Valentine, D. (1982). The experience of pregnancy: A developmental process. *Family Relations, 31*(2), 243–248.

Valsiner, J. (1997). *Čovekov razvoj i kultura*. Zavod za udžbenike i nastavna sredstva.

Valsiner, J. (2002). Forms of dialogical relations and semiotic autoregulation within the self. *Theory & Psychology, 12*(2), 251–265.

Valsiner, J. (2004). Culture in psychology: Between social positioning and producing new knowledge. *Culture & Psychology, 10*(1), 5–27. https://doi.org/10.1177/1354067X04040925

Valsiner, J. (2007). *Culture in minds and societies: Foundations of cultural psychology*. Sage Publications.

Valsiner, J. (2012). Introduction: Culture in psychology: A renewed encounter of inquisitive minds. In J. Valsiner (Ed.), *The Oxford handbook of culture and psychology* (pp. 3–16). Oxford University Press.

van der Gucht, N., & Lewis, K. (2015). Women's experiences of coping with pain during childbirth: A critical review of qualitative research. *Midwifery, 31*, 349–358.

van der Ploeg, I. (2004). 'Only angels can do without skin': On reproductive technology's hybrids and the politics of body boundaries. *Body & Society, 10*(2–3), 153–181. https://doi.org/10.1177/1357034X04042941

van Langenhove, L., & Harré, R. (1999). Introducing positioning theory. In R. Harré & L. van Langenhove (Eds.), *Positioning theory: Moral contexts of international action*. Blackwell Publishers.

van Nistelrooij, I., & Visse, M. (2019). Me? The invisible call of responsibility and its promise for care ethics: A phenomenological view. *Medicine, Health Care, and Philosophy, 22*(2), 275–285. https://doi.org/10.1007/s11019-018-9873-7

Venn, C. (1998). The subject of psychology. In J. Henriques, W. Hollway, C. Urwin, C. Venn, & V. Walkerdine (Eds.), *Changing the subject: Psychology, social regulation and subjectivity* (pp. 115–147).

Verbeek, P. (2005). *What things do: Philosophical reflections on technology, agency, and design*. The Pennsylvania State University Press.

Verdery, K. (1996). *What was socialism and what comes next*. Princeton University Press.

Vidić, J., Stanković, B., & Džamonja Ignjatović, T. (2022). Iskustva medicinske tranzicije transrodnih osoba u Srbiji: Od afirmacije identiteta do institucionalnog nasilja. *Sociologija, LXIV*(3), 401–427. https://doi.org/10.2298/SOC2203401V

Vilenica, A. (2013). Postajanje majkom: Od neoliberalnog režima materinstva ka radikalnoj političkoj subjektivizaciji. In A. Vilenica (Ed.), *Postajanje majkom u vreme neoliberalnog kapitalizma* (pp. 9–31). uz)bu))na))).

Vujadinović, D., & Stanimirović, V. (2017). Rodni odnosi u Srbiji u doba tranzicije—Između emancipacije i retradicionalizacije. In *Studije roda* (pp. 151–177). Pravni fakultet Univerziteta u Beogradu.

Vygotsky, L. S. (1997). The history of the development of higher mental functions. In *The collected works of L. S. Vygotsky* (Vol. 4). Springer.

Waldenström, U., Hildingsson, I., Rubertsson, C., & Rådestad, I. (2004). A negative birth experience: Prevalence and risk factors in a national sample. *Birth, 31*(1), 17–27.

Walker, M. B. (1998). *Philosophy and the maternal body: Reading silence.* Routledge.

Wehrle, M. (2017). The normative body and the embodiment of norms: Bridging the gap between phenomenological and Foucauldian approaches. *Yearbook for Eastern and Western Philosophy, 2017*(2), 323–337. https://doi.org/10.1515/yewph-2017-0023

Weiss, G., & Haber, H. F. (1999). Introduction. In G. Weiss & H. F. Haber (Eds.), *Perspectives on embodiment: The intersections of nature and culture* (pp. xiii–xvii).

Weisstein, N. (1968). *Kinder, Küche, Kirche as scientific law: Psychology constructs the female.* New England Free Press. Retrieved from http://www.cwluherstory.com/psychology-constructs-the-female.html

Wilson, E. A. (1998). *Neural geographies: Feminism and the microstructure of cognition.* Routledge.

Wilson, A. (2003). Participant or patient? Seventeenth century childbirth from the mother's point of view. In R. Porter (Ed.), *Patients and practitioners: Lay perceptions of medicine in pre-industrial society* (pp. 129–144). Cambridge University Press.

Woollett, A., & Marshall, H. (1997). Discourses of pregnancy and childbirth. In L. Yardley (Ed.), *Material discourses of health and illness* (pp. 176–198). Routledge.

World Health Organization (WHO). (1996). *Care in normal birth: A practical guide.* Department of Reproductive Health & Research, WHO.

World Health Organization (WHO). (2018). *WHO recommendations: Intrapartum care for a positive childbirth experience.* World Health Organization.

Yardley, L. (1996). Reconciling discursive and materialist perspectives on health and illness: A reconstruction of the biopsychosocial approach. *Theory & Psychology, 6*(3), 485–508. https://doi.org/10.1177/0959354396063008

Yardley, L. (1997). Introducing material-discursive approaches to health and illness. In L. Yardley (Ed.), *Material discourses of health and illness* (pp. 1–24). Routledge.
Young, I. M. (2005a). Throwing like a girl: A phenomenology of feminine body comportment, motility, and spatiality. In *On female body experience: 'Throwing like a girl' and other essays* (pp. 27–45). Oxford University Press.
Young, I. M. (2005b). Pregnant embodiment: Subjectivity and alienation. In *On female body experience: 'Throwing like a girl' and other essays* (pp. 46–61). Oxford University Press.
Zahavi, D. (2018). Getting it quite wrong: Van Manen and Smith on phenomenology. *Qualitative Health Research, 28*(6), 854–863. https://doi.org/10.1177/1049732318817547
Zerilli, L. M. G. (1992). A process without a subject: Simone de Beauvoir and Julia Kristeva on maternity. *Signs, 18*(1), 111–135. https://doi.org/10.1086/494781
Zittoun, T. (2006). *Transitions: Development through symbolic resources.* Information Age Publishing.
Zlotogorski, Z., Tadmor, O., Rabinovitz, R., & Diamant, Y. (1997). Parental attitudes toward obstetric ultrasound examination. *The Journal of Obstetrics and Gynaecology Research, 23*(1), 25–28. https://doi.org/10.1111/j.1447-0756.1997.tb00800.x

Index[1]

A

Activity theory, 27, 28
Actor-network theory (ANT), 26, 26n24, 28, 28n26, 29, 30n28, 328n13
Aesthetic relationship with the body, 307, 308n2
Agency
 as distributed, 46, 49, 221–295, 341
 as inherent property, 333, 335, 337, 339, 340
Alienation, x, 13, 119, 162–167, 215, 232, 242, 251, 252, 271, 307, 317, 325, 328, 329, 331, 333, 336
Ambiguous transcendence, 7, 7n3
Androcentrism in psychology, 15
Autobiographical self, x, 31

B

Baby's movements
 early detection of, 169
 embodied experience of, 96, 156, 159, 160, 168–176, 180, 181, 184, 189, 192, 195, 196, 292, 319, 321n6, 324
 changes over pregnancy, 173, 182, 322
Biomedical model, 21, 22
Biopsychosocial model, 20, 21
Birth, *see* Childbirth

[1] Note: Page numbers followed by 'n' refer to notes.

B. Stanković, *Giving Birth To A Subject*, Sociocultural Psychology of the Lifecourse,
https://doi.org/10.1007/978-3-031-77236-8

Bodily socialisation, 193, 308, 310, 341
Body image in pregnancy, 165, 166
Body schema in pregnancy, 165, 166
Body Story: The Takeover (documentary), 187
Butler, Judith, 25, 164, 338

C

Caesarean section, 83, 212, 232, 232n9, 263, 279, 281–283, 295, 330n16
Cartesian dualism in medicine, 69, 278, 331
Chadwick, Rachelle, 15, 18, 31, 42, 44, 73, 123, 254n24, 313–315
Chaos narrative, 46
Childbirth
  cultural representations and practices surrounding childbirth, 4, 5, 47, 48
  emergence of body-in-labour, 222–228, 289
  institutional treatment of childbirth, 44
  loss of control during childbirth, 221, 251
  monitoring during childbirth, 75, 109, 228, 255
  reproductive choices in childbirth, 35, 36, 38, 44, 91, 101n29, 102, 109, 110, 118, 122n54, 336
  technocratic approach to childbirth, 38
Childbirth preparation classes, 214n43, 267, 270n31, 284, 285, 288n39
  Soviet psychoprophylactic method, 104
Civic initiatives in maternal healthcare, 93
Contractions
  artificial contractions, 252, 256
  natural contractions, 252, 254, 256, 257, 259
Critical-discursive analysis, x, 29, 45
Critical health psychology, 20, 20n16
CTG (cardiotocography), 72n4, 96, 96n21, 211–215, 211n39, 211n40, 213n41, 214n43, 223–225, 227, 245, 256
Cultural psychology, xi, xii, 24, 24n18

D

Davis-Floyd, Robbie, 5, 72, 83, 84, 87, 88, 118, 330, 330n17, 331, 331n19, 337n22, 342
de Beauvoir, Simone, 5, 13, 14, 45, 119n51
Decline in birth rate, 39
DeLee, Joseph B., 73–75, 75n8
Desubjectification, 210, 228, 229, 232, 233, 235, 236, 272, 331, 333
Dick-Read, Grantly, 101, 101n30, 104, 104n34, 108, 120
Discourse of risk, 74–83, 96, 111, 111n43, 151, 196, 263, 307
Duden, Barbara, 5n2, 8n6, 9, 120, 120–121n52, 148, 169, 169n25, 320, 324, 325, 330
Dys-appearance, 251, 251n23, 252, 254, 303
Dys-embodiment, 251–265, 292, 295, 306, 317, 329, 329n15, 335

E
Embodiment
body as subject & body as object, 136, 308
disrupted body-embodied self relationship, 265, 291, 317
gendered embodiment, 2
lived body, 7n3, 31, 136n5, 188, 306
role of tools in embodiment, 25–26n21, 119, 136n4
Emotional regulation during pregnancy, 81–83
Empowerment, 15, 102, 335
Engel, George L., 20, 21
Epidural anaesthesia, 109, 110, 110n42, 112n46, 113–116, 115n47, 115n48, 263, 284, 291, 293–295, 294n40, 316
Episiotomy, 38n42, 75n8, 83, 85–89, 85n11, 85n12, 86n13, 91, 92, 109n40, 232n8, 232n9, 290, 295, 331n18
husband stitch, 91
Epistemological shift in medicine, 10
Epistemological uncertainties in pregnancy and birth, 142, 148, 155, 193, 206
Ethnography, 34, 36, 37, 39n43
Expert and lay knowledge, 92

F
Fetish Mother, 68
First-person perspective, ix, x, 2, 15, 29, 31, 133, 136
Flint, Austin, 73
Forceps delivery, 83, 287
Foucault, Michel, xi, 5n2, 10, 11n9, 27, 69, 70, 233, 243, 245n17, 338, 338n23, 338n24, 339
Frank, Arthur, 46, 313

G
Gadow, Sally, 252, 307, 308n2, 316, 331, 331n18
Gender and sexual difference, 3

H
Haraway, Donna, 26, 42n46, 305, 311, 333n20, 342
Harré, Rom, 27
Hermeneutic role of medical knowledge and technology, 140, 311–315
Home birth, 36, 44n49, 102, 102n31, 121n53, 124, 124n57, 197, 226n3, 279, 281, 281n37, 330n16
Home Doppler devices, 196
Hunter, William, 99

I
Ihde, Don, 325, 326, 326n10, 342
Individuation of the baby, 48, 134, 155–193, 319, 321, 322, 324
Induction of labour, 112n45, 212, 254, 255n25
Informed consent, 38, 84, 242, 242n14
Institutional embeddedness of technology, *see* Medical technology, situated medical technology

Integrity, 116n50, 210n38, 222, 264–266, 268, 273, 276, 284, 285, 287, 294, 295, 306, 315–317, 333, 333n20, 334n21, 337
Intensive mothering ideology, 75–83, 115, 117
Interoception, 137
  qualitative reduction of, 138
  spatial ambiguity of, 138
  spatio-temporal discontinuity of, 138
Interpretative phenomenological analysis (IPA), 45
Intersubjectivity, 167–193
Interview methodology, 40

K

Kitzinger, Sheila, 90, 101, 120, 280
Kristeva, Julia, 12, 14n10, 156, 304, 305
Kukla, Rebecca, 5n2, 8, 9, 31, 32, 42, 67, 68, 73, 74, 77, 99n25, 122, 122n55, 124, 157n21, 310, 322, 334, 334n21, 338, 343

L

Latour, Bruno, xi, 7, 26, 28n26, 29, 69, 328n13, 335, 339, 339n25, 342
Leder, Drew, 25, 26, 26n21, 30, 31, 135, 135n2, 135n3, 136, 138–140, 138n11, 182n27, 251, 252, 258, 261, 262, 264, 303, 304, 311, 315, 328, 329n15, 331
Leontyev, Aleksei N., 27, 28
Local and global medical knowledge, 92

M

Male body as normative ideal, 72
Material-discursive approach, 22
Material turn in social sciences, ix
Maternal sensitivity, 192
Medical gaze, 243, 245n17
Medicalisation, *see* Reproductive body, medicalisation of the reproductive body
Medical model of pregnancy and birth, 68, 116
Medical practitioners
  role of medical practitioners, 93n18, 140, 201, 204, 284, 327, 328n13
  triadic relationship in medicine, 328, 328n14, 329
Medical record, 227, 236, 237, 240, 241, 288n39
Medical technology
  feminist critique of medical technology, 118, 325, 332
  situated medical technology, 222
  utopian *vs*. dystopian views of medical technology, 326, 336
Merleau-Ponty, Maurice, 25, 30, 31, 135
Mind-body separation, *see* Cartesian dualism in medicine
Modernist conception of subjectivity, 49, 333, 334
Motherhood
  cultural representations of motherhood, 47

feminist theory on motherhood, 14
intersectionality and motherhood, 15
motherhood and self-sacrifice, 115
neoliberal discourses on motherhood, 117
patriarchal discourses on motherhood, 13, 14
Motherhood studies, 14–15

N

Natural model of pregnancy and birth, 68, 100, 116, 336
Naturalness ideal, 109–116, 263, 342
Neoliberal values in health care, 123, 123n56, 124
Normalisation of problematic medical and institutional practices, 87

O

Oakley, Ann, 1, 40, 48, 118
Objectification, 8–12, 72n4, 136, 215, 216, 229, 235, 252, 254, 307, 316, 329, 335, 336
Ontological choreography, 279

P

Pain, 47n53
coping with pain, 101n30, 103–105, 110, 254, 282
dissociation as a reaction to pain, 251, 261, 262, 266
experience of time and pain, 258
pain and the destruction of language, 260
Panopticon, 243
Passivity, 7
Pathologisation, *see* Reproductive body, pathologisation of the reproductive body
Patient-centred care, 124, 330
Phenomenology, ix, 3, 30, 45, 47, 133–141
Plath, Sylvia, 264
Postphenomenology, 326
Pregnancy
bodily boundaries in pregnancy, 162, 163
bodily changes in pregnancy, 5, 31, 41, 47, 141, 142, 146, 162, 164, 188, 194, 197, 301
cultural beliefs and practices surrounding pregnancy, 4–8
epistemic uncertainty in pregnancy, 146, 155
hybrid nature of pregnancy, 7
identification with pregnancy, 134, 155–193, 197
institutional management of pregnancy, 9
loss of private space in pregnancy, 81–83
Pregnancy test, 121n52, 133, 144, 144n15, 145, 149, 150, 152
Prenatal courses, *see* Childbirth preparation classes
Prenatal diagnostics, 157, 157n21, 320
Pre-reflective experience, 25, 26
Privacy violation, 234, 235, 243n15

Privatisation of female experience, 8–12
Pronatalist population policy, 39
Proto-interaction and proto-communication, 324
Psychology of women, 16–18, 20, 20n16
Pushing stage of labour, 105

Q

Quickening, 167–193, 169n25, 320

R

Re-embodiment, 295, 306, 315
Relational aspects of care
  assembly line care, 205, 249, 255
  distanced relationship with caregivers, 243, 245
  information withholding, 237, 239, 239n13, 241
  lack of communication, 237, 285
Reproductive body
  dissociative representation of the reproductive body, 67, 68, 124, 310
  essentialist understanding of the reproductive body, 123
  historical representations of the reproductive body, 5, 5n2, 8–12, 110
  mechanisation of reproductive body, 69–75
  medicalisation of the reproductive body, 73, 74n7, 333
  pathologisation of the reproductive body, 17, 69–75, 99
Reproductive care
  evidence-based medicine in reproductive care, 84
  guidelines for good clinical practice in reproductive care, 36, 84, 242n14
  interventionism as the norm in reproductive care, 74, 75, 83–99
  privatisation of reproductive care, 8–12, 123, 124
  unequal distribution of power and authority in reproductive care, 38, 98, 208, 239n13, 277
Reproductive politics, 17, 39, 122n54
Reproductive processes
  clinical psychology on reproductive processes, 16, 18
  developmental psychology on reproductive processes, 17, 18, 341
Resistance, 1, 23, 37n36, 94, 96, 97, 211, 231, 306, 339, 339n25, 342, 343
Rich, Adrienne, 5, 6, 8, 14, 15, 31, 42, 67, 77, 118, 176, 276, 310, 320
Rothman, Barbara Katz, 75, 101, 102, 120, 320, 321
Routinisation of medical interventions, 278

S

Sartre, Jean-Paul, 30, 135, 135n1
Scarry, Elaine, 260, 263, 264, 291
Sedative use in childbirth, 265, 266, 268, 287

Serbian maternal healthcare system, 35
Simpson, James Young, 70
Smellie, William, 70, 71n3, 99
Sociocultural psychology, vii–ix, xi, xii, 3, 25, 340
Socio-material network of birth, 281, 288, 290, 330n16

T

Technologically mediated experience, viii, 175, 180, 215, 318, 319, 323, 330n17
Temporality, 134, 156, 321
Theoretical sampling, 43
Third-person perspective, ix, x, 28, 29, 31, 136, 187
Thompson, Charis, 42, 232, 235, 279, 321, 336, 339, 340
Trust, in medical authority, 83, 87, 98, 154, 201

U

Ultrasound technology
  medical *vs.* non-medical uses, 198, 199
  role of expertise in understanding ultrasound images, 201, 325
  role of ultrasound in pregnancy, 152, 198, 204, 322
  visual *vs.* kinaesthetic experience, 320, 323
Uncritical use of hormones in childbirth, 83
Unruly Mother, 68
Ussher, Jane, 1n1, 17, 18, 21, 22, 23n17, 164

V

Valsiner, Jaan, vii, viii, xi, 24, 24n18, 30n29, 151n18
Visceral body, 135, 135n3, 136, 138n11, 139, 222
Vow of silence surrounding traumatic childbirth, 42
Vygotsky, Lev, 192n30

W

Women as active users of maternity care, 92–99, 208

Y

Yardley, Lucy, 21, 22
Young, Iris Marion, 7, 7n3, 12, 14, 25, 30, 31, 45, 76, 118, 156, 165, 304, 307, 320, 324, 331

The manufacturer's authorised representative in the EU is Springer Nature Customer Service Centre GmbH, Europaplatz 3, 69115 Heidelberg, Germany. If you have any concerns regarding our products, please contact ProductSafety@springernature.com

Printed and bound by CPI Group (UK) Ltd, Croydon, CR0 4YY
30/09/2026
02225595-0010